Cancers of the Head and Neck: From Diagnosis to Treatment

Cancers of the Head and Neck: From Diagnosis to Treatment

Edited by Bishop Hill

STATES
ACADEMIC PRESS
www.statesacademicpress.com

States Academic Press,
109 South 5th Street,
Brooklyn, NY 11249, USA

Visit us on the World Wide Web at:
www.statesacademicpress.com

ISBN: 978-1-63989-094-1

Cataloging-in-Publication Data

Cancers of the head and neck : from diagnosis to treatment / edited by Bishop Hill.
p. cm.
Includes bibliographical references and index.
ISBN 978-1-63989-094-1
1. Head--Cancer. 2. Neck--Cancer. 3. Head--Cancer--Diagnosis. 4. Neck--Cancer--Diagnosis.
5. Head--Cancer--Treatment. 6. Neck--Cancer--Treatment. I. Hill, Bishop.
RC280.H4 C36 2022
616.994 91--dc23

Table of Contents

Preface

The numerous types of tumors which are malignant in nature, and which occur in and around the nose, throat, larynx and mouth are termed as cancers of the head and neck. Most of the cancers which belong to this category are squamous cell carcinomas. Some of the major types of head and neck cancers are laryngeal and hypopharyngeal cancer, nasopharyngeal cancer, salivary gland cancer, and nasal cavity and paranasal sinus cancer. The diagnosis of these cancers can be done through various methods such as MRI, CT scan, ultrasound, physical examination, biopsy, endoscopy and X-ray. The major ways in which these cancers can be treated are through surgery, radiation therapy, and medications such as chemotherapy, targeted therapy and immunotherapy. This book includes some of the vital pieces of work being conducted across the world, on various topics related to the cancers of the head and neck. It provides significant information of this discipline to help develop a good understanding of the diagnosis and treatment of these diseases. Those in search of information to further their knowledge will be greatly assisted by this book.

The information shared in this book is based on empirical researches made by veterans in this field of study. The elaborative information provided in this book will help the readers further their scope of knowledge leading to advancements in this field.

Finally, I would like to thank my fellow researchers who gave constructive feedback and my family members who supported me at every step of my research.

Editor

1

Epigenetic Mechanisms in Head and Neck Cancer

Julio Cesar Osorio and Andres Castillo

Abstract

Head and neck cancer (HNC) is one of the most prevalent human malignancies, affecting different anatomic sites of the upper aerodigestive tract (UADT) such as the oral cavity, larynx, and naso-, oro-, and hypopharynx. HNC develops through the accumulation of multiple genetic and epigenetic alterations in a multistep process. In this issue, the aim is to describe epigenetic mechanisms behind HNC. The main mechanisms evaluated are DNA methylation, posttranslational histone modification, and noncoding RNAs.

Keywords: Methylation, Histone modification, microRNA, Long non-coding RNAs

1. Introduction

Genetic information flow (transcription, translation, and subsequent protein modification) in a normal cell represents the machine of cell gene expression.[1] Each cell has the same information, but its expression change between different types of cells. The control of gene expression is therefore at the heart of differentiation and development.[1]

In addition to inheriting genetic information, cells inherit chemical modifications that are not encoded in the nucleotide sequence of DNA, and this modification impacts the program of gene expression. This type of modification has been termed epigenetic information.[1]

Epigenetic refers specifically to the study of mitotically and meiotically heritable changes in the control of gene expression that occur without changes in the nucleotide sequence of genome and chromatin.[2]

In both genetic and epigenetic heritage, mitosis distributes genetic information or the chemical modification through the ontogeny. Meiosis distributes genetic information or chemical modification through the formation of gametes. This means that sperm and egg carry genetic and epigenetic information. When the embryo is formed, this information is distributed through the all the cells by mitosis (Figure 1). When it comes to population level, natural selection determines which genetically and epigenetically inherited information is present.

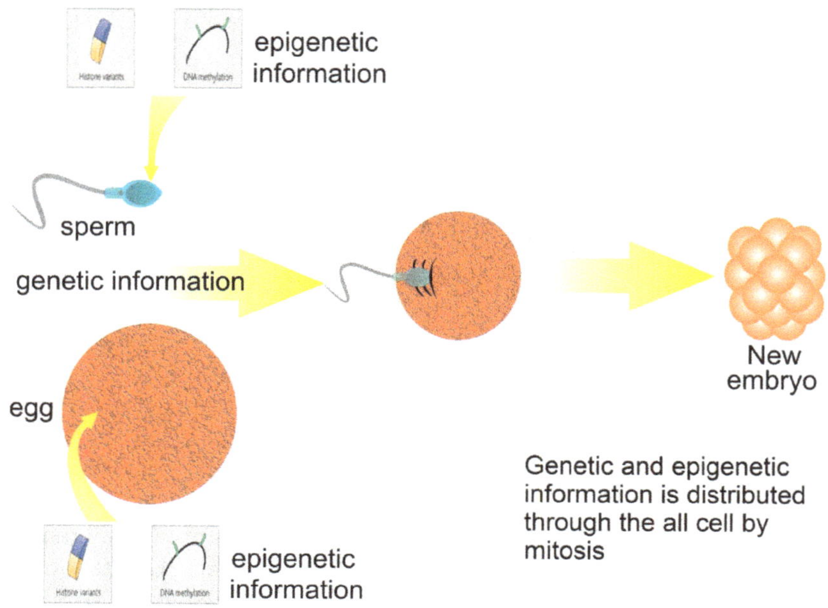

Figure 1. Genetic and epigenetic information in gametes and a new embryo.

Gene regulation and genome function are intimately related to the physical organization of genomic DNA and, in particular, to the way it is packaged into chromatin.[3] There are many chemical modifications affecting DNA, RNA, and proteins that create different epigenetic process.[4] These modifications are related to DNA methylation, histone modifications, chromatin remodeling factors (associated with nucleosome positioning), and noncoding RNAs.[4] The changes will influence the chromatin states and impact gene expression patterns (Figure 2).[5] Epigenetic alterations are associated with chromosomal instability and changes in transcriptional control, which influence the overall gene expression differences seen in many human malignancies.[5]

The carcinogenesis of head and neck cancer (HNC) is a human malignancy influenced by genetic factors, age, geography, and lifestyles, among which include smoking, oral hygiene, and human papillomavirus.[6, 7] In general, different types of carcinogens attack the oral mucosa through the accumulation of multiple genetic and epigenetic alterations in a multistep process.[8] The clinical appearance of HNC preoncogenic lesion of the mucosal surfaces include leukoplakia, erythroplakia, or speckled leukoplakia reflecting the presence of white, red, or mixed white/red lesion, respectively.[9]

HNC is one of the most prevalent human malignancies, affecting different anatomic sites of the upper aerodigestive tract (UADT) such as the oral cavity, larynx, and naso-, oro-, and hypopharynx.[10] The most common histologic type among the head and neck tumors are the squamous cell carcinomas (head and neck squamous cell carcinomas [HNSCCs]).[7]

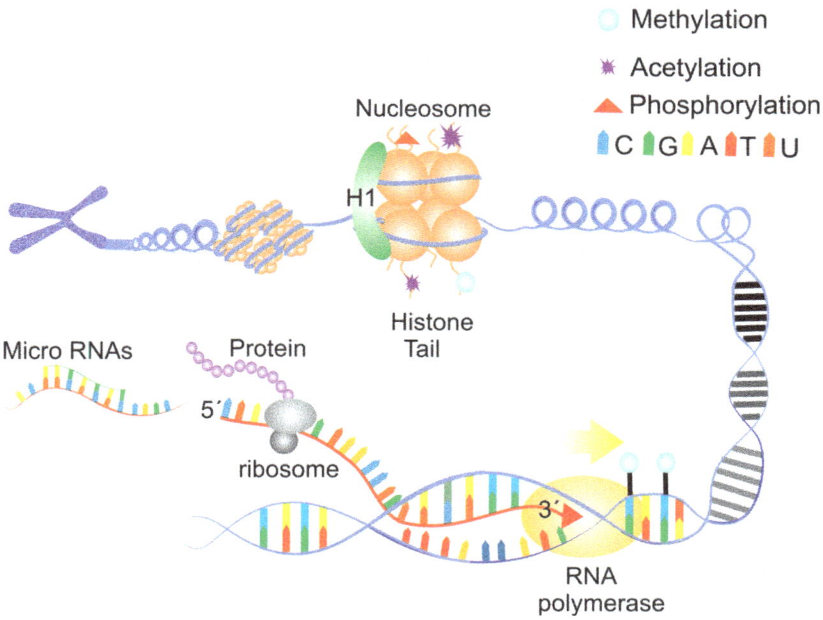

Figure 2. Genetic and epigenetic information.

It was reported that 42,440 new cases of HNSCCs were diagnosed in the United States in 2014, and 8,390 deaths were due to this disease.[11] The mortality rate (from 2003 to 2007) was of 2.5 per 100,000 persons per year. U.S. incidence and mortality rates are about 2.5 and 2.8 in men and women, respectively.[12]

Generally, the highest HNSCC rates are found in Melanesia, South-Central Asia, and Central and Eastern Europe and the lowest in Africa, Central America, and Eastern Asia for both males and females.[13]

The incidence rates for HNSCC related to HPV infections, such as oropharynx, tonsil, and tongue base, are increasing in young adults in the United States and in some countries in Europe, which is hypothesized to be in part due to changes in oral sexual behavior.[14]

In this issue, the aim is to describe epigenetic mechanisms behind HNSCC. The main mechanisms evaluated are DNA methylation, posttranslational histone modification, and noncoding RNAs

2. Epigenetic mechanisms

2.1. DNA methylation

DNA methylation is a chemical marking system for annotating genetic information by causing gene repression through its ability to affect factor binding and chromatin structure.[14] This system has gene expression patterns that are regulated in a spatial and time-dependent manner.[5] Heritable information is carried by chemical modifications of both DNA and chromatin-associated proteins and modulates chromatin structure and DNA accessibility.[5]

DNA methylation refers to the methylation of DNA cytosine residues at the carbon 5 position.[15, 16] DNA methyltransferases (DNMTs) catalyze the transfer of a methyl group to position 5 of a cytosine, generating 5-methylcytosine (5mC).[17] This chemical modification affects gene expression when CpG-rich areas are present inside promoter regions (figure 3).[16, 18] This is accomplished by the activities of one or more DNA methyltransferases (DNMTs), which use S-adenosylmethionine (AdoMet) as a cofactor.[19]

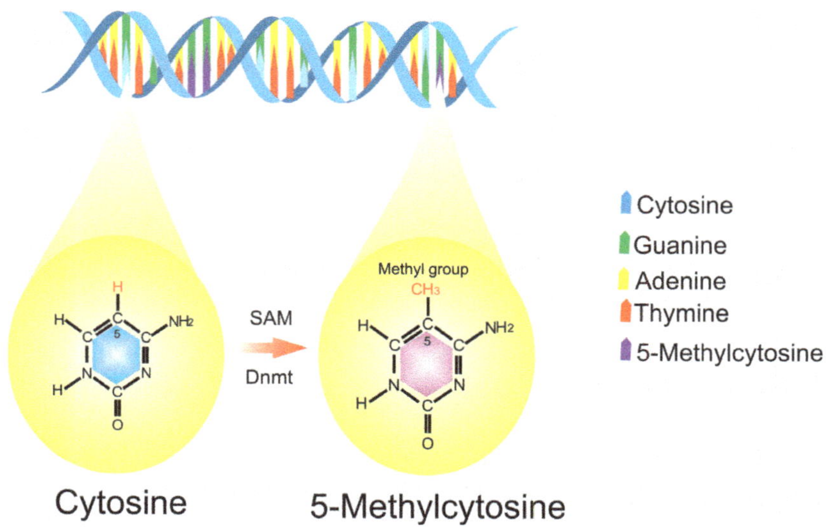

Figure 3. DNA methylation.

About 60% of human gene promoters are associated with CpG islands and are usually unmethylated in normal cells, although some of them (~6%) become methylated in a tissue-specific manner during early development or in differentiated tissues.[20]

Recent findings also suggest that extensive DNA methylation changes caused by differentiation take place at CpG island "shores," regions of comparatively low CpG density close to CpG islands.[2]

A relationship between DNA methylation and cancer has been found, given that DNA methyltransferases can be genetically altered in malignancies, that is, occur with DNMT3A20 and DNMT3B.[21] Aberrant DNA methylation is an epigenetic mechanism that contributes to the development of a wide variety of human cancers, either in the form of promoter-specific hypermethylation or genome-wide hypomethylation.[22] Hypermethylation in gene promoter regions is usually associated with expression suppression[23] and is the most common alterations in human cancers, leading to the abnormal expression of a broad spectrum of genes.[22] On the other hand, hypomethylation occurs in a large percentage in repetitive DNA elements.[24]

2.2. Posttranslational covalent histone modifications

Chromatin is the state in which DNA is packaged within the cell.[25] The chromatin architecture can be remodeled by a network of protein mediators called histones that play an important role in gene regulation by compacting DNA.[26] The nucleosome is the fundamental unit of chromatin, and it is composed of an octamer of histones (H2A, H2B, H3, and H4) around which 147 base pairs of DNA are wrapped.[25] Dynamic variations in the organization of chromatin structure are mediated by histone acetylation and deacetylation (figure 4).[25]

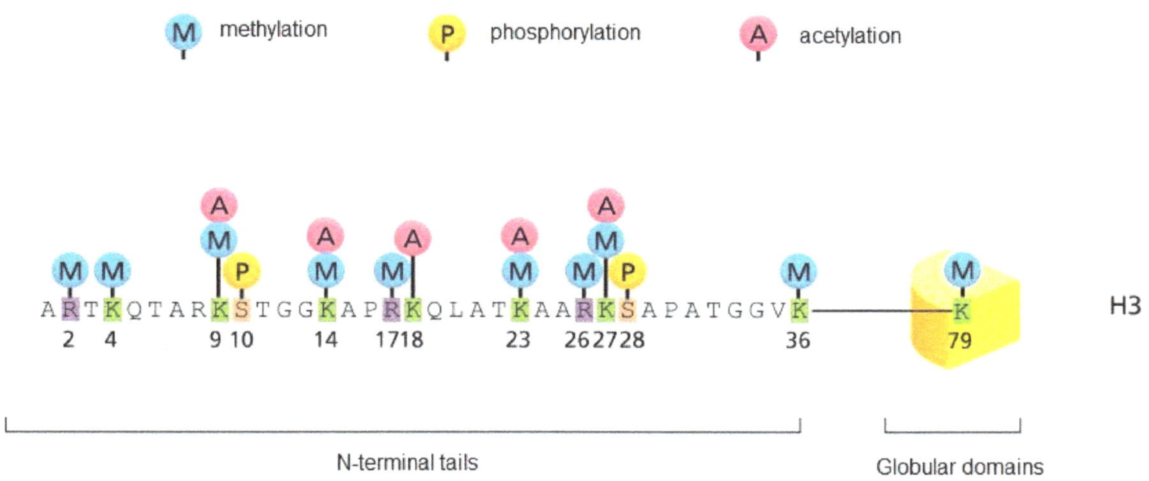

Figure 4. Posttranslational covalent histone modifications.

Acetylation neutralizes the positive charge of lysine residues, weakening charge-dependent interactions between histone and nucleosomal DNA, linker DNA, or adjacent histones, thus increasing the accessibility of DNA to the transcription machinery. Histone lysine acetylation also functions in other cellular processes that require DNA access.[27]

The posttranslational modification of histones by methylation is an important and widespread type of chromatin modification that is known to influence biological processes in the context of development and cellular responses.[28] Other modifications can be performed through lysine ubiquitination, serine phosphorylation, sumoylation, and methylation of lysines and arginines.[29]

Sumoylation is a process in which proteins are functionally or structurally similar to ubiquitin and are termed ubiquitin-like proteins (UBLs). UBLs include SUMO, NEDD8, ISG15, and FAT10.[30]

Histone acetyltransferases (HAT) catalyze the transfer of an acetyl group from acetyl-CoA to ε-amino group of a histone lysine residue.[31] The action of histone deacetylases (HDAC) is different because the effect is on the lysine residues. The first process involves chromatin decondensation, and the second process involves chromatin compaction. Either one or the other affects the gene transcription due to conformation changes in the chromatin.[31]

2.3. Noncoding RNAs

The noncoding RNAs are another level of epigenetic control for their capacity to establish other epigenetic marks and control gene expression.[4] Noncoding RNA (ncRNA) is a type of RNA that does not code for protein but has enzymatic, structural, or regulatory function.[32] ncRNAs can be classed as either small or long ncRNA, based on their transcript length.[33, 34]

2.4. MicroRNAs

MicroRNAs (miRNAs) are a set of non-protein-coding RNAs that bind to partially complementary sites in the 3′-untranslated regions of their messenger RNA targets.[35] MicroRNAs are the 21–23 nucleotide single-stranded RNA molecules found in eukaryotic cells.[36] The miRNAs interfere with messenger RNA translation or cause messenger RNA degradation, thereby repressing gene expression posttranscriptionally (Figure 5).[37] This is possible through imperfect base pairing with the 3′-untranslated region (3′-UTR) of target mRNAs of protein-coding genes, leading to the cleavage of homologous mRNA or translational inhibition.[38]

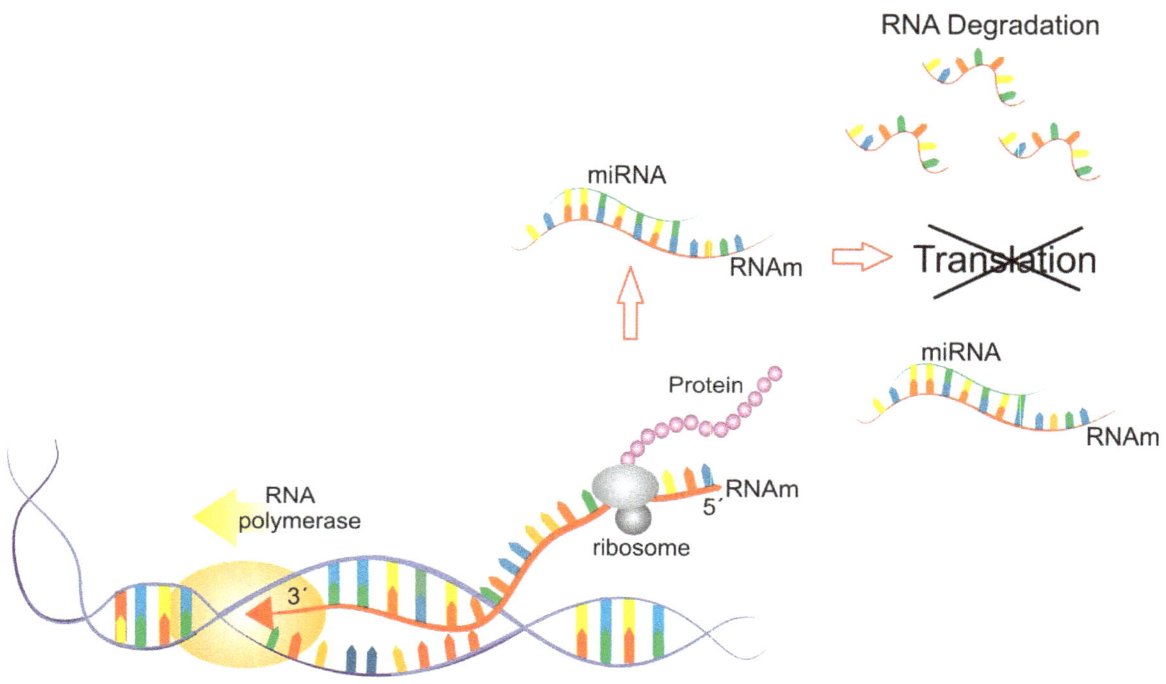

Figure 5. RNA degradation by miRNA.

miRNAs are transcribed for the most part by RNA polymerase II as long primary transcripts characterized by hairpin structures (pri-miRNA) and are processed in the nucleus by RNase III Drosha into 70–100 nucleotide long precursor miRNAs (pre-miRNAs).[39]

MicroRNAs are partial complementarity between their target transcripts. A single microRNA is capable of simultaneously regulating up to hundreds of genes, giving rise to an enormous modulatory potential.[40]

MicroRNAs are involved in a variety of cellular processes, including the regulation of cellular differentiation, proliferation, and apoptosis, and an aberrant expression of miRNA is known to induce various human malignancies.[41] New evidence suggests that miRNAs can act as oncogenes or tumor suppressors, exerting a key function in tumorigenesis.[42] Recently, a new function mediating tumor metastasis in breast cancer has been assigned to miRNAs, by which this malignant step is promoted or suppressed.[42]

2.5. Long noncoding RNAs

Long noncoding RNAs (lncRNAs) are generated by the same transcriptional machinery as are other mRNAs. These lncRNAs have a 5′ terminal methylguanosine cap and are often spliced and polyadenylated.[45] lncRNAs have length greater than 200 nucleotides without protein-coding potential but with a wide range of structural and functional roles.[34] Some of this process can include the chromatin remodeling and transcriptional control assemblies.[31] They are generally transcriptionally activated or repressed by associated transcription factors and function as molecular mediators of gene expression.[43] When the lncRNAs act as molecular scaffolds, they can guide the chromatin-modifying complexes to bind into specific genomic loci. This way, they impart a repressive or activating effect on gene expression (Figure 6).[43]

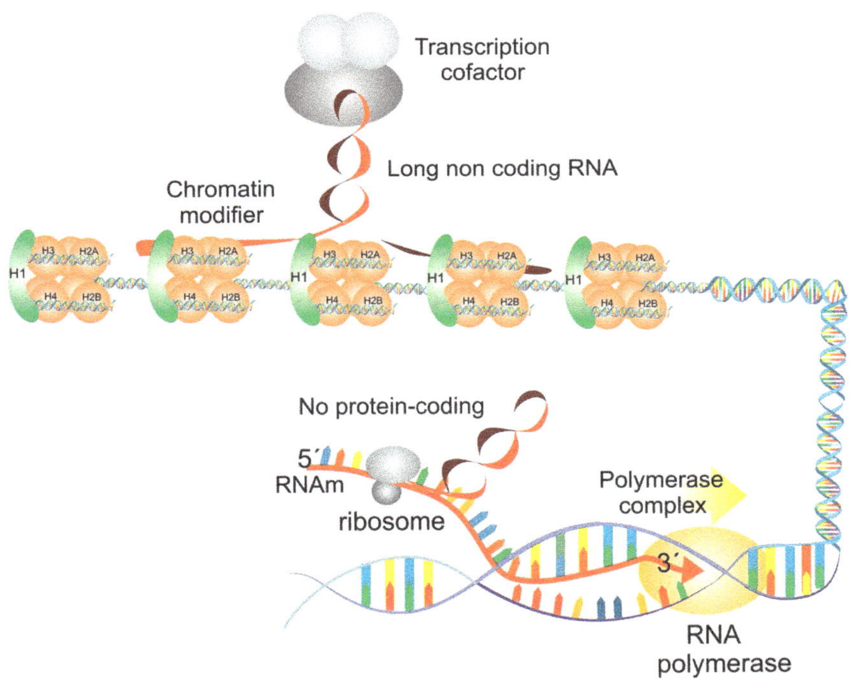

Figure 6. Long noncoding RNA.

According to their association with mRNA, the LncRNAs can be divided in different categories[44]: this can overlap with coding regions of a transcript on the same strand and with coding regions of a transcript on the opposite strand. This can be intronic lncRNAs from other transcript and can be intergenic lncRNAs between two genes on the same strand.[45]

The functions of the RNA in regulation of gene expression can be summarizing at transcriptional levels, RNA processing, and translation. Furthermore, they can protect genomes from foreign nucleic acids. At chromatin level, they can modulate the genome rearrangement.

Finally, the ncRNAs can operate as RNA–protein complexes, including ribosomes, snRNPs, snoRNPs, telomerase, microRNAs, and long ncRNAs.[46]

Long noncoding RNAs have also been shown to be necessary for targeting histone-modifying activities. Histone methylation is the end result of the transcription of long noncoding RNAs and the subsequent nucleation and targeting of histone modifying completes.[27]

The aberrant expression of lncRNAs has been associated with human cancers, suggesting a critical role in tumorigenesis.[47, 48] It has been demonstrated that a novel lncRNA, HOTAIR, was up-regulated and promoted cancer metastasis and predicted poor prognosis in ESCC.[34] Additionally, the association of dysregulated lncRNAs with specific developmental stages and clinical outcomes indicates their potential as strong diagnostic and prognostic predictors as well as therapeutic targets.[49]

3. Epigenetic changes in head and neck cancer

3.1. DNA methylation in head and neck cancer

The DNA methylation events in HNSCC include genes involved in cell cycle regulation, signal transduction, secreted protein, transmembrane protein, transcription factors, prostaglandin metabolism, metal ion homeostasis, oxidative stress, and oncoviruses.[50] Additionally, HNSCCs have genes involved in DNA damage repair, apoptosis, Wnt signaling, signal transduction, tissue invasion/metastasis, tumor suppression, and others (Figure 7, Table 1). [13, 51]

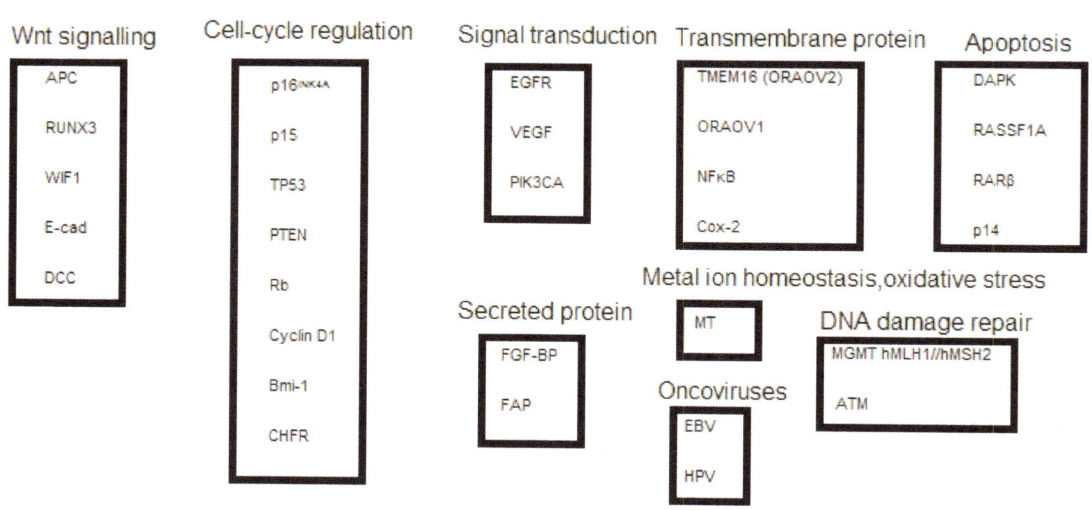

Figure 7. Genes and DNA methylation in HNSCC. Modified from Magić et al.,[13] Polanska et al.,[50] and Kaabi et al.[51]

Major classes	Member	Function
Cell cycle regulation	p16^{INK4A}	A tumor suppressor gene regulating senescence and cell cycle progression
	p15	Cyclin-dependent kinase inhibitor
	TP53	A tumor suppressor gene regulating cell cycle progression and cell survival
	PTEN	A tumor suppressor gene regulating signaling pathways controlling cell proliferation and apoptosis
	Rb	A proto-oncogene regulating cell cycle progression
	Cyclin D1	Controls cell cycle and self-renewal of tissue stem cells
	Bmi-1	Transmembrane TK that acts as a central transducer of multiple signaling pathways
	CHFR	Early G2/M checkpoint
Signal transduction	EGFR	A transmembrane TK that acts as a central transducer of multiple signaling pathways
	VEGF	A transmembrane TK that promotes proliferation, migration, and survival of endothelial cells during tumor growth
	PIK3CA	A gene encoding the p110a subunit of phosphoinositide 3-kinase (PI3K) α
Secreted protein	FGF-BP	Fibroblast growth factors binding protein
	FAP	Protein secreted by cancer-associated stroma
Transmembrane protein	TMEM16 (ORAOV2)	Calcium-activated chloride channel
	ORAOV1	A regulator of cell growth and tumor angiogenesis
	NFκB	Proinflammatory transcription factor
	Cox-2	Catalyzes prostaglandin synthesis from arachidonic acid
Metal ion homeostasis, oxidative stress	MT	Low molecular weight proteins involved in heavy metal detoxification, essential metal ion homeostasis, and cell protection against free radicals
Oncoviruses	EBV	A causative agent for most nasopharyngeal carcinomas, plasma EBV DNA load is an independent prognostic factor
	HPV	A causative agent for most oropharyngeal cancers
DNA damage repair	MGMT	DNA repair for alkylated guanine
	hMLH1//hMS	DNA mismatch repair
	H2 ATM	DNA double-strand breaks

Major classes	Member	Function
Apoptosis	DAPK	p53-dependent apoptosis
	RASSF1A	RAS pathway regulation and tumor suppression
	RARβ	Regulatory protein and apoptosis
	p14	Proapoptosis
Wnt signaling	APC	Wnt signaling and adhesion
	RUNX3	Wnt signaling inhibitor, TGF-β-induced tumor sup pression
	WIF1	Secreted Wnt antagonist
	E-cad	Cell adhesion, forming adherens junctions
	DCC	Cell–cell adhesion
Signal transduction	SFRP1	Antagonists of the Wnt pathway
	EDNRB	Endothelin receptor type B
	RUNX3	Wnt pathway antagonist
Tumor suppression	HIN1	Inhibitor Ras pathway
	DAPK1	Proapoptosis
	DCC	Proapoptosis
	RASSF1A/RASSF2	Negative RAS effector, proapoptotic, microtubule stabilization
Others	KIF1A	Cell division and microtubule-dependent intracellular organelle transport

Table 1. Genes and DNA methylation in HNSCC. Modified from Magić et al.,[13] Polanska et al.,[50] and Kaabi et al.[51]

The primary risk factors for the development of HNSCC include tobacco use, alcohol consumption, human papillomavirus (HPV) infections (mainly for oropharyngeal cancers), and Epstein–Barr virus (EBV) infections (for nasopharyngeal cancer).[52]

In promoter methylation, the p16 and p15 genes are commonly observed in human epithelial malignancies, including HNSCC. Histologically normal surgical margin epithelium of HNSCC patients with chronic smoking and drinking habits has a significantly higher prevalence of p15 methylation compared with nonsmokers and nondrinkers.[53]

Between genes that have been associated with hypermethylation, the p16 and the p14 genes undergo inactivation due to promoter hypermethylation.[13] Encoded by the CDKN2A gene, p16 inhibits cyclin-dependent kinases 4 and 6, thus blocking the promotion of cells from the G1 to the S phase of the cell cycle.[54] CDKN2A (p16) inactivation is common in lung cancer and occurs via homozygous deletions, methylation of promoter region, or point mutations.[55] CDKN2A (p16) disruption is reported as a frequent event in head and neck squamous cell carcinomas that confers poor prognosis.[56] Other genes as DAP-K, RASSF1A, RARß2, and MGMT have been reported as genes under hypermethylation promotor but with functions in DNA repair. These genes removed mutagenic (O6-guanine) adducts from DNA.[57]

DAPK and RASSF1A genes have shown methylation in HNSCC.[58] The methylation of p16 could be an initial process that might address abnormalities or deregulation of cell cycle controls.[59]

The ataxia-telangiectasia-mutated (*ATM*) gene produces a protein kinase that functions as a tumor suppressor by triggering appropriate cellular response to genome damage resulting from ionizing radiation or chemical carcinogen exposure.[60] It is currently unknown whether ATM is lost in HNSCCs displaying the deletion in the 11q22–23 locus.[61]

Aggressive HNSCC has been linked to expression loss of E-cadherin (ECAD) protein.[51] The protein ECAD can be inactivated by promoter hypermethylation.[62] In patients with HNSCC who are low smokers, the hypermethylation of CDH1 occurs more commonly, suggesting that an additional factor may be driving this epigenetic alteration.[62]

Cyclooxygenase-2 (Cox-2) is presumed to contribute to cancer progression through its multifaceted function, and recently its inverse relationship with E-cadherin was suggested. Increased expression of Cox-2 has been found in a variety of human malignancies, including HNSCC. [63]

The death-associated protein kinase (DAPk) family contains three closely related serine/threonine kinases, namely, DAPk, ZIPk, and DRP-1, which display a high degree of homology in their catalytic domains.[64] The methylation profile of DAPK in HNSCC (including oral squamous cell carcinoma) is a promising biomarker for the follow-up and early detection of head and neck cancer recurrence.[65]

The Ras association domain family protein 1A (RASSF1A) is arguably one of the most frequently inactivated tumor suppressors in human cancer. RASSF1A modulates apoptosis via the Hippo and Bax pathways but also modulates the cell cycle.[66] The epigenetic inactivation of RASSF1A plays an important role in the development of cancer.[67]

TP53, once activated, leads to apoptosis and growth arrest (either cell cycle arrest or senescence). It is clear that TP53 mutation is common in HNSCC.[68] The p53 transcription factor stands out as a key tumor suppressor and a master regulator of various signaling pathways involved in this process.[69] Tobacco smoke is the best known and studied mutagen involved in lung carcinogenesis, and TP53 mutational patterns differ between smokers and nonsmokers, with an excess of G to T transversions in smoking-associated cancer.[69]

The Cancer Genome Atlas has informed about smoking-related HNSCCs and its relations with the universal loss of function of TP53 mutations and CDKN2A. This inactivation is accompanied with frequent copy number alterations, including amplification of 3q26/28 and 11q13/22.[70]

The phosphatidylinositol 3-kinase (PI3K)/AKT/mTOR pathway is antagonized by phosphatase and tensin homologue (PTEN). PTEN protein is a tumor suppressor frequently disrupted in cancer, altering tumor cell growth and survival.[71] The decrease in PTEN function in HNSCC is due to several genetic and epigenetic alterations. Recently, promoter hypermethylation has been implicated in the down-regulation of PTEN in HNSCC cell lines.[72]

HNSCCs also exhibit many chromosomal abnormalities, including amplifications of the 11q13 region containing the cyclin D1 gene and the 7p11 region encoding EGFR, which lead to proto-oncogene activation.[73] The most critical point in regulation of the cell cycle is the G1 checkpoint. Cyclin D1, a G1 cyclin, has been implicated in the regulation of the G1 to S phase progression in many different cell types. Cyclin D1 forms active complexes that promote the phosphorylation of retinoblastoma protein (RB) and the activation of E2F-responsive gene.[74]

PIK3CA is a human gene that regulates various cellular functions, including proliferation and invasion. Because it is an oncogene, its activation by either gene amplification or mutation results in a cellular growth advantage contributing toward cancer formation and progression.[75] Mutations in PIK3CA have cases displayed of concurrent amplification. Additionally, some tumors (20%) contain focal amplification without evidence of mutation. The largest mutation proportions of PIK3CA are localized to hotspots that promote activation.[70] PIK3CA is an active mutation that is common in conjunction with infrequent copy number alteration, and it forms part of a subgroup of oral cavity tumors with favorable clinical outcomes.[70]

Bmi1 (B-cell-specific Moloney Murine Leukemia virus insertion site 1) is a transcription repressor for cell senescence, implicated in the self-renewal of stem cell. Bmi1 is highly expressed in the CD44+ cell population sorted from oral SCC tumors.[76]

E3 ubiquitin-protein ligase (CHFR) is a gene involved in a checkpoint regulating entry to mitosis.[77] Loss of CHFR leads to mitotic catastrophe and apoptosis due to mitotic spindle alteration. Aberrant methylation of the gene has been reported in several primary tumor genes. EGFR is a potential prognostic biomarker.[78]

Epidermal growth factor receptor (erb-B1) is a member of the erbB family of tyrosine kinase receptor proteins.[79] Previous studies have shown that EGFR is expressed or highly expressed in various human tumor cells.[79] The overexpression of EGFR is attributed to gene amplification, which is noted to be about 12 copies per cell in relation to head and neck squamous cell carcinomas. The constitutive EGFR activation caused via autocrine stimulation and through the coexpression of EGFR with its ligands, TGFα, has been observed and is indicative of its poor prognosis.[72] EGFR-targeted therapy is commonly used for the treatment of advanced HNSCC due to numerous findings that describe overexpression and/or high activity of EGFR in the majority of HNSCC.[80]

Various factors are known to regulate angiogenesis; for example, vascular endothelial cell growth factor (VEGF) has potent angiogenic effects. The presence of VEGF has been reported in approximately 40% of head and neck squamous cell carcinomas (HNSCCs), and its presence is associated with a poor prognosis.[72]

Other mechanisms included in the tumorous angiogenesis lie in the intake and utilization of locally stored fibroblast growth factors (FGFs).[50] FGF-1 (aFGF) and FGF-2 (bFGF) are found in most embryonic and adult normal and tumor tissues, where they are immobilized in the extracellular matrix (ECM).[81]

Fibroblast activation protein (FAP) is a member of the serine protease family that is selectively expressed in the stromal fibroblasts associated with epithelial cancers and is expressed at low or undetectable levels in the resting fibroblasts of normal adult tissues. FAP is expressed in more than 90% of epithelial carcinomas, which makes it a promising target.[82]

Oral cancer overexpressed 1 and 2 (ORAOV1-ORAOV2) overexpression was reported in HNSCC.[50, 83] The first is required for cell growth and tumor angiogenesis,[84] and the second is required in the modulation of TMEM16A activity in various epithelial tissues.[85]

Multiple signaling pathways have been linked to tumor resistance, including activation of nuclear factor kappa B (NFκB).[86] NFκB is an epigenetic modifier that plays a major role in malignant transformation, and this pathway serves as a target for epigenetic drugs.[26] The constitutive activation of NFκB signaling is often observed in HNSCC, suggesting a common epigenetic mechanism in HNSCC biology. Indeed, the activation of NFκB signaling in HNSCC induced chromatin compaction and acquisition of resistance to chemotherapy.[26]

Metallothionein (MT) is a family of cysteine-rich, low molecular weight (500–14,000 Da) proteins. MTs have been proposed to play important roles in protecting against DNA damage, apoptosis, and oxidative stress. MT is a tumor suppressor reported to show promoter hypermethylated in various cancers.[87]

Human mismatch repair genes (hMMR) have the ability to repair both mismatched bases and insertion loop errors during DNA replication.[88] Suboptimal DNA repair could result in disrupting the pattern of repeat sequences, causing chromosomal aberrations in the genome of patients suffering from instability syndromes. Significant proportions of carcinomas develop through DNA mismatch repair genes (MMR) deficiency and exhibit frequent microsatellite alteration (MA).[88]

The hypermethylated adenomatosis polyposis coli (APC) tumor suppressor gene has reduced expression levels along with loss of heterozygosity (LOH), leading to the altered functioning of the APC tumor suppressor proteins, which play a role for the integrity and function of the β-catenin destruction complex.[72] The APC protein, a negative regulator of this pathway, has been strongly implicated in the development of colon cancer but still has an undetermined role in the formation of oral cancer.[89]

Loss of heterozygosity of the APC gene and epigenetic events lead to the decreased expression of APC and the Wnt antagonists, the secreted frizzled-related proteins (SFRPs), Wnt inhibitory factors (WIFs), and Dickkopf family members (DKKs), primarily by promoter hypermethylation.[90] The persistent β-catenin signaling contributes to increased growth, metastatic potential, and resistance to chemotherapy in HNSCC and their tumor-initiating cells.[90] The methylation of WIF-1 correlated with shorter survival in oral cancer patients. The methylation of WIF1 may be considered a prognostic marker in oral cancers.[91]

Wnt pathway stimulates several intracellular signal transduction cascades (canonical and noncanonical).[92] The possible role of RUNX3 as a tumor suppressor in HNSCC has been reported. The promoter hypermethylation of antagonist's genes to Wnt (RUNX3) has been identified as a common event in cancer.[93]

Deleted in colorectal cancer (DCC) is a candidate tumor suppressor gene located at chromosome 18q21.[94] DCC promoter region hypermethylation was found in 75% of primary HNSCC. There was a significant correlation between DCC promoter region hypermethylation and DCC expression.[94] DCC is a putative conditional tumor suppressor gene that is epigenetically inactivated by promoter hypermethylation in a majority of HNSCC.[94, 95]

Secreted frizzled-related protein (SFRP1) is epigenetically silenced and functions as a tumor suppressor in oral squamous cell carcinoma (OSCC). The loss of SFRP2 expression is associated with hypermethylation of its promoter.[96]

The methylation of the *KIF1A* and *EDNRB* gene promoters is a frequent event in HNSCC.[97] KIF1A (kinesin family member 1A) encodes a protein that is a microtubule-dependent molecular motor involved in important intracellular functions such as organelle transport and cell division.[98] Endothelin receptor type B (EDNRB) is a G-protein-coupled receptor that activates a phosphatidylinositol calcium second messenger system.[97, 99]

Runt domain transcription factors (RUNXs) are homologous to products encoded by the Drosophila segmentation genes runt and lozenge.[100] The *RUNX3* gene is located on human chromosome 1p36, a region that has long been suspected to harbor one or more suppressors of various tumors.[101] Inactivation of RUNX3, which is caused mainly by epigenetic alteration, is closely associated with bladder tumor development, recurrence, and progression.[100, 101]

HIN-1 (high in normal-1) is a putative cytokine with growth inhibitory activities and is down-regulated by aberrant methylation in breast cancers.[102] Evidence suggests that HIN-1 is a potential tumor suppressor gene in non-small cell lung cancer (NSCLC), silenced by promoter hypermethylation and negatively regulated by AKT signaling pathway.[103] Silencing of HIN-1 expression and methylation of its promoter occurs in multiple human cancer types, suggesting that the elimination of HIN-1 function may contribute to several forms of epithelial tumorigenesis.[104]

3.2. Histone modifications in head and neck cancer

Aberrant regulation of the demethylases controlling H3K9me3 and H4K20me3 levels could contribute to the oncogenic potential. For instance, levels of H3K4me2 and me3 are significantly different in oral squamous cell carcinoma in comparison with cells of the healthy tissues; the level of H3K4me2 is increased while that of H3K4me3 is decreased.[102, 105]

A similar trend was observed in tongue squamous cell carcinoma (SCC) cells where the levels of the H3K27me3 marks at chromatin near homeobox genes were inversely correlated with the transcript levels in nontumorigenic, immortalized human oral keratinocytes (OKF6-TERT1R) and tumorigenic oral SCC-9 cells.[25] This investigation found that the levels of the H3K27me3 marks at chromatin near homeobox genes were inversely correlated with the transcript levels in nontumorigenic, immortalized human oral keratinocytes (OKF6- TERT1R) and tumorigenic oral SCC-9 cells.[25]

The emerging importance of the regulation of the H3K27me3 mark as a driver of squamous differentiation suggests that SCCs may harbor defects in the epigenetic regulation of squamous differentiation.[106] The dysregulation of squamous differentiation is fundamental to the development of SCC and has been reported to occur early in premalignant lesions.[107]

On the other hand, serine phosphorylation plays an important role in assembling the DNA damage response complex by identifying DNA double-strand breaks (DSB) in the chromatin. Upon DSB, ATM induces the phosphorylation of γH2AX at serine 139, resulting in the recruitment of BRCA1, BRCA2, Rad51, Mre11, NBS1, FANCD2, and p53 repair proteins to sites of DNA damage.[108]

In addition, the phosphorylation of serine 536 involved in the phosphorylation of RELA has also been reported. RELA, also known as p65, is an REL-associated protein involved in NF-κB heterodimer formation, nuclear translocation, and activation.[109] The phosphorylation of serine 468 is also associated with RELA.[109]

Regarding sumoylation, there are also desumoylating enzymes called SENPs, which remove the SUMO residues from the sumoylated proteins. Two molecules involved in the SUMO pathway, Ubc9 and SENP5, are up-regulated in SCCs. The up-regulation of SENP5 is found in oral SCCs, and strong SENP5 expression is correlated with poor prognosis.[110]

Finally, the lysine methylation of HSP90AB1 is important for its homodimerization and its interaction with stress-induced phosphoprotein 1 (STIP1) and cell division cycle 37 (CDC37), which are co-chaperones of HSP90AB1 in human cancer cells, resulting in enhancement of cancer cell growth.[111]

3.3. miRNAs in head and neck cancer

DNA copy number variations or deregulation of miRNA expression has been shown to contribute to carcinogenesis, including carcinogenesis of HNSCC.[112] Several studies have reported global miRNA expression changes in carcinogenesis of HNSCC, using various samples sizes, anatomical sites, and profiling methodologies.[113]

It has been demonstrated the differential expression patterns of miRNAs in numerous types of cancer. MiR-92a, miR-103/107, miR-21, miR143, miR145, miR-205 and miR-296, among others, have been confirmed to be involved in the development of esophageal squamous cell carcinoma (ESCC).[34]

It has been reported that members of the miR-17-92 cluster were deregulated in 15 patients with OSCC (tongue and floor of the mouth) and 35 patients with HNSCC. The miR-19a and the miR-19b were strongly up-regulated. The miR-17-3p/miR-17-5p and the miR-92b were moderately up-regulated. Evidence has been found that the miR-17-92 cluster is up-regulated in many cancer types.[114] Furthermore, the miR-196a and the miR-10b, not previously associated with HNSCC, may play an oncogenic role in this disease through the deregulation of cell proliferation.[114]

Other studies informed that miR-21, miR-31, miR-504, and miR-10b are target tumor suppressor genes. These miRNAs are involved in HNSCC.[115] Many studies have confirmed the tumor suppressor roles of the let-7 family (the miR-99 family, miR-107, miR-133a, miR-137, miR-138, and miR-375). Other miRNAs such as miR-21, let-7, miR-107, miR-138, and miR-200c are involved in regulating stemness or the epithelial–mesenchymal transition of tumor cells.[115]

It has also been evaluated that miR-34a is significantly down-regulated in HNSCC tumors and cell lines.[116] The ectopic expression of miR-34a in HNSCC cell lines significantly inhibited tumor cell proliferation, colony formation, and migration. Tumor samples from HNSCC patients showed an inverse relationship between miR-34a and survival as well as between miR-34a and E2F3 levels.[116]

In silico analysis identified three putative microRNA-107 (miR-107) binding sites in the 3′-untranslated region (UTR) of PKCε.[117] An inverse relationship was revealed between miR-107 and PKCε in HNSCC cell lines. These data demonstrated that PKCε is directly regulated by miR-107 and, moreover, suggest that miR-107 may be a potential anticancer therapeutic for HNSCC.[117]

New computational approach strategies complementary to microRNA profiling are capable of simultaneously predicting tumor suppressor microRNAs as well as their functional targets from gene expression.[118] It provided a plausible mechanism that loss of the tumor suppressor function of miR-204 as a result of allelic imbalance at 9q21.1–q22.3 may significantly increase genetic susceptibility to HNSCC oncogenesis and progression.[118] The complete suppression of miR-204 and its host gene TRPM3 has become possible that the mRNA expression may serve as a marker the expression status in HNSCC.[118]

3.4. lncRNAs in head and neck cancer

LncRNAs have been linked to essential growth-promoting activities, and their deregulation contributes to tumor cell survival. A prominent example is the Hox transcript antisense intergenic lncRNA, HOTAIR.[119] The HOTAIR gene controls gene expression, and its expression is deregulated in a spectrum of cancers. Furthermore, HOTAIR expression correlates with patient survival.[119, 120]

HOTAIR serves as a scaffold for at least two distinct histone modification complexes. A 5′ domain of HOTAIR binds Polycomb Repressive Complex 2 (PRC2), while a 3′ domain of HOTAIR binds the LSD1/CoREST/REST complex. lncRNAPCAT-1, a target gene of polycomb repressive complex 2, has been implicated in disease progression by promoting cell proliferation.[121] The ability to link two distinct complexes enables RNA-mediated assembly of PRC2 and LSD1 and coordinates targeting of PRC2 and LSD1 to chromatin for coupled histone H3 lysine 27 methylation and lysine 4 demethylation.[122]

In prostate cancer, the up-regulation of antisense noncoding RNA in the INK4 locus (ANRIL) is required for the expression of the tumor suppressors INK4a/p16 and INK4b/p15.[121]

Some examples of lncRNAs that has a role in chromatin remolding include *XIST*, which acts by recruiting the PRC2 complex to initiate X-chromosome inactivation as well as *MALAT* and *NEAT1*, both of which play a role in mRNA processing and nuclear organization.[123]

The expression of LINC00312 in nasopharyngeal carcinoma has a tumor-suppressive function. Under physiological conditions, LINC00312 inhibits proliferation in nasopharyngeal epithelium by preventing cell cycle passage from the G1 into S phase but increases cell adhesion, motility, and invasion by down-regulating the expression of estrogen receptor alpha (ERα).[124]

Other genes regulated by lncRNAs that have been implicated in cancer include NDM29, BACE1AS, and Drosophila hsr-ω gene.[125] Neuroblastoma differentiation Marker 29 (NDM29) is an RNA polymerase (pol) III-transcribed noncoding (nc) RNA whose synthesis drives neuroblastoma (NB) cell differentiation to a nonmalignant neuron-like phenotype.[126] BACE1 plays a pivotal role in the accumulation of β-amyloid plaques and has been shown to regulate the expression of BACE1 by increasing BACE1 mRNA stability.[127] The heat shock RNA omega (hsrω) gene of *Drosophila melanogaster* is inducible by cell stress and provides structural base for sequestering diverse RNA-processing/regulatory proteins.[128]

4. Clinical applications in head and neck cancer

To date, four epigenetic inhibitors have been approved by the U.S. Food and Drug Administration (FDA) for cancer treatment.[129] The DNMT inhibitors as 5-aza-cytidine and 5-aza-2′-deoxycytidine are widely used in in vitro in research. The cytosine analogs are converted to deoxynucleotide triphosphates inside the cell and then incorporated into the DNA during replication in the original C positions.[130]

Other inhibitors of HATs approved by FDA are p300, lysine methyltransferases (H3K79 methyltransferase DOT1L, or the polycomb complex member EZH2), and lysine demethylases (LSd1). Furthermore, small molecule inhibitors targeting the histone reader, BRD4, have also shown promise as therapeutic agent in many cancer types.[131]

The effects of an epigenetic inhibitor as lysine residues on histone tails are HDAC inhibitors that counteract the global overexpression of HDACs in cancer and reinstate a more permissive nucleosome structure for transcription.[132] Vorinostat (a pan-HDAC inhibitor) and romidepsin (a class I HDAC inhibitor) have each shown >30% response rates against cutaneous T-cell lymphoma (CTCL) in phase II trials.[132]

Cetuximab is an inhibitor of the epidermal growth factor receptor (EGFR) that is used in radiation therapy. It was found to enhance HNSCC patient survival compared with radiation therapy alone.[133] The FDA has approved cetuximab to treat HNSCC; the drug has a response rate of about 10% when used as a single agent in recurrent/metastatic disease.[134] However, despite approval of cetuximab, improvement in patient survival with the use of this agent has been only modestly incremental.[133]

Advances in oncogenomics have also identified mutations in epigenetic-associated genes that encode histones and their linkers, proteins associated with the recruitment of DNA-binding proteins, HDAC I and II interacting proteins, corepressor proteins, and transcriptional activators and coactivators.[135]

The understanding of which gene mutations, DNA methylation, posttranslational histone modification, and noncoding RNAs drive the carcinogenesis may help us understand how tumor susceptibility guides the development of new combination therapies. However, it is important remember that not all cancers are equally susceptible to epigenetic therapies. The biology underpinning this observation urgently warrants our attention if epigenetic therapies are to be more widely applicable.[136]

5. Conclusions

Understanding the complexity of the epigenome, the different dynamics, and the different subunits is complex and intimidating. Gene mutations, DNA methylation, posttranslational histone modification, and noncoding RNAs are actors involved in modulating its interactions with genomic sequences, and this is fundamental for health and disease.

Only our hope and desire can continue creating new ways to interact with the epigenome, and it will be possible to build a new world where the HNSCC and other types of cancer will be able to have new therapies and new opportunities for a better life.

Author details

Julio Cesar Osorio[1] and Andres Castillo[2*]

*Address all correspondence to: acastillo.doc@gmail.com

1 School of Biomedical Sciences, Universidad del Valle, Cali, Colombia

2 Biology Department, Faculty of Exact and Natural Sciences of Universidad del Valle, Cali, Colombia

References

[1] Gibney ER, Nolan CM. Epigenetics and gene expression. Heredity. 2010 07//print; 105(1):4–13.

[2] Rodriguez-Paredes M, Esteller M. Nature Medicine. 2011;17(null):330.

[3] Bernstein BE, Stamatoyannopoulos JA, Costello JF, Ren B, Milosavljevic A, Meissner A, et al. The NIH roadmap epigenomics mapping consortium. Nat Biotechnol. 2010 Oct;28(10):1045–8.

[4] Esteller M. Cancer epigenetics for the 21st century: what's next? Genes and Cancer. 2011 Jun;2(6):604–6.

[5] Park YJ, Claus R, Weichenhan D, Plass C. Genome-wide epigenetic modifications in cancer. Progress in Drug Research. 2011;67:25–49.

[6] Ragin CC, Taioli E. Survival of squamous cell carcinoma of the head and neck in relation to human papillomavirus infection: review and meta-analysis. International Journal of Cancer. 2007 Oct 15;121(8):1813–20.

[7] Magić Z, Supić G, Branković-Magić M, Jović N. DNA Methylation in the Pathogenesis of Head and Neck Cancer. 2012 2012-11-28.

[8] Mao L, Hong WK, Papadimitrakopoulou VA. Focus on head and neck cancer. Cancer Cell. 5(4):311–6.

[9] Harrison LB, Sessions RB, Hong WK. Head and Neck Cancer: A Multidisciplinary Approach. Lipppincott Williams & Wilkins; 2009.

[10] Koffler J, Sharma S, Hess J. Predictive value of epigenetic alterations in head and neck squamous cell carcinoma. Molecular and Cellular Oncology. 2014 2014/06/16;1(2):e954827.

[11] American Cancer Society. Cancer Facts & Figures 2014. Atlanta: American Cancer Society; 2014.

[12] Ferlay J, Shin HR, Bray F, Forman D, Mathers C, Parkin DM. Estimates of worldwide burden of cancer in 2008: GLOBOCAN 2008. International journal of cancer. 2010;127(12):2893–917.

[13] Jemal A, Bray F, Center MM, Ferlay J, Ward E, Forman D. Global cancer statistics. CA Cancer J Clin. 2011 Mar–Apr;61(2):69–90.

[14] Bergman Y, Cedar H. DNA methylation dynamics in health and disease. Nature Structural and Molecular Biology. 2013;20(3):274–81.

[15] O'Sullivan E, Goggins M. DNA methylation analysis in human cancer. Methods in Molecular Biology. 2013;980:131–156.

[16] Herman JG, Graff JR, Myöhänen S, Nelkin BD, Baylin SB. Methylation-specific PCR: a novel PCR assay for methylation status of CpG islands. Proceedings of the National Academy of Sciences of the United States of America. 1996;93(18):9821–6.

[17] Witte T, Plass C, Gerhauser C. Pan-cancer patterns of DNA methylation. Genome Medicine. 2014;6(8):66.

[18] Dantas Machado AC, Zhou T, Rao S, et al. Evolving insights on how cytosine methylation affects protein–DNA binding. Briefings in Functional Genomics. 2015;14(1):61–73.

[19] Weisenberger DJ, Campan M, Long TI, Kim M, Woods C, Fiala E, et al. Analysis of repetitive element DNA methylation by MethyLight. Nucleic Acids Research. 2005;33(21):6823–36.

[20] Portela A, Esteller M. Epigenetic modifications and human disease. Nature Biotechnology. 2010;28(10):1057–68.

[21] Fernandez AF, Assenov Y, Martin-Subero JI, Balint B, Siebert R, Taniguchi H, et al. A DNA methylation fingerprint of 1628 human samples. Genome Research. 2012;22(2): 407–19.

[22] Lima SC, Hernandez-Vargas H, Simao T, Durand G, Kruel CD, Le Calvez-Kelm F, et al. Identification of a DNA methylome signature of esophageal squamous cell carcinoma and potential epigenetic biomarkers. Epigenetics. 2011 Oct 1;6(10):1217–27.

[23] Adorján P, Distler J, Lipscher E, Model F, Müller J, Pelet C, et al. Tumour class prediction and discovery by microarray-based DNA methylation analysis. Nucleic Acids Research. 2002 Mar 1, 2002;30(5):e21.

[24] Richards KL, Zhang B, Baggerly KA, Colella S, Lang JC, Schuller DE, et al. Genome-wide hypomethylation in head and neck cancer is more pronounced in HPV-negative tumors and is associated with genomic instability. PloS One. 2009;4(3):e4941.

[25] Marcinkiewicz KM, Gudas LJ. Altered histone mark deposition and DNA methylation at homeobox genes in human oral squamous cell carcinoma cells. Journal of Cellular Physiology. 2014;229(10):1405–16.

[26] Le JM, Squarize CH, Castilho RM. Histone modifications: targeting head and neck cancer stem cells. World Journal of Stem Cells. 2014 11/26;6(5):511–25. PubMed PMID: PMC4178252.

[27] Zentner GE, Henikoff S. Regulation of nucleosome dynamics by histone modifications. Nature Structural and Molecular Biology. 2013;20(3):259–66.

[28] Greer EL, Shi Y. Histone methylation: a dynamic mark in health, disease and inheritance. Nature Reviews. Genetics. 2012;13(5):343–57.

[29] Spotswood HT, Turner BM. An increasingly complex code. Journal of Clinical Investigation. 2002 Sep;110(5):577–82.

[30] Welchman RL, Gordon C, Mayer RJ. Ubiquitin and ubiquitin-like proteins as multifunctional signals. Nature Reviews. Molecular Cell Biology. 2005 Aug;6(8):599–609.

[31] Giudice FS, Pinto DS, Nör JE, Squarize CH, Castilho RM. Inhibition of histone deacetylase impacts cancer stem cells and induces epithelial-mesenchyme transition of head and neck cancer. PloS One. 2013 03/20;8(3):e58672.

[32] Kugel JF, Goodrich JA. Non-coding RNAs: key regulators of mammalian transcription. Trends in Biochemical Sciences. 2012 Apr;37(4):144–51.

[33] Costa FF. Non-coding RNAs: meet thy masters. Bioessays. 2010 Jul;32(7):599–608.

[34] Li SQ, Li F, Xiao Y, Wang CM, Tuo L, Hu J, et al. Comparison of long noncoding RNAs, microRNAs and messenger RNAs involved in initiation and progression of esophageal squamous cell carcinoma. Molecular Medicine Reports. 2014 Aug;10(2): 652–62.

[35] Schickel R, Boyerinas B, Park SM, Peter ME. MicroRNAs: key players in the immune system, differentiation, tumorigenesis and cell death. Oncogene. 2008 Oct 6;27(45): 5959–74.

[36] Zhou X, Yang PC. MicroRNA: a small molecule with a big biological impact. Micro-RNA (Shariqah, United Arab Emirates). 2012;1(1):1.

[37] Avissar M, McClean MD, Kelsey KT, Marsit CJ. MicroRNA expression in head and neck cancer associates with alcohol consumption and survival. Carcinogenesis. 2009 Dec 1, 2009;30(12):2059–63.

[38] Shiiba M, Uzawa K, Tanzawa H. MicroRNAs in head and neck squamous cell carcinoma (HNSCC) and oral squamous cell carcinoma (OSCC). Cancers. 2010;2(2):653–69.

[39] Takahashi R-u, Miyazaki H, Ochiya T. The role of microRNAs in the regulation of cancer stem cells. Frontiers in Genetics. 2013;4:295.

[40] Avissar M, Christensen BC, Kelsey KT, Marsit CJ. MicroRNA expression ratio is predictive of head and neck squamous cell carcinoma. Clinical Cancer Research. 2009;15(8):2850–5.

[41] Kimura S, Naganuma S, Susuki D, Hirono Y, Yamaguchi A, Fujieda S, et al. Expression of microRNAs in squamous cell carcinoma of human head and neck and the esophagus: miR-205 and miR-21 are specific markers for HNSCC and ESCC. Oncology Reports. 2010 Jun;23(6):1625–33.

[42] Lujambio A, Calin GA, Villanueva A, Ropero S, Sánchez-Céspedes M, Blanco D, et al. A microRNA DNA methylation signature for human cancer metastasis. Proceedings of the National Academy of Sciences. 2008 Sept 9, 2008;105(36):13556–61.

[43] Ghosal S, Das S, Chakrabarti J. Long noncoding RNAs: new players in the molecular mechanism for maintenance and differentiation of pluripotent stem cells. Stem Cells and Development. 2013 Aug 15;22(16):2240–53.

[44] Quan M, Chen J, Zhang D. Exploring the secrets of long noncoding RNAs. Pichler M, editor. International Journal of Molecular Sciences. 2015;16(3):5467–5496.

[45] Mercer TR, Mattick JS. Structure and function of long noncoding RNAs in epigenetic regulation. Nature Structural and Molecular Biology. 2013;20(3):300–7.

[46] Cech Thomas R, Steitz Joan A. The noncoding RNA revolution—trashing old rules to forge new ones. Cell.157(1):77–94.

[47] Gibb EA, Enfield KS, Stewart GL, Lonergan KM, Chari R, Ng RT, et al. Long non-coding RNAs are expressed in oral mucosa and altered in oral premalignant lesions. Oral Oncology. 2011 Nov;47(11):1055–61.

[48] Qi P, Du X. The long non-coding RNAs, a new cancer diagnostic and therapeutic gold mine. Modern Pathology. 2013;26(2):155–65.

[49] Xu M-d, Qi P, Du X. Long non-coding RNAs in colorectal cancer: implications for pathogenesis and clinical application. Modern Pathology. 2014;27(10):1310–20.

[50] Polanska H, Raudenska M, Gumulec J, Sztalmachova M, Adam V, Kizek R, et al. Clinical significance of head and neck squamous cell cancer biomarkers. Oral Oncology. 2014;50(3):168–77.

[51] Al-Kaabi A, van Bockel LW, Pothen AJ, Willems SM. p16INK4A and p14ARF gene promoter hypermethylation as prognostic biomarker in oral and oropharyngeal squamous cell carcinoma: a review. Disease Markers. 2014;2014:8.

[52] Ovchinnikov DA, Wan Y, Coman WB, Pandit P, Cooper-White JJ, Herman JG, et al. DNA methylation at the novel CpG sites in the promoter of MED15/PCQAP gene as a biomarker for head and neck cancers. Biomarker Insights. 2014;9:53–60.

[53] Wong TS, Man MW, Lam AK, Wei WI, Kwong YL, Yuen AP. The study of p16 and p15 gene methylation in head and neck squamous cell carcinoma and their quantitative evaluation in plasma by real-time PCR. European Journal of Cancer. 2003 Sept; 39(13):1881–7.

[54] Pierini S, Jordanov SH, Mitkova AV, Chalakov IJ, Melnicharov MB, Kunev KV, et al. Promoter hypermethylation of CDKN2A, MGMT, MLH1, and DAPK genes in laryngeal squamous cell carcinoma and their associations with clinical profiles of the patients. Head and Neck. 2014;36(8):1103–8.

[55] Tam KW, Zhang W, Soh J, Stastny V, Chen M, Sun H, et al. CDKN2A/p16 inactivation mechanisms and their relationship to smoke exposure and molecular features in non-small-cell lung cancer. Journal of Thoracic Oncology. 2013 Nov;8(11):1378–88.

[56] Lim AM, Do H, Young RJ, Wong SQ, Angel C, Collins M, et al. Differential mechanisms of CDKN2A (p16) alteration in oral tongue squamous cell carcinomas and correlation with patient outcome. International Journal of Cancer. 2014;135(4):887–95.

[57] Worsham MJ, Stephen JK, Chen KM, Havard S, Shah V, Gardner G, et al. Delineating an epigenetic continuum in head and neck cancer. Cancer Letters. 2014 Jan 28;342(2): 178–84.

[58] Supic G, Kozomara R, Brankovic-Magic M, Jovic N, Magic Z. Gene hypermethylation in tumor tissue of advanced oral squamous cell carcinoma patients. Oral Oncology. 2009 Dec;45(12):1051–7.

[59] Laytragoon-Lewin N, Chen F, Castro J, Elmberger G, Rutqvist LE, Lewin F, et al. DNA content and methylation of p16, DAPK and RASSF1A Gene in tumour and dis-

tant, normal mucosal tissue of head and neck squamous cell carcinoma patients. Anticancer Research. 2010 Nov 1, 2010;30(11):4643–8.

[60] Ai L, Vo QN, Zuo C, Li L, Ling W, Suen JY, et al. Ataxia-telangiectasia-mutated (ATM) gene in head and neck squamous cell carcinoma: promoter hypermethylation with clinical correlation in 100 cases. Cancer Epidemiology Biomarkers and Prevention. 2004 Jan 1, 2004;13(1):150–6.

[61] Chen Y, Chen C. DNA copy number variation and loss of heterozygosity in relation to recurrence of and survival from head and neck squamous cell carcinoma: a review. Head and Neck. 2008 Oct;30(10):1361–83.

[62] Marsit CJ, Posner MR, McClean MD, Kelsey KT. Hypermethylation of E-cadherin is an independent predictor of improved survival in head and neck squamous cell carcinoma. Cancer. 2008 Oct 1;113(7):1566–71.

[63] Fujii R, Imanishi Y, Shibata K, Sakai N, Sakamoto K, Shigetomi S, et al. Restoration of E-cadherin expression by selective Cox-2 inhibition and the clinical relevance of the epithelial-to-mesenchymal transition in head and neck squamous cell carcinoma. Journal of Experimental and Clinical Cancer Research. 2014;33(1):40.

[64] Gozuacik D, Kimchi A. DAPk protein family and cancer. Autophagy. 2006 Apr–Jun; 2(2):74–9.

[65] Liu M, Feng L, Tang X, Guo X. Gene promoter hypermethylation in leukoplakia of the oral mucosa. Pathology and Laboratory Medicine International. 2010;2:71–7.

[66] Donninger H, Clark JA, Monaghan MK, Schmidt ML, Vos M, Clark GJ. Cell cycle restriction is more important than apoptosis induction for RASSF1A protein tumor suppression. Journal of Biological Chemistry. 2014 Nov 7;289(45):31287–95.

[67] Koutsimpelas D, Pongsapich W, Heinrich ULF, Mann S, Mann WJ, Brieger J. Promoter methylation of MGMT, MLH1 and RASSF1A tumor suppressor genes in head and neck squamous cell carcinoma: pharmacological genome demethylation reduces proliferation of head and neck squamous carcinoma cells. Oncology Reports. 2012;27(4): 1135–41.

[68] Mitra S, Mukherjee N, Das S, Das P, Panda CK, Chakrabarti J. Anomalous altered expressions of downstream gene-targets in TP53-miRNA pathways in head and neck cancer. Scientific Reports. 2014 09/04/online;4.

[69] Rivlin N, Brosh R, Oren M, Rotter V. Mutations in the p53 tumor suppressor gene: important milestones at the various steps of tumorigenesis. Genes and Cancer. 2011;2(4):466–74.

[70] The Cancer Genome Atlas N. Comprehensive genomic characterization of head and neck squamous cell carcinomas. Nature. 2015;517(7536):576–82.

[71] M. Dillon L, W. Miller T. Therapeutic targeting of cancers with loss of PTEN function. Current Drug Targets. 2014 //;15(1):65–79.

[72] Grover J, Rakheja M, Rao NN, Singh A, Solomon MC. Emerging strategies against head and neck cancer—a review. IOSR Journal of Dental and Medical Sciences. 2014;13(9):138–47.

[73] Guerrero-Preston R, Michailidi C, Marchionni L, Pickering CR, Frederick MJ, Myers JN, et al. Key tumor suppressor genes inactivated by "greater promoter" methylation and somatic mutations in head and neck cancer. Epigenetics. 2014;9(7):1031–46.

[74] Iizuka S, Oridate N, Nashimoto M, Fukuda S, Tamura M. Growth Inhibition of head and neck squamous cell carcinoma cells by sgRNA targeting the cyclin D1 mRNA based on TRUE gene silencing. PloS One. 2014;9(12):e114121.

[75] Park B. PIK3CA Oncogene. In: Schwab M, editor. Encyclopedia of Cancer. Springer Berlin Heidelberg; 2009. pp. 2342–3.

[76] Li C-C, Woo S-B. Understanding the pathobiology of head and neck squamous cell carcinoma. Current Oral Health Reports. 2014;1(3):196–203.

[77] van Kempen PMW, van Bockel L, Braunius WW, Moelans CB, van Olst M, de Jong R, et al. HPV-positive oropharyngeal squamous cell carcinoma is associated with TIMP3 and CADM1 promoter hypermethylation. Cancer Medicine. 2014;3(5):1185–96.

[78] Pelosof L, Yerram SR, Ahuja N, Delmas A, Danilova L, Herman JG, et al. CHFR silencing or microsatellite instability is associated with increased antitumor activity of docetaxel or gemcitabine in colorectal cancer. International Journal of Cancer. 2014;134(3):596–605.

[79] Han YH, Hamid MRA, Telisinghe PU, Hussin JBH, Mabruk M. Overexpression of EGFR protein in Bruneian lung cancer patients. Asian Pacific Journal of Cancer Prevention. 2015;16(1):233.

[80] Tepper SR, Zuo Z, Khattri A, Heitmann J, Heß J, Seiwert T. Abstract 1847: Influence of growth factors on resistance to EGFR inhibitor treatment in HNSCC—Temsirolimus as a potential concept. Cancer Research. 2014;74(19 Supplement):1847.

[81] Aigner A, Butscheid M, Kunkel P, Krause E, Lamszus K, Wellstein A, et al. An FGF-binding protein (FGF-BP) exerts its biological function by parallel paracrine stimulation of tumor cell and endothelial cell proliferation through FGF-2 release. International Journal of Cancer. 2001;15;92(4):510–7.

[82] Rettig WJ, Garin-Chesa P, Healey JH, Su SL, Ozer HL, Schwab M, et al. Regulation and heteromeric structure of the fibroblast activation protein in normal and transformed cells of mesenchymal and neuroectodermal origin. Cancer Research. 1993 Jul 15;53(14):3327–35.

[83] Kashyap MK, Marimuthu A, Kishore CJH, Peri S, Keerthikumar S, Prasad TSK, et al. Genomewide mRNA profiling of esophageal squamous cell carcinoma for identification of cancer biomarkers. Cancer Biology and Therapy. 2009;8(1):36–46.

[84] Ayoub C, Wasylyk C, Li Y, Thomas E, Marisa L, Robe A, et al. ANO1 amplification and expression in HNSCC with a high propensity for future distant metastasis and its functions in HNSCC cell lines. British Journal of Cancer. 2010;103(5):715–26.

[85] Huang F, Wong X, Jan LY. International union of basic and clinical pharmacology. LXXXV: calcium-activated chloride channels. *Pharmacological Reviews*. 2012;64(1):1–15.

[86] Almeida LO, Abrahao AC, Rosselli-Murai LK, Giudice FS, Zagni C, Leopoldino AM, et al. NFkappaB mediates cisplatin resistance through histone modifications in head and neck squamous cell carcinoma (HNSCC). FEBS Open Bio. 2014;4:96–104.

[87] Tao Y-F, Xu L-X, Lu J, Cao L, Li Z-H, Hu S-Y, et al. Metallothionein III (MT3) is a putative tumor suppressor gene that is frequently inactivated in pediatric acute myeloid leukemia by promoter hypermethylation. Journal of Translational Medicine. 2014;12(1):182.

[88] Panda S, Beena V, Sivakumar R, Choudhary K, Nalinakumari K, Sathyan S, et al. Microsatellite instability in D2S123 flanking the hMSH2 gene in oral squamous cell carcinoma in South India. Clinical Cancer Investigation Journal. 2015;4(1):22.

[89] de Souza MVR, Servato JPS, Loyola AM, Cardoso SV, Chammas R, Liu F-T, et al. Expression of APC protein during tongue malignant transformation in galectin-3-deficient mice challenged by the carcinogen 4-nitroquniline-n-oxide. International Journal of Clinical and Experimental Pathology. 2014;7(6):3255–63.

[90] Castilho RM, Gutkind JS. The Wnt/β-catenin signaling circuitry in head and neck cancer. In: Burtness B, Golemis EA, editors. Molecular Determinants of Head and Neck Cancer. Current Cancer Research. New York: Springer; 2014. pp. 199–214.

[91] Paluszczak J, Sarbak J, Kostrzewska-Poczekaj M, Kiwerska K, Jarmuż-Szymczak M, Grenman R, et al. The negative regulators of Wnt pathway—DACH1, DKK1, and WIF1 are methylated in oral and oropharyngeal cancer and WIF1 methylation predicts shorter survival. Tumour Biology. 2014 2014/12/07:1–7.

[92] Komiya Y, Habas R. Wnt signal transduction pathways. Organogenesis. 2008;4(2):68–75.

[93] Supic G, Kozomara R, Jovic N, Zeljic K, Magic Z. Hypermethylation of RUNX3 but not WIF1 gene and its association with stage and nodal status of tongue cancers. Oral Diseases. 2011 Nov;17(8):794–800.

[94] Carvalho AL, Chuang A, Jiang W-W, Lee J, Begum S, Poeta L, et al. Deleted in colorectal cancer is a putative conditional tumor-suppressor gene inactivated by promoter

hypermethylation in head and neck squamous cell carcinoma. Cancer Research. 2006 Oct 1, 2006;66(19):9401–7.

[95] Kaur J, Demokan S, Tripathi SC, Macha MA, Begum S, Califano JA, et al. Promoter hypermethylation in Indian primary oral squamous cell carcinoma. International Journal of Cancer. 2010;127(10):2367–73.

[96] Xiao C, Wang L, Zhu L, Zhang C, Zhou J. Secreted frizzled-related protein 2 is epigenetically silenced and functions as a tumor suppressor in oral squamous cell carcinoma. Molecular Medicine Reports. 2014;10(5):2293–8.

[97] Demokan S, Chang X, Chuang A, Mydlarz WK, Kaur J, Huang P, et al. KIF1A and EDNRB are differentially methylated in primary HNSCC and salivary rinses. International Journal of Cancer. 2010;127(10):2351–9.

[98] Okada Y, Yamazaki H, Sekine-Aizawa Y, Hirokawa N. The neuron-specific kinesin superfamily protein KIF1A is a unique monomeric motor for anterograde axonal transport of synaptic vesicle precursors. Cell. 1995;81(5):769–80.

[99] Smollich M, Wulfing P. Targeting the endothelin system: novel therapeutic options in gynecological, urological and breast cancers. Expert Review of Anticancer Therapy. 2008 Sept;8(9):1481–93.

[100] Yan C, Kim YW, Ha YS, Kim IY, Kim YJ, Yun SJ, et al. RUNX3 methylation as a predictor for disease progression in patients with non-muscle-invasive bladder cancer. Journal of Surgical Oncology. 2012 Mar 15;105(4):425–30.

[101] Kim W-J, Kim E-J, Jeong P, Quan C, Kim J, Li Q-L, et al. RUNX3 inactivation by point mutations and aberrant DNA methylation in bladder tumors. Cancer Research. 2005;65(20):9347–54.

[102] Shigematsu H, Suzuki M, Takahashi T, Miyajima K, Toyooka S, Shivapurkar N, et al. Aberrant methylation of HIN-1 (high in normal-1) is a frequent event in many human malignancies. International Journal of Cancer. 2005 Feb 10;113(4):600–4.

[103] Yu Y, Yin D, Hoque MO, Cao B, Jia Y, Yang Y, et al. AKT signaling pathway activated by HIN-1 methylation in non-small cell lung cancer. Tumour Biology. 2012 Apr; 33(2):307–14.

[104] Krop I, Player A, Tablante A, Taylor-Parker M, Lahti-Domenici J, Fukuoka J, et al. Frequent HIN-1 promoter methylation and lack of expression in multiple human tumor types. Molecular Cancer Res. 2004 Sep;2(9):489–94.

[105] Mancuso M, Matassa DS, Conte M, Colella G, Rana G, Fucci L, et al. H3K4 histone methylation in oral squamous cell carcinoma. Acta Biochimica Polonica. 2009;56(3): 405–10.

[106] Gannon OM, Merida de Long L, Endo-Munoz L, Hazar-Rethinam M, Saunders NA. Dysregulation of the repressive H3K27 trimethylation mark in head and neck squa-

mous cell carcinoma contributes to dysregulated squamous differentiation. Clinical Cancer Research.2013;19(2):428–41.

[107] Dicker AJ, Serewko MM, Dahler AL, Khanna KK, Kaur P, Li A, et al. Functional characterization of cultured cells derived from an intraepidermal carcinoma of the skin (IEC-1). Experimental Cell Research. 2000 Aug 1;258(2):352–60.

[108] Almeida LO, Abrahao AC, Rosselli-Murai LK, Giudice FS, Zagni C, Leopoldino AM, et al. NFκB mediates cisplatin resistance through histone modifications in head and neck squamous cell carcinoma (HNSCC). FEBS Open Bio. 2014;4(0):96–104.

[109] Huang B, Yang X-D, Lamb A, Chen L-F. Posttranslational modifications of NF-kappaB: another layer of regulation for NF-kappaB signaling pathway. Cell Signalling. 2010;22(9):1282–90.

[110] Nakayama K. Growth and progression of melanoma and non-melanoma skin cancers regulated by ubiquitination. Pigment Cell and Melanoma Research. 2010;23(3):338–51.

[111] Hamamoto R, Saloura V, Nakamura Y. Critical roles of non-histone protein lysine methylation in human tumorigenesis. Nature Reviews. Cancer. 2015;15(2):110–24.

[112] Nohata N, Hanazawa T, Kinoshita T, Okamoto Y, Seki N. MicroRNAs function as tumor suppressors or oncogenes: aberrant expression of microRNAs in head and neck squamous cell carcinoma. Auris, Nasus, Larynx. 2013 Apr;40(2):143–9.

[113] Yan B, Broek R, Saleh A, Mehta A, Waes C. Signaling networks of activated oncogenic and altered tumor suppressor genes in head and neck cancer. Journal of Carcinogenesis and Mutagenesis. 2013;7:21–3.

[114] Severino P, Bruggemann H, Andreghetto FM, Camps C, KlingbeilMde F, de Pereira WO, et al. MicroRNA expression profile in head and neck cancer: HOX-cluster embedded microRNA-196a and microRNA-10b dysregulation implicated in cell proliferation. BMC Cancer. 2013;13:533.

[115] Tu HF, Lin SC, Chang KW. MicroRNA aberrances in head and neck cancer: pathogenetic and clinical significance. Current Opinion in Otolaryngology and Head and Neck Surgery. 2013 Apr;21(2):104–11.

[116] Kumar B, Yadav A, Lang J, Teknos TN, Kumar P. Dysregulation of microRNA-34a expression in head and neck squamous cell carcinoma promotes tumor growth and tumor angiogenesis. PloS One. 2012;7(5):e37601.

[117] Datta J, Smith A, Lang JC, Islam M, Dutt D, Teknos TN, et al. microRNA-107 functions as a candidate tumor-suppressor gene in head and neck squamous cell carcinoma by downregulation of protein kinase Cvarepsilon. Oncogene. 2012 Sept 6;31(36):4045–53.

[118] Lee Y, Yang X, Huang Y, Fan H, Zhang Q, Wu Y, et al. Network modeling identifies molecular functions targeted by mir-204 to suppress head and neck tumor metastasis. PLoS Computational Biology. 2010;6(4):e1000730.

[119] Malek E, Jagannathan S, Driscoll JJ. Correlation of long non-coding RNA expression with metastasis, drug resistance and clinical outcome in cancer. Oncotarget. 2014;5(18):8027–38.

[120] Yao Y, Li J, Wang L. Large intervening non-coding RNA HOTAIR is an indicator of poor prognosis and a therapeutic target in human cancers. International Journal of Molecular Sciences. 2014;15(10):18985–99.

[121] Frith M, Bailey T, Kasukawa T, Mignone F, Kummerfeld S, Madera M, et al. Discrimination of non-protein-coding transcripts from protein-coding mRNA. RNA Biol. 2006;3:40–8.

[122] Tsai M-C, Manor O, Wan Y, Mosammaparast N, Wang JK, Lan F, et al. Long noncoding RNA as modular scaffold of histone modification complexes. Science. 2010;329(5992):689–93.

[123] Marques Howarth M, Simpson D, Ngok SP, Nieves B, Chen R, Siprashvili Z, et al. Long noncoding RNA EWSAT1-mediated gene repression facilitates Ewing sarcoma oncogenesis. Journal of Clinical Investigation. 2014;124(12):5275–90.

[124] Smolle M, Uranitsch S, Gerger A, Pichler M, Haybaeck J. Current status of long non-coding RNAs in human cancer with specific focus on colorectal cancer. International Journal of Molecular Sciences. 2014;15(8):13993–4013.

[125] Amaral PP, Clark MB, Gascoigne DK, Dinger ME, Mattick JS. lncRNAdb: a reference database for long noncoding RNAs. Nucleic Acids Research. 2011;39(Database issue):D146-D51.

[126] Massone S, Ciarlo E, Vella S, Nizzari M, Florio T, Russo C, et al. NDM29, a RNA polymerase III-dependent non coding RNA, promotes amyloidogenic processing of APP and amyloid beta secretion. Biochimica et Biophysica Acta. 2012 Jul;1823(7):1170–7.

[127] Sánchez Y, Huarte M. Long non-coding RNAs: challenges for diagnosis and therapies. Nucleic Acid Therapeutics. 2013;23(1):15–20.

[128] Lakhotia SC. Long non-coding RNAs coordinate cellular responses to stress. Wiley Interdisciplinary Reviews RNA. 2012 Nov–Dec;3(6):779–96.

[129] Verma M. Epigenome-Wide Association Studies (EWAS) in cancer. Current Genomics. 2012;13(4):308–13.

[130] Brait M, Sidransky D. Cancer epigenetics: above and beyond. Toxicology Mechanisms and Methods. 2011;21(4):275–88. PubMed PMID: PMC3309610.

[131] Hoke HA. Enhancers and super-enhancers in human disease and therapy. Massachusetts Institute of Technology; 2014.

[132] Ho AS, Turcan S, Chan TA. Epigenetic therapy: use of agents targeting deacetylation and methylation in cancer management. Onco Targets and Therapy. 2013 03/21;6:223–32.

[133] Li C, Zang Y, Sen M, Leeman-Neill RJ, Grandis JR, Johnson DE. Bortezomib up-regulates activated signal transducer and activator of transcription-3 and synergizes with inhibitors of signal transducer and activator of transcription-3 to promote head and neck squamous cell carcinoma cell death. Molecular Cancer Therapeutics. 2009 07/28;8(8):2211–20.

[134] Nelson NJ. Genetic Events in head and neck squamous cell carcinoma revealed. Journal of the National Cancer Institute. 2013 Dec 4, 2013;105(23):1766–8.

[135] Martins MD, Castilho RM. Histones: controlling tumor signaling circuitry. Journal of Carcinogenesis and Mutagenesis. 2013;1(Suppl 5):1.

[136] Dawson Mark A, Kouzarides T. Cancer epigenetics: from mechanism to therapy. Cell. 2012 7/6/;150(1):12–27.

2

Health-Related Quality of Life in Maxillectomy Patients Rehabilitated with Obturator Prostheses

Kadriye Peker

Abstract

The prosthetic rehabilitation of the maxillectomy defect is important to restore oral functions and facial contours as well as to improve patients' health-related quality of life (HRQOL). This literature review aims to assess the HRQOL of maxillectomy patients rehabilitated with obturator prostheses and their determinants as well as to identify the most commonly used HRQOL measures. A literature search has been performed using PubMed, EMBASE, and Google Scholar to identify studies published before October 10, 2016. Twenty-three studies were identified. Most studies are cross-sectional. The most frequently used HRQOL measures were the Obturator Functioning Scale and the University of Washington Quality of Life scale version 4. Studies showed that postoperative radiation therapy, residual dentition, obturator functioning, impairment of ingestion, speech, appearance, the extent of therapy, and pain were important factors affecting patients' HRQOL. This review provides valuable information for clinicians and researchers in determining patients' needs, selecting HRQOL measure, planning future studies, as well as planning and developing comprehensive prosthetic rehabilitation programs. Well-designed clinical, multicenter, longitudinal studies with a larger sample are needed to evaluate the impacts of different reconstruction and retention methods as well as several determinants including sociodemographic, clinical, and psychological on patients' HRQOL.

Keywords: maxillectomy patients, health-related quality of life, obturator prosthesis, obturator functioning

1. Introduction

As a patient reported outcome, the assessment and monitoring of the health-related quality of life (HRQOL) in patients with head and neck cancer play a critical role in the treatment of decision-making process and developing treatment protocols as well as providing supportive care [1, 2].

Globally, cancer burden are increased due to population growth, aging, and an increasing prevalence of risk factors such as smoking, obesity, and dietary patterns [3].

Oral cavity cancer is the most common type of head and neck cancer [4]. Despite significant advances in its treatments, oral cancer has a poor prognosis and a low survival rate [5].

The Global Burden of Disease Study [6] reported that the global burden of periodontal disease, oral cancer, and dental caries increased markedly by an average of 45.6% from 1990 to 2010. Oral cancer is the eighth most common cancer worldwide. When compared with high-income countries, oral cancer is common in low-income countries [7]. In 2012, lip, oral cavity, and pharyngeal cancers were responsible for 529,500 incident cases and 292,300 deaths, accounting for approximately 3.8% of all cases and 3.6% of cancer deaths. Maxillary cancer is a rare tumor with increased mortality and 10% of all oral cancers occur in the oral cavity subsites of the upper gingiva and hard palate [8].

Oral cancer and its treatment have a direct impact on patients' physical, psychological, and social well-being. After resection of maxillofacial tumor, these patients experience orofacial functional changes and social and emotional issues that can have significant negative effects on their HRQOL and obturator functioning. The prosthetic rehabilitation of the maxillectomy defect is important to restore oral functions and facial contours as well as to improve HRQOL of patients. Following maxillectomy, patients experience severe problems in oral functioning, including speech, swallowing, mastication, and orofacial esthetics, all of which consequently affect their HRQOL and well-being. Therefore, prosthetic rehabilitation by the multidisciplinary team is a critical element to restore both oral function and facial form [9].

Maxillary defects after tumor resection can be reconstructed by using an obturator prosthesis or by a surgical reconstruction according to the extent of the maxillectomy defect and the need for radiation therapy [9, 10]. Although there is no consensus regarding the more effective treatment option, obturator prosthesis is the most widely used noninvasive approach and the recommended treatment modality to restore the patient's oral functions, aesthetics, and resocialization in the management of maxillary defects [10–15] because it provides a quick and adequate prosthetic rehabilitation in older patients, patients with a high morbidity rate, and patients with an unfavorable life expectancy [11]. Obturator rehabilitation is an equivalent reconstructive option for improving HRQOL and reducing complications in patients undergoing total or extended maxillectomy for advanced malignancy [16]. The comprehensive oral rehabilitation management is crucial for improving survival and oral functions in patients with advanced-stage disease and large defect which are treated by combination therapy, including preoperative irradiation, chemotherapy, surgery, and immediate reconstruction.

Besides clinical parameters, the subjective assessment by patients gives more information about patients' needs, expectations, and treatment effectiveness. To assess the HRQOL, many HRQOL instruments have been used by researchers, which are categorized into five groups: patient performance questionnaires, generic quality of life questionnaires, generic cancer questionnaires, head and neck cancer questionnaires, and head and neck functional questionnaires [17]. However, most studies used different questionnaires and study design to measure patients' HRQOL which hinders the ability to make direct comparison among studies. In addition, the existing studies reported several factors affecting patients' HRQOL and obturator functioning. Recent systematic review on the HRQOL of patients with maxillary defects who had undergone restoration with obturator prostheses and/or free tissue reported that prospective, blinded, randomized, multicenter studies with standardized methods are needed to reach definitive conclusions about the best method and the related factors with these treatment options [18].

This review provides an outline of existing literature on HRQOL of maxillectomy patients rehabilitated with obturator prostheses. Additionally, it provides valuable information for clinicians and researchers in determining patients 'needs, selecting an existing validated measure, planning future studies, as well as planning and developing comprehensive prosthetic rehabilitation programs.

The aim of this literature review was to assess the HRQOL in maxillectomy patients rehabilitated with obturator prostheses and its determinants as well as to identify the most commonly used HRQOL measures.

2. Methods

A literature search has been performed in PubMed, EMBASE, and Google Scholar to identify studies published in the period July 1996–October 10, 2016. The following keywords such as maxillectomy patients, palatal obturators, patient satisfaction, HRQOL, and obturator function in diverse combinations with MeSH search were used to identify all relevant studies. In addition, the reference lists of these manuscripts and all included chapters were checked for eligible articles.

3. Selection criteria

3.1. Inclusion criteria

Titles and abstracts were screened by the author, according to the following inclusion criterion: studies published in English; quantitative studies; study sample consisted of maxillectomy patients who had undergone restoration with obturator prostheses; studies published in the period July 1996–October 10, 2016; studies used at least one validated HRQOL measure; studies reported determinants related to HRQOL and patient satisfaction; and studies compared HRQOL outcomes of patients who had undergone maxillectomy followed by different prosthetic modalities.

3.2. Exclusion criteria

Case reports or case series, qualitative studies, studies used self-reported HRQOL factors, validation studies, systematic reviews, unpublished theses, and dissertations were excluded.

3.3. Data extraction

Data were extracted on study design, characteristics of participants, outcome measure(s), and findings.

4. Findings

Screening of the titles and abstracts resulted in a selection of 23 articles. Of the 23 selected studies, 13 were retrospective cross-sectional studies, 1 was case-control study, 4 were experimental studies, and 5 were cohort studies.

4.1. Study characteristics

Of the 23 studies included in this review were conducted in the United States (n = 4), China (n = 4), Pakistan (n = 3), UK (n = 2), the Netherlands (n = 2), Denmark (n = 1), Germany (n = 2), Egypt (n = 1), Brazil (n = 1), India (n = 1), and Canada (n = 2).

Sample sizes of the studies varied widely, between 8 and 73 participants. Selected characteristics of the 23 studies are presented in **Table 1**.

4.2. Measurement of HRQOL

The most frequently used HRQOL measures were the Obturator Functioning Scale (OFS) (n = 14) and the University of Washington Quality of Life scale version 4 (UW-QoLv4) (n = 6). Twelve studies used more than one instrument to measure HRQOL and only three studies used an oral health-related quality of life measure. Five studies used only one measure, namely, OFS. Five studies used a head and neck cancer-specific measure besides a generic measure.

The most frequently used head and neck cancer-specific instruments were: the European Organization for Research and Treatment of Cancer general form (EORTC C-30), head-neck specific version (EORTC HN35), the UW-QoLv4, the Performance Status Scale for Head and Neck Cancer Patients (PSS-HN), the OFS, the Swallowing Quality Of Life (SWAL-QOL), and the Eastern Cooperative Oncology Group performance score (ECOG).

Only two region-specific HRQOL measures [The Disabilities of the Arm, Shoulder and Hand (DASH) and the American Academy of Orthopedic Surgeons (AOSS) Hip and Knee Questionnaire] were used in combination with a head and neck cancer function-specific HRQOL measure [19]. Only one study used a questionnaire which is originally developed for DOESAK (a German, Austrian, and Swiss cooperative group on tumors of the maxillofacial region) in combination with head and neck cancer specific measures [14].

Author (year)/ country	Title	Study design	Patient information	HRQOL	General results
Chen et al. (2016)/ China [28]	Quality of Life in Patients After Maxillectomy and Placement of Prosthetic Obturator	Retrospective cross-sectional study	$N = 29$ (16 male, 13 female); mean age = 48.8 years; 29 OP	UWQOLv4 OFS	Postoperative radiotherapy was the strongest variable affecting HRQOL in patients with maxillectomy and prosthetic obturator reconstruction. The size of the defect affected the obturator function.
Chen et al. (2016)/ China [25]	Function of obturator prosthesis after maxillectomy and prosthetic obturator rehabilitation	Retrospective cohort study (10 years)	$N = 28$ (19 male, 9 female); mean age= 62.05 years; 9 COP 11 AOP 8 MOP	OFS	Obturator prosthesis improves oral function of maxillectomy patients; the retention of the obturator prosthesis enhanced by the addition of attachments showed more benefits in oral function. There was significant difference in functions such as speech, swallowing and chewing among these three sub-groups.
Breeze et al. (2016)/ England [12]	Health-related quality of life after maxillectomy: obturator rehabilitation compared with flap reconstruction	A prospective study two-group pretest-posttest design	$N = 39$ (22 male, 17 female); mean age= 64 ± 7 years; 18 flap reconstruction 21 OP	UWQOLv4	There was a significant decrease in HRQOL after treatment compared with before, but there was no significant difference in the effects of these treatment methods on HRQOL. Obturators remain an important option for rehabilitation in selected patients in addition to reconstruction with a flap. The size of the vertical defect and the use of postoperative radiotherapy had no adverse effect on HRQOL.
Wang et al. (2016)/ China [27]	Functional outcome and quality of life after a maxillectomy: a comparison between an implant supported obturator and implant supported fixed prostheses in a free vascularized flap	Comparative cross-sectional study	$N = 38$ (23 male, 15 female); 18 implant supported OP (mean age of 56.2 years) 20 vascularized free flap transfer with implant supported fixed prostheses (mean age 45.6 years)	OFS EORTC HN 35 MHI	There is no difference in oral function between these patient groups. Patients wearing obturator had poorer mental health than did patients with fixed prostheses.

Table 1. (continued).

Author (year)/ country	Title	Study design	Patient information	HRQOL	General results
Gotfredsen and Abdullah (2015)/ Denmark [21]	Oral prosthetic rehabilitation with and without implants after radiation therapy and ablative surgery	Quasi Experimental Designs One group before after study	*N* = 51 (35 male, 16 female); mean age= 66 years; 10 OP 16 fixed prosthesis 5 fixed combined with removable prostheses 30 had only removable prostheses	OHIP-49	After oral rehabilitation with fixed and removable dental prosthesis, a significant improvement in oral health related quality of life was found in all patients. The oral rehabilitation resulted in better appearance and chewing function. No significant effect between fixed versus removable prostheses and no significant effect of implant on the OHIP-score were found.
Salem et al. (2015)/ Egypt [20]	Evaluation of Zygomatic implant retained obturator in rehabilitation of partial palato-maxillectomy patients	A prospective comparative study	*N* = 8 (5 female, 3 male); age range 20 to 58 years conventional OP Implant retained OP	OHIP 14	For the abutment teeth, there was no statistically significant difference in gingival index, tooth mobility, and bone level between these patients groups. The implant retained obturator highly improved the masticatory function and oral health-related quality of life in comparison to conventional obturator.
Seignemartin et al. (2015)/Brazil [26]	Understandability of Speech Predicts Quality of Life Among Maxillectomy Patients Restored With Obturator Prosthesis	Retrospective cross-sectional study	*N* = 73 (37 male, 36 female); mean age= 62.2 years; 52 total upper OP and 21 upper partial OP	PSS-HN UWQOLv4 OFS	The understandability of speech was the only predictor of HRQOL Classification of the defect, eating in public, and understandability of speech were predictors of worse obturator functioning. Patients wearing partial removable prostheses had better HRQOL than those with total removable prostheses. There were no statistical associations of age, gender, maxillary teeth status, and tumor stage with total HRQOL and OFS scores.
Murphy et al. (2015)/USA [16]	Quality of life factors and survival after total or extended maxillectomy for sinonasal malignancies	Retrospective cohort study	*N* = 25 (12 male,13 female); mean age= 67.8 years; 13 free flap 11 OP 1 regional flap	ECOG performance score	The inevitable morbidity could be deemed acceptable by patients. Obturator rehabilitation was found to be an equivalent reconstructive option in these patients in terms of the HRQOL factors and complications.

Table 1. (continued).

Author (year)/ country	Title	Study design	Patient information	HRQOL	General results
Hussain et al. (2014)/Pakistan [22]	Quality of life in oral cancer patients after provision of maxillary obturators	Before-after study One group Pretest, Posttest	*N* = 32 (25 male, 7 female); age range of 15–74 years 32 OP	OHIP-14	After provision of obturators, there was significantly improvement in oral health quality of life in these patients, especially in speech, mastication and self-confidence.
Khan et al./Pakistan [35]	Subjective assessment of obturator functioning in patients with hemimaxillectomy	Cross-sectional study	*N* = 50 (37 male,13 female); mean age = 41.7 years. 50 OP	OFS	Obturator prosthesis provides better functioning in speech and esthetics but it is not very efficient in terms of mastication and swallowing.
Jiao et al. (2014)/ China [23]	Rehabilitation of maxillectomy defects with obturator prostheses fabricated using computer-aided design and rapid prototyping: a pilot study	Quasi Experimental Designs	*N* = 11 (7 male, 4 female); age range 25–68 years.	OFS	These methods improve oral function and social acceptance. It has shown significant clinical value, especially for use in developing countries.
Chigurupati et al. (2013)/USA [32]	Quality of life after maxillectomy and prosthetic obturator rehabilitation	Retrospective, cross-sectional study	*N* = 23 (14 male,9 female); mean age = 61 years	UWQOLv4 OFS MHI	Postoperative radiation therapy was the most important predictors of HRQOL in patients with maxillectomy and prosthetic obturator reconstruction. Further multicenter trials with large sample size are needed to identify how factors affecting HRQOL of patients after maxillectomy might influence the choice of reconstruction.
Kumar et al. (2013)/ India [13]	Assessment of the quality of life in maxillectomy patients: a longitudinal study	A longitudinal study Before after treatment	*N* = 30 (20 male, 10 female); mean age=46.83 years	EORTC QLQ-H &N 35v1	Obturator prosthesis is a highly positive and non-invasive approach to improve patients' HRQOL. A statistically significant improvement was found in some functions such as problems in swallowing solid food, problem in opening mouth wide, trouble in eating, difficulty in eating food in front of family and other people, problem in enjoying food, difficulty in conversation to people and on the telephone, problem in making social contacts with friends, trouble in making public appearance and difficulty in making physical contacts with others.

Table 1. (continued).

Author (year)/ country	Title	Study design	Patient information	HRQOL	General results
Kreeft et al. (2012)/ Netherlands [31]	Oral function after maxillectomy and reconstruction with an obturator	Retrospective cohort study	$N = 32$ (13 male, 19 female); mean age=49 years 32 OB	EORTC-H&N 35 OFS	Size of the maxillectomy defect did not significantly influence functional outcome, but adjuvant radiotherapy resulted in worse mouth opening and self-reported oral and swallowing problems. Residual dentition had a significant effect on both mastication and HRQOL.
Depprich et al. (2011)/Germany [14]	Evaluation of the quality of life of patients with maxillofacial defects after prosthodontics therapy with obturator prostheses	Cross-sectional study	$N = 31$ (14 male, 17 female); mean age=67.6 years; 31 OB	DOESAK EORTC QLQ-H&N35 OFS	Obturator functioning, impairment of ingestion, speech, appearance, the extent of therapy, and the existence of pain had significant impact on the HRQOL. Orofacial rehabilitation of patients with maxillofacial defects using obturator prostheses is an appropriate treatment modality. To improve the situation of patients prior to and after maxillectomy sufficient information about the treatment, adequate psychological care and speech therapy should be provided.
Riaz and Warriach (2010)/Pakistan [15]	Quality of life in patients with obturator prostheses	Cross-sectional study	30 (19 male, 11 female); mean age=57.6 years; 30 OB	UW-QOLv4 OFS	Obturator functioning, impairment of ingestion, speech and appearance, the extent of therapy, and the existence of pain had significant impact on the HRQOL. Orofacial rehabilitation using obturator prostheses is an appropriate treatment modality. To improve the situation of patients prior to and after maxillectomy sufficient information about the treatment, adequate psychological care and speech therapy should be provided.
Lethaus et al. (2010)/Netherlands [11]	Surgical and prosthetic reconsiderations in patients with maxillectomy	Retrospective cohort study	11 (6 male, 5 female); mean age=60 years; a computer-aided design/computer-aided manufacturing designed prosthesis	OFS	Obturator prosthesis fabricated with CAD/CAM techniques improves oral function and social acceptance.

Table 1. (continued).

Author (year)/ country	Title	Study design	Patient information	HRQOL	General results
Irish et al. (2009)/ Canada [33]	Quality of life in patients with maxillectomy prostheses	Cross-sectional study	$N = 42$ (12 male, 30 female); mean age=60.7 years; 42 OB	OFS MHI IES IIRS CES-D	Leakage when swallowing foods was the most frequently reported problem. Difficulty with speech and eating resulted in an increase in avoidance of social life. The surgical approach had a significant effect on the OFS, IES, and MHI subscales. Good obturator function is associated with a better HRQOL.
Hertrampf et al. (2004)/Germany [34]	Quality of life of patients with maxillofacial defects after treatment for malignancy	Case-control study	Patients with defects who received prosthetic treatment ($n = 17$, mean age 61.7 years); Persons affected with a nonmalignant condition (control; $n = 17$, mean age 53.4 years) German population reference data ($n = 2028$)	EORTC QLQ-C30 EORTC-H&N 35	Tumor patients did not significantly differ from nontumor patients in terms of the total HRQOL. Tumor patients had worse scores in role functioning, speech, mouth opening, and dry mouth, as well as pain and swallowing. In comparison with the reference data of the German population, tumor patients had more deficits regarding role functioning, dyspnea, financial difficulties, fatigue, insomnia, and appetite. Tumor patients rated the diagnosis as the most stressful event and reported that the family was most instrumental in the recovery process. Patients with maxillofacial defects suffer from many symptoms and problems, even after prosthodontic treatment. These patients need psychologic care at the time of diagnosis and after completion of the prosthodontic treatment, therapy options for pain or speech problems should be offered.

Table 1. (continued).

Author (year)/ country	Title	Study design	Patient information	HRQOL	General results
Rieger et al. (2003)/ Canada [29]	Maxillary obturators: the relationship between patient satisfaction and speech outcome	Cross – sectional	*N* = 20(12 female, 8 male); mean age 55 years 20 OP	OFS	The poorer aeromechanical speech were associated with the avoidance of social events, whereas lower speech intelligibility outcomes were related to worse speech function on the OFS. Background patient characteristics such as gender, degree of resection, type of prosthesis retention, history of orbital exenteration, history of radiation therapy, and the wearing time of definitive obturator are most important determinants of functional speech functions and patient satisfaction.
Rogers et al. (2003)/ England [24]	Health-related quality of life after maxillectomy: a comparison between prosthetic obturation and free flap	Cross sectional study	*N* = 28 (18 male, 10 female); mean age = 64 years; 10 OB 18 SR	UW-QOL EORTC QLQ C30 -EORTC HN 35 HAD	No significant differences were identified between obturator and free flap groups. Obturator patients were more concerned about their appearance, more aware of their upper teeth, more self-conscious, less satisfied with their upper dentures, and less satisfied with function. They had more pain and soreness in their mouths.
Genden et al. (2003)/USA [19]	Comparison of functional and quality-of-life outcomes in patients with and without palatomaxillary reconstruction: a preliminary report	Comparative cross sectional	*N* = 8 (5 male, 3 female); mean age=42 years; 4 OB with a tissue-borne prosthetic obturator; 4 vascularized bone-containing free flap	DASH AAOS Hip and Knee Questionnaire SWALQOL	Patients with free flap had higher scores on mastication and speech than those with a prosthetic obturator. Compared with their prosthetic counterparts, flap patients enjoyed a better HRQOL without incurring significant donor site morbidity. Although free flaps requires a second operative site, this method can provide better functional and HRQOL outcomes than prosthetic obturator.

Table 1. (continued).

Author (year)/ country	Title	Study design	Patient information	HRQOL	General results
Kornblith et al. (1996)/USA [30]	Quality of life of maxillectomy patients using an obturator prosthesis	Retrospective cross-sectional	*N* = 47 (31 male, 16 female); mean age = 59.5 years; 47 OP	OFS, PAIS, MHI, IES, Family Functioning Scale, Perceived Negative Socioeconomic Impact of Cancer Index	Obturator functioning are associated with better adjustment and an improvement in pronouncing words, chewing and swallowing food, and voice quality after surgery. The most important predictors of obturator functioning were the extent of resection of their soft palate (one third or less) and hard palate (one fourth or less). Well-functioning obturator is important for improving the HRQOL of maxillectomy patients.

Note: OP, obturators; COP, conventional retained obturator prosthesis; AOP, enhanced retentive obturator prosthesis with stud attachment; MOP, enhanced retentive obturator prosthesis with magnetic attachment; HRQOL, health-related quality of life; UWQOLv4, the University of Washington Quality of Life scale version 4; OFS, the Obturator Functioning Scale; EORTC QLQ-C30, the European Organization for Research and Treatment of Cancer general form; EORTC HN 35, the European Organization for Research and Treatment of Cancer general form, head-neck specific version; MHI, the Mental Health Inventory; OHIP-49, the 49 items of the Oral Health Impact Profile; OHIP 14, the short version OHIP; PSS-HN, the Performance Status Scale for Head and Neck Cancer Patients; ECOG (the Eastern Cooperative Oncology Group) performance score; DOESAK, a German, Austrian and Swiss cooperative group on tumors of the maxillofacial region; IES, Impact of Events Scale; IIRS, Illness Intrusiveness Ratings Scale; CES-D, Centre for Epidemiologic Studies Depression Scale; HAD, Hospital Anxiety Depression; DASH, The Disabilities of the Arm, Shoulder and Hand; AAOS (American Academy of Orthopaedic Surgeons) Hip and Knee Questionnaire; SWALQOL, the Swallowing Quality of Life; PAIS, the Psychosocial Adjustment to Illness Scale.

Table 1. Characteristics of selected studies.

The used general quality of life measures were: Mental Health Inventory (MHI; n = 4), Impact of Events Scale (IES; n = 2), Illness Intrusiveness Ratings Scale (IIRS; n = 1), Centre for Epidemiologic Studies Depression Scale (CES-D; n = 1), the Psychosocial Adjustment to Illness Scale (PAIS; n = 1), the Family Function Scale (n = 1), the Perceived Negative Socioeconomic Impact Index (n = 1), and the Hospital Anxiety and Depression Scale (HAD; n = 1).

There are only three studies using an oral health-related quality of life [20–22]. Of the three studies identified, one used the forty-nine items of the Oral Health Impact Profile (OHIP-49), and two used the short version OHIP-14.

Two studies evaluated the effects of different technologies used in manufacturing individualized obturators on patients' HRQOL [11, 23], three compared the HRQOL after maxillectomy between obturators and flaps [12, 16, 24], and three compared patients' HRQOL who used obturator prosthesis with different retention mechanism [20, 21, 25], one compared the HRQOL between patients with an upper denture obturator and upper partial obturator [26], and one evaluated the differences in obturator functioning and HRQOL between patients with implant-supported obturators and implant-supported fixed prostheses in free vascularized flaps [27].

4.3. Studies on the effects of different technologies used for manufacturing individualized obturators

Studies about comparing different technologies used for manufacturing individualized obturators showed that the computer-aided design with rapid prototyping technology is an alternative and feasible method for manufacturing individualized obturators for patients after maxillary resection [23]. In other study, the treatment protocol which incorporates the use of standard dental implants in combination with a computer-aided design/computer-aided manufacturing showed good functional and social outcomes [11].

4.4. Studies on the effects of different retention mechanism

Studies on the effects of different retention mechanism on patients' HRQOL reported that the retention of the obturator prosthesis enhanced by the addition of attachments showed some improvements in oral function such as speech, swallowing, and chewing. Patients treated with an enhanced retentive obturator prosthesis with stud attachment reported higher scores in the domains of speech and swallowing than patients treated with conventional and magnetic retentive prosthesis. Patients who were treated with an enhanced retentive obturator prosthesis with stud attachment and with an enhanced retentive obturator prosthesis with magnetic attachment had better scores in "swallowing-leakage with solid" and "chewing/eating" domains of HRQOL than patients with a conventional retained obturator prosthesis. The large one-side defect and gender were found to be important factor for enhancing retention and improving patient's confidence and esthetics [25].

Study on the evaluation of zygomatic implant retained obturator in rehabilitation of partial palato-maxillectomy patients showed that rehabilitation of maxillectomy patients with conventional or implant retained obturator had significant improvement in the functional impairment, psychological disability, and social disability domains of the oral health-related quality of life in comparison to patients without obturator. Significant improvements were found in patients' oral health-related quality of life as well as their masticatory function after converting the conventional obturator to implant retained obturator. For the abutment teeth, there was no statistically significant difference in some clinical parameters such as gingival index, tooth mobility, and bone level between conventional obturator and implant retained obturator [20].

Another study [21] conducted on patients treated with radiation therapy and/or ablative surgery reported a significant improvement in appearance and chewing function after oral rehabilitation with fixed and removable dental prosthesis. In this study, no significant effect between fixed versus removable prostheses and no significant effect of implant on the oral health-related quality of life of patients were found. Seignemartin et al. [26] reported that patients wearing partial removable prostheses had higher HRQOL than those with total removable prostheses.

4.5. Studies comparing the obturator replacement with free flap

There are a small number of studies comparing the HRQOL of patients wearing obturator prostheses with those who underwent free flap reconstruction. The cross-sectional study by Rogers et al. [24] found no statistically significant difference in HRQOL between these groups, but obturator patients were more concerned about their appearance, more aware of their upper teeth, more self-conscious, less satisfied with their upper dentures, less satisfied with function, and they reported more pain and soreness in their mouths. Similarly, Wang et al. [27] found no differences in HRQOL and oral functioning between patients with implant-supported obturators and implant-supported fixed prostheses in free vascularized flaps after a maxillectomy but obturator patients had worse mental health than those with fixed prostheses. Consistent with these findings, Breeze et al. [12] found no significant difference in the effects of these treatments on patients' HRQOL.

In contrast, another cross-sectional study reported that palatomaxillary reconstruction with vascularized bone-containing free flaps may improve the functional and HRQOL outcomes relative to defect-matched patients rehabilitated with a prosthetic obturator although this method requires a second operative site [19].

In a 5-year retrospective cohort study [16], obturator placement was found to be an equivalent reconstructive option with respect to the HRQOL factors and complications, because inevitable morbidity caused by the disfiguring effects of maxillectomy (total or extended) could be deemed acceptable by these patients. In another longitudinal study conducted by Breeze et al. [12] reported similar findings. They found no significant difference in the effects of these treatment options on patients' HRQOL.

4.6. Studies assessing obturator functioning among patients wearing an obturator prosthesis

There were 11 cross-sectional studies that examined the HRQOL among patients wearing an obturator prosthesis. Existing studies showed that obturator functioning is associated with the size of defect [26, 28, 29], the extent of resection in the soft palate and hard palate [30], the grade of impairment of speech [14, 29], ingestion [14], eating in public, and understandability of speech [26]. Some studies reported conflicting results with regards to the impact of defect size [14, 31]. Depprich et al. [14] reported that the prosthesis form, the former wearing of dentures, and the existence of maxillary teeth or dental implants had no significant effects on the obturator functioning. Kreeft et al. [31] reported that obturator functioning is not related to the history of adjuvant radiotherapy and the presence of residual dentition. Rieger et al. [29] reported that background patient characteristics such as gender, type of prosthesis retention, history of orbital exenteration, history of radiation therapy, and the wearing time of the definitive obturator are important predictors of obturator functioning and satisfaction. Seignemartin et al. [26] found no statistical associations of age, salivary flow, tooth in the maxilla, and tumor stage with obturator function.

4.7. Studies assessing HRQOL among patients wearing an obturator prosthesis

Studies of maxillectomy patients rehabilitated with obturator prostheses reported that post-operative radiotherapy [26, 28, 31, 32], the size of defect [26], the degree of hyposalivation [15, 26], understandability of speech [26], functioning of the obturator prosthesis [14, 15, 30, 33], impairment of ingestion, speech, and appearance [14, 15], the extent of therapy [14, 15], the existence of pain [14, 15, 24, 34], the type of surgery [33], and residual dentition [31] had significant impacts on patients' HRQOL. Some studies have reported conflicting results. Depprich et al. [14] found that the classification of maxillary defects and the type of surgery (transoral vs. transfacial) had no significant influence on HRQOL. Seignemartin et al. [26] found no statistical associations of salivary flow, tooth in the maxilla, and tumor stage with the HRQOL. Breeze et al. [12] reported that there are no adverse effects of both the size of the vertical defect and postoperative radiotherapy on HRQOL.

There are conflicting findings concerning demographic characteristics. Some researchers reported that gender [15] and the level of education [14] were associated with HRQOL, while others did not find any relationships between these variables and patients' HRQOL [14, 15, 26, 33]. No significant association was found between HRQOL and age [14, 15, 26].

4.8. The self-reported problems among patients wearing an obturator prosthesis

In general, the most common problems reported by patients wearing an obturator prosthesis include: leakage when swallowing foods, impairment of speech, chewing, swallowing, and pain [14, 30, 33, 35]. Difficulties in pronouncing words, chewing and swallowing food, and voice changes after surgery were found to be related with worse adjustment [30].

The longitudinal study conducted by Kumar et al. [13] reported that there was a significant increase in some items scores of the EORTC QLQ-H&N35 after treatment compared with before (e.g., problems in swallowing solid food, opening mouth, eating, enjoying food, conversation with people, talking over the telephone, making social and physical contacts with friends and others). These findings are consistent with previous cross-sectional studies conducted by Depprich et al. [14], Irish et al. [33], and Kornblith et al. [30].

Another longitudinal study using the OHIP-14 showed that there was significant improvement in speech, mastication, and self-confidence domains of oral health-related quality of life in maxillectomy patients after prosthodontic rehabilitation [22].

5. Discussion

In recent years, there has been a growing interest in evaluating HRQOL and patient satisfaction as patient-reported outcome measures among maxillectomy patients rehabilitated with obturator prostheses.

Patients who underwent radiotherapy due to oral cavity cancer showed worse oral health-related quality of life than patients with other tumor sites and the population average. In head and cancer patients, tumor site is a more important factor affecting HRQOL than the number of remaining teeth or type of prosthesis [36].

Only, one study compared the HRQOL in maxillectomy patients with that of the general population. Compared to nontumor patients, tumor patients showed a significant decrease in oral functions such as speech, mouth opening, dry mouth, pain, and swallowing. Comparison with the reference data of the German population, tumor patients experienced some problems regarding role functioning, dyspnea, and financial difficulties [34].

Due to additional radiotherapy and chemotherapy, maxillectomy patients with advanced malignancy and large defect size tend to have more fear of the future and to be depressed because they are at a higher risk of relapse and survival [15]. It is known that patients' HRQOL depends on the extent and location of the resection, the types of cancer treatment, patients' coping strategies besides the functionality of dentures, and the type of rehabilitation [37].

In general, the most common problems reported by patients wearing an obturator prosthesis were leakage when swallowing foods, impairment of speech, chewing, swallowing, and pain [14, 30, 33, 35]. Prosthodontic rehabilitation using maxillary obturator improves speech, mastication, esthetics, swallowing, and self-confidence [22, 30, 35]. In these patients, difficulties with speech, eating, and swallowing may lead to avoid social life [13–15, 26, 29, 33]. Obturator functioning are associated with better psychosocial adjustment and improvement in pronouncing words, chewing and swallowing food, and voice quality after surgery [30].

Even after prosthodontic treatment, these patients suffered from psychological, functional, or behavioral problems [26, 27, 30, 33, 34]. After assessing the information about patient-related clinical factors, needs, and personality, comprehensive oral health rehabilitation including psychological care, speech therapy, and pain management should be given by the multidisciplinary team for improving patients' HRQOL [14, 15, 19, 21, 26, 29–31, 33, 34].

Obturator prosthesis improves oral function of patients after surgery. The retention of the obturator prosthesis enhanced by the addition of attachments may provide more benefits in oral function [25]. Implant retained obturator showed significant improvement over conventional obturator in the social and psychological aspects of HRQOL of these patients because additional retention provides the opportunity to prevent obturator movement during speech [20].

To date, there are few studies comparing obturators to free flap reconstructions of maxillectomy defects [12, 16, 19, 21, 24, 27]. Some studies reported that there was no significant difference in HRQOL after treatment between flaps and obturators [12, 21, 24], whereas others reported a significant difference in the functional and HRQOL outcomes between these patients [19, 27]. In the future, large multicenter studies are needed to compare the effects of different types of flaps and alternative reconstruction methods (i.e., stem cells) on patients' HRQOL [12, 14, 15, 19]. Large prospective and longitudinal studies are needed to compare the HRQOL of patients wearing obturator prostheses with those who underwent free flap reconstruction and to understand the effects of functional factors and patient-perceived symptoms on the selection of appropriate treatment [24, 29]. In addition, large and multicenter trials are required to identify the factors affecting HRQOL after maxillectomy which might influence the choice of reconstruction [26, 32].

Only two studies examined the effects of different technologies used in manufacturing individualized obturators on patients' HRQOL. These studies suggest the integration of the combination of three-dimensional (3-D) technology, implant insertion, and resection into treatment protocol for improving patients' HRQOL and obturator functioning, especially in developing countries, because obturator prosthesis fabricated with CAD/CAM techniques or rapid prototyping improves oral function and social acceptance as well as reduce the treatment cost, time, and effort [11, 23]. Future studies using additional assessment for the classification of maxillary defect and soft palate junction are needed to evaluate the validity of these methods.

There were 11 cross-sectional studies that examined the HRQOL among patients using an obturator prosthesis. Studies using multivariate analysis method reported that the most important factors affecting HRQOL in patients using obturator prosthesis were the postoperative radiotherapy [28, 32], understandability of speech [26], obturator functioning, impairment of ingestion, appearance, the extent of therapy, the existence of pain [15], and residual dentition [31]. The most frequently reported factors regarding obturator functioning were defect size [28], surgical approach [33], postoperative radiotherapy, and premorbid dentition [25]. More longitudinal studies are needed to evaluate temporal changes in HRQOL and obturator functioning because most studies used cross-sectional design. These studies may provide valuable information about the likely effects of the various phases of illness, treatment, and rehabilitation on patients' HRQOL.

The most frequently used head and neck-specific HRQOL measures were the OFS [11, 14, 15, 20, 23, 25–27, 29, 30–33, 35] and the UW-QoLv4 [12, 15, 24, 26, 28, 32]. The OFS subsite-specific questionnaire has been most frequently used in studies of maxillectomy patients wearing obturator prosthesis. Although this measure may be used by clinicians to identify the patients who are likely to have a poor HRQOL for improving the outcomes of prosthodontic rehabilitation [33], more studies are needed to assess the clinical utility of the OFS as a screening measure.

There are only three studies using oral health-related quality of life [20–22]. Although oral health-related quality of life measures has been used mainly in studies evaluating different oral rehabilitation treatment modalities, the validity of these measure may be questioned in head and neck patients with a compromised functional status for assessing the effect of oral rehabilitation on HRQOL [21]. Comparison studies showed that the OHIP-49 was a better method for measuring the impact of treatment, whereas the individual systematic interview method was more appropriate for gaining detailed information for decision making than the OHIP-49 [38]. Most HRQOL instruments do not capture all relevant determinants [39]. Thus, combined HRQOL measures (head and neck cancer specific and general) were used in five studies [24, 27, 30, 32, 33]. Some studies reported that patients adjusted favorably after maxillectomy and rehabilitation with obturator prostheses [15, 30].

The life contexts and psychosocial factors are most important determinants of HRQOL [21, 24, 27, 30, 32, 33]. Thus, future studies should examine the impacts of the personal resources and life context-related factors such as having a loving family, socioeconomic advantages, absence of psychologically independent stressful life events, and social support on these patients' HRQOL.

It is known that many generic, cancer-specific, and head and neck cancer-specific measures have overlapping content. Researchers and clinicians should consider the factors such as study objectives, research question, study sample, instrument properties, content/HRQOL domains, disease subsite, treatment, the pitfalls, and benefits of combining measures, and the time frame of the questions when selecting HRQOL instrument [17, 39].

There are conflicting findings concerning demographic characteristics [14, 15, 26, 32, 33]. Considering the findings and suggestions of these previous studies, future studies should be planned to assess the impacts of patients' sociodemographic and clinical factors on HRQOL and obturator functioning.

There were a relatively small number of studies that used the additional clinical test such as nasometry, salivary flow test, chewing performance, and mixing ability test [19, 20, 26, 29, 31]. Using both clinical and patients' subjective evaluation may provide a better judgment for prosthodontic management of these patients [31]. More attention should be paid by clinicians for integrated use of clinical tests together with HRQOL instruments in clinical practice. More studies are needed to assess the associations between functional status and HRQOL outcomes for successful prosthodontic management in these patients.

The most commonly used classification system for maxillary defects is the Brown classification in these studies [12, 14, 15, 25, 26, 28, 31, 32]. Further comparative studies are needed to evaluate the effects of different classification systems of defect size (such as Armany and Okay) on patients' HRQOL.

Studies on HRQOL in maxillectomy patients rehabilitated with obturator prostheses had small sample size because maxillary cancer is a rare tumor with increased mortality. In these studies, different study design and HRQOL measures were used. Because of these reasons, comparisons across studies were difficult. To date, there is no gold standard method for measuring head and neck cancer patients' HRQOL. By reviewing existing HRQOL measures, HRQOL studies, and its results, I hope this review provides an opportunity to improve future HRQOL studies in maxillectomy patients rehabilitated with obturator prostheses maxillectomy.

6. Conclusion

The main findings of this review revealed that the obturator prosthesis had a significant influence on patients' HRQOL and functioning. Studies showed that postoperative radiation therapy, residual dentition, functioning of the obturator prosthesis, impairment of ingestion, speech, appearance, the extent of therapy, and the existence of pain were important factors affecting patients' HRQOL. This review provides valuable information for clinicians and researchers in determining patients' needs, selecting an existing validated measure, planning future studies, as well as in planning and developing comprehensive prosthetic rehabilitation programs. Well-designed clinical, multicenter, longitudinal studies are necessary to evaluate the impacts of different reconstruction and retention methods on patients' HRQOL. There is further need for multicenter and comprehensive studies with a larger sample to identify several determinants including sociodemographic, clinical, and psychological that may affect patients' HRQOL and satisfaction.

Author details

Kadriye Peker

Address all correspondence to: kpeker@istanbul.edu.tr

Department of Dental Public Health, Faculty of Dentistry, Istanbul University, Capa Istanbul, Turkey

References

[1] Rogers SN. Quality of life for head and neck cancer patients—has treatment planning altered? Oral Oncology. 2009;**45**(4-5):435-439. DOI: 10.1016/j.oraloncology.2008.11.006

[2] Rogers SN, Semple C, Babb M, Humphris G. Quality of life considerations in head and neck cancer: United Kingdom National Multidisciplinary Guidelines. The Journal of Laryngology and Otology. 2016;**130**(Suppl 2):49-52. DOI: 10.1017/S0022215116000438

[3] Global Burden of Disease Cancer Collaboration, Fitzmaurice C, Dicker D, et al. The Global Burden of Cancer 2013. JAMA Oncology. 2015;**1**(4):505-527. DOI: 10.1001/jamaoncol.2015.0735

[4] Ayaz B, Saleem K, Azim W, Shaikh A. A clinico-pathological study of oral cancers. Biomedica. 2011;**27**:29-32

[5] Noguti J, De Moura CF, De Jesus GP, Da Silva VH, Hossaka TA, Oshima CT, Ribeiro DA. Metastasis from oral cancer: An overview. Cancer Genomics Proteomics. 2012;**9**(5):329-335

[6] Murray CJ, Vos T, Lozano R et al. Disability-adjusted life years (DALYs) for 291 diseases and injuries in 21 regions, 1990-2010: A systematic analysis for the Global Burden of Disease Study 2010. Lancet. 2012;**380**(9859):2197-2223. DOI: 10.1016/S0140-6736(12)61689-4

[7] FDI World Dental Federation. Oral Health Worldwide—A report by FDI. Geneva: The FDI World Dental Federation; 2014

[8] Nagy J, Braunitzer G, Antal M, Berkovits C, Novák P, Nagy K. QOL in head and neck cancer patients after tumor therapy and subsequent rehabilitation: An exploratory study. Quality of Life Research. 2014;**23**(1):135-143. DOI: 10.1007/s11136-013-0446-1

[9] Pace-Balzan A, Shaw RJ, Butterworth C. Oral rehabilitation following treatment for oral cancer. Periodontology 2000. 2011;**57**(1):102-117. DOI: 10.1111/j.1600-0757.2011.00384.x

[10] Andrades P, Militsakh O, Hanasono MM, Rieger J, Rosenthal EL. Current strategies in reconstruction of maxillectomy defects. Archives of Otolaryngology Head Neck Surgery. 2011;**137**(8):806-812. DOI: 10.1001/archoto.2011.132

[11] Lethaus B, Lie N, de Beer F, Kessler P, de Baat C, Verdonck HW. Surgical and prosthetic reconsiderations in patients with maxillectomy. Journal of Oral Rehabilitation. 2010;**37**(2):138-142. DOI: 10.1111/j.1365-2842.2009.02031.x

[12] Breeze J, Rennie A, Morrison A, Dawson D, Tipper J, Rehman K, Grew N, Snee D, Pigadas N. Health-related quality of life after maxillectomy: Obturator rehabilitation compared with flap reconstruction. British Journal of Oral and Maxillofacial Surgery. 2016;**54**(8):857-862. DOI: 10.1016/j.bjoms.2016.05.024

[13] Kumar P, Alvi HA, Rao J, Singh BP, Jurel SK, Kumar L, Aggarwal H. Assessment of the quality of life in maxillectomy patients: A longitudinal study. Journal of Advanced Prosthodontics. 2013;**5**(1):29-35. DOI: 10.4047/jap.2013.5.1.29

[14] Depprich R, Naujoks C, Lind D, Ommerborn M, Meyer U, Kübler NR, Handschel J. Evaluation of the quality of life of patients with maxillofacial defects after prosthodontic therapy with obturator prostheses. International Journal of Oral and Maxillofacial Surgery. 2011;**40**(1):71-79. DOI: 10.1016/j.ijom.2010.09.019

[15] Riaz N, Warriach RA. Quality of life in patients with obturator prostheses. Journal of Ayub Medical College, Abbottabad. 2010;**22**(2):121-125

[16] Murphy J, Isaiah A, Wolf JS, Lubek JE. Quality of life factors and survival after total or extended maxillectomy for sinonasal malignancies. Journal of Oral and Maxillofacial Surgery. 2015;**73**(4):759-763. DOI: 10.1016/j.joms.2014.11.002

[17] Kanatas AN, Rogers SN. A guide of the questionnaires used in the measurement of health-related quality of life in head and neck oncology. Tumori. 2008;**94**(5):724-731

[18] Brandão TB, Vechiato Filho AJ, Batista VE, de Oliveira MC, Santos-Silva AR. Obturator prostheses versus free tissue transfers: A systematic review of the optimal approach to improving the quality of life for patients with maxillary defects. The Journal of Prosthetic Dentistry. 2016;**115**(2):247-253.e4. DOI: 10.1016/j.prosdent.2015.08.002

[19] Genden EM, Okay D, Stepp MT, Rezaee RP, Mojica JS, Buchbinder D, Urken ML. Comparison of functional and quality-of-life outcomes in patients with and without palatomaxillary reconstruction: A preliminary report. Archives of Otolaryngology Head Neck Surgery. 2003;**129**(7):775-780. DOI: 10.1001/archotol.129.7.775

[20] Salem AA, Shakel EA, Sadakha AA, Kassem EM, El-Segai AA. Evaluation of Zygomatic implant retained obturator in rehabilitation of partial palato-maxillectomy patients. Tanta Dental Journal. 2015;**12**(1):35-40. DOI: http://dx.doi.org/10.1016/j.tdj.2014.10.003

[21] Gotfredsen K, Abdullah S. Oral prosthetic rehabilitation with and without implants after radiation therapy and ablative surgery. International Journal of Dentistry Oral Science. 2015;**2**(4):21-25. DOI: http://dx.doi. org/10.19070/2377-8075-SI02004

[22] Hussain M, Naqvi SK, Ali SA, Yazdanie N, Khan MY, Khan M. Quality of life in oral cancer patients after provision of maxillary obturators. Pakistan Oral and Dental Journal. 2014;**34**(4):761-764

[23] Jiao T, Zhu C, Dong X, Gu X. Rehabilitation of maxillectomy defects with obturator prostheses fabricated using computer-aided design and rapid prototyping: A pilot study. International Journal of Prosthodontics. 2014;**27**(5):480-486. DOI:10.11607/ijp.3733

[24] Rogers SN, Lowe D, McNally D, Brown JS, Vaughan ED. Health-related QOL after maxillectomy: A comparison between prosthetic obturation and free flap. Journal of Oral and Maxillofacial Surgery. 2003;**61**(2):174-181. DOI: 10.1053/joms.2003.50044

[25] Chen C, Ren W, Gao L, Cheng Z, Zhang L, Li S, Zhi PK.Function of obturator prosthesis after maxillectomy and prosthetic obturator rehabilitation. Brazilian Journal of Otorhinolaryngology. 2016;**82**(2):177-183. DOI: 10.1016/j.bjorl.2015.10.006

[26] Seignemartin CP, Miranda ME, Luz JG, Teixeira RG. Understandability of speech predicts quality of life among maxillectomy patients restored with obturator prosthesis. Journal of Oral and Maxillofacial Surgery. 2015;**73**(10):2040-2048. DOI: 10.1016/j.joms.2015.04.031

[27] Wang F, Huang W, Zhang C, Sun J, Qu X, Wu Y. Functional outcome and quality of life after a maxillectomy:A comparison between an implant supported obturator and implant supported fixed prostheses in a free vascularized flap. Clinical Oral Implants Research. 2016:1-7. DOI: 10.1111/clr.12771

[28] Chen C, Ren WH, Huang RZ, Gao L, Hu ZP, Zhang LM, Li SM, Dong K, Qi H, Zhi KQ. Quality of life in patients after maxillectomy and placement of prosthetic obturator. International Journal of Prosthodontics. 2016;**29**(4):363-368. DOI: 10.11607/ijp.4608

[29] Rieger JM, Wolfaardt JF, Jha N, Seikaly H. Maxillary obturators: The relationship between patient satisfaction and speech outcome. Head Neck. 2003;**25**(11):895-903. DOI: 10.1002/hed.10299

[30] Kornblith AB, Zlotolow IM, Gooen J, Huryn JM, Lerner T, Strong EW, Shah JP, Spiro RH, Holland JC. Quality of life of maxillectomy patients using an obturator prosthesis. Head

Neck. 1996;**18**(4):323-334. DOI: 10.1002/(SICI)1097-0347(199607/08)18:4<323:AID-HED3>3.0.CO;2-#

[31] Kreeft AM, Krap M, Wismeijer D, Speksnijder CM, Smeele LE, Bosch SD, Muijen MS, Balm AJ. Oral function after maxillectomy and reconstruction with an obturator. International Journal of Oral and Maxillofacial Surgery. 2012;**41**(11):1387-1392. DOI: 10.1016/j.ijom.2012.07.014

[32] Chigurupati R, Aloor N, Salas R, Schmidt BL. Quality of life after maxillectomy and prosthetic obturator rehabilitation. Journal of Oral and Maxillofacial Surgery. 2013;**71**(8):1471-1478. DOI: 10.1016/j.joms.2013.02.002

[33] Irish J, Sandhu N, Simpson C, Wood R, Gilbert R, Gullane P, Brown D, Goldstein D, Devins G, Barker E. Quality of life in patients with maxillectomy prostheses. Head Neck. 2009;**31**(6):813-821. DOI: 10.1002/hed.21042

[34] Hertrampf K, Wenz HJ, Lehmann KM, Lorenz W, Koller M. Quality of life of patients with maxillofacial defects after treatment for malignancy. International Journal of Prosthodontics. 2004;**17**(6):657-665

[35] Khan MWU,Shah AA, Fatima A, Hanıf A. Subjective assessment of obturator functioning in patients with hemimaxillectomy. Pakistan Journal of Medical and Health Sciences. 2014;**8**(3):694-697

[36] Schweyen R, Kuhnt T, Wienke A, Eckert A, Hey J. The impact of oral rehabilitation on oral health-related quality of life in patients receiving radiotherapy for the treatment of head and neck cancer. Clinical and Oral Investigation. 2017;**21**(4):1123-1130. DOI: 10.1007/s00784-016

[37] Hahn TR, Krüskemper G, Enkling N, Kübler NR. Zur Lebensqualität nach chirurgischer Therapie von Mundhöhlenkarzinomen—eine retrospektive Multicenterstudie. Mund-, Kiefer- und Gesichtschirurgie. 2007;**11**(1):27-33. DOI: 10.1007/s10006-006-0038-0

[38] Ozhayat EB, Gotfredsen K, Elverdam B, Owall B. Patient-generated aspects in oral rehabilitation decision making. II. Comparison of an individual systematic interview method and the oral health impact profile. International Journal of Prosthodontics. 2010;**23**(5):421-428

[39] Ojo B, Genden EM, Teng MS, Milbury K, Misiukiewicz KJ, Badr H. A systematic review of head and neck cancer quality of life assessment instruments. Oral Oncology. 2012;**48**(10):923-937. DOI: 10.1016/j.oraloncology.2012.03.025

3

Salivary Gland Cancers: A Survey through History, Classifications and Managements

Mohammad Hossein Khosravi, Ali Bagherihagh,
Masoumeh Saeedi, Payman Dabirmoghaddam,
Ali Kouhi and Mohammad Hosein Amirzade-Iranaq

Abstract

In this chapter, we are going to discuss about salivary glands cancers, their clinical manifestations and categories, pathogenesis, diagnosis and treatment. We will go through details in each part in both clinical and surgical aspects based on recently prominent published studies and research in prestigious journals. After a short review on clinical features, epidemiology, pathogenesis, diagnosis and treatment, we will show staging and tumor node metastasis (TNM) classification of major salivary gland tumors and also basic principles of approach to salivary gland cancers. A little will be explained about basic surgical procedures for removal of cancers and benign tumors.

Keywords: cancer, salivary gland, classification, benign tumors

1. Embryology, anatomy and structure of salivary glands

There are three pairs of salivary glands in human: parotid (PG), submandibular (SMG) and sublingual gland (SLG). They all have the same architecture; an arborized duct which opens into the oral cavity with secretary end pieces called acini which produce the saliva [1]. A mixed structure of extracellular matrix, myoepithelial cells, myofibroblasts, immune cells, endothelial cells, stromal cells, and nerve fibers surround the acinar cells. The main excretory duct of PG is Stensen's duct which opens in buccal mucosa near the second maxillary molar after crossing the masseter muscle and penetrating buccinators muscle. Submandibular glands secrete the saliva through their main excretory duct, called Wharton's, which opens into the oral cavity under the tongue by the lingual frenum at a structure called the sublingual caruncule. In contrast, sublingual gland has small ducts called ducts of Rivinus and a common duct, Bartholin's duct, which connects with Wharton's duct at the sublingual caruncle [1].

Blood supply of parotid gland is mainly provided by the transverse facial artery and SMG by the facial artery. Postganglionic nerves from the otic and submandibular ganglia provide parasympathetic innervation. Superior cervical ganglion makes sympathetic postganglionic nerves which innervate the glands along blood vessels [1, 2]. Facial nerve is closely associated with PG capsule and facial nerve injury resulting in hemifacial paralysis is a major complication of parotid gland surgery. Lingual nerve accompanies Wharton's duct and then lingual nerve injury may be a complication of surgical exploration of floor of mouth for salivary stones removal.

Major salivary glands produce over 90% of saliva in a healthy adult. Saliva excretion is stimulated by both parasympathetic and sympathetic autonomic nervous system necessary for lubricating the oral cavity to enable eating, talking, swallowing, dental health and maintaining oral homeostasis, tasting, while also providing protective functions and aiding in digestion. Different types of saliva are produced by two types of acinar cells. Parotid gland secretes watery serous saliva produced by serous acini. SMGs and SLGs contain both serous and mucous acinar cells. Most of the acinar cells in SMGs are serous, while the majority of SLG is composed by mucous acinar cells. In addition to major salivary glands, there are several minor glands which are widely distributed across the oral mucosa [3].

Major salivary glands start to develop at 6–8 weeks of gestation. Oral ectoderm starts thickening to produce placodes of major glands. Growth factors and other necessary molecular cues for epithelial branching morphogenesis are provided by neural crest-derived mesenchyme. SMGs seem well differentiated with desmosomes and microvilli projected from cells along lumens by 13–16 weeks of gestation. At 16 weeks, the striated and intercalated ducts can be recognized and acinar cells begin to predominate tissue by 20–24 weeks [4]. Salivary glands continue to develop up to 28 weeks and glands can secret saliva at birth.

2. Salivary gland neoplasms

Salivary gland tumors are a diverse group of neoplasms in terms of both morphology and clinical manifestations. These tumors have an incidence of approximately 2.5 cases to 3.0 cases per 100,000 per year [5]. Salivary gland malignancies consist more than 0.5% of all malignancies and approximately 3–5% of all head and neck cancers [6]. Salivary gland tumors usually involve people in their sixth or seventh decade of life [7, 8]. Recent studies have indicated that incidence of major salivary glands are increasing [9].

The exact etiology of salivary gland malignancies has not been determined; however ionizing radiation is indicated as a cause of salivary gland cancer [6, 7, 10, 11].

Tumors of salivary gland are related to both major and minor salivary glands. Minor salivary gland lesions are more frequently seen in palate; however, they can be found throughout oral cavity as oral mucosa, posterior tongue, larynx, pharynx, paranasal sinuses, retromolar and peritonsillar areas, uvula and floor of mouth [6, 12]. More than 50% of salivary gland tumors are benign and about 70–80% of all salivary gland neoplasms originate from parotid gland [13]. Different sites have different rate of malignancy so that 20–25% of parotid, 35–40% of submandibular, 50% of palate and more than 90% of sublingual gland tumors are malignant [14].

Comprising about 50% of all salivary gland tumors and 65% of parotid gland tumors, pleomorphic adenoma is the most common benign minor and major salivary gland tumor. On the other hand, mucoepidermoid carcinoma is the most prevalent major and minor salivary gland tumor comprising 10% of all salivary gland and about 35% of malignant salivary neoplasms [15]. This neoplasm mostly occurs in parotid gland [15, 16].

Most benign major and minor salivary gland tumors present with painless swelling of the parotid, submandibular or sublingual glands. Numbness or weakness which are signs of nerve involvement, typically indicate malignancy. Facial nerve weakness accompanied by parotid tumor is not a pleasant sign. A majority of benign and malignant tumors of parotid gland present as asymptomatic mass in the gland [13].

Tumors have more favorable prognosis when present in major salivary glands; parotid gland tumors have the best prognosis followed by submandibular gland. On the other hand, sublingual and minor salivary gland tumors have less favorable prognosis. Adequate surgical resection is enough for curing early-stage low-grade major and minor salivary gland tumors. In contrary, high-grade tumors have poorer prognosis and may need postoperative radiation therapy [17]. In addition, histology, grade, extent of primary tumor (stage), facial nerve involvement, fixation to skin or deep structures and lymph node or distant metastasis are among other factors involved in prognosis [18, 19].

3. Classification of tumors

Several pathological classifications have been proposed for salivary gland tumors since 50 years by several authorities such as Armed Forces Institute of Pathology and the World Health Organization (WHO). In 1954, there were only 16 salivary gland epithelial tumor entities in pathological classification which increased to 36 entities in 1996 showing an evident progress [20]. **Table 1** shows WHO histological classification of epithelial tumors of the salivary glands.

3.1. Acinic cell carcinoma

Acinic cell carcinoma (AcCC) comprises one of six parotid cancers which is supported by a nationwide study in the Netherlands where 15% of parotid malignancies were AcCC [21–23]. Based on 1973–2009 Surveillance, Epidemiology, and End Results (SEER) analysis AcCC comprises 11% of salivary malignancies [24]. AcCC has an average annual incidence of 0.13 cases per 100,000 patients per year. Also approved by other studies, SEER program indicated that AcCC has a higher average incidence for females than males (0.15 cases vs. 0.11 cases per

Malignant epithelial (n = 24)

Acinic cell carcinoma

Oncocytic carcinoma

Mucoepidermoid carcinoma

Salivary duct carcinoma

Adenoid cystic carcinoma

Adenocarcinoma (NOS)

Polymorphous (LG)

Adenocarcinoma

Myoepithelial carcinoma

Epithelial-myoepithelial carcinoma

Carcinoma ex pleomorphic adenoma

Clear cell carcinoma (NOS)

Carcinosarcoma

Basal cell adenocarcinoma

Metastasising pleomorphic adenoma

Sebaceous carcinoma

Squamous cell carcinoma

Sebaceous lymphadenocarcinoma

Small-cell carcinoma

Cystadenocarcinoma

Large cell carcinoma

LG cribriform cystadenocarcinoma

Lymphoepithelial carcinoma

Mucinous adenocarcinoma

Sialoblastoma

Benign epithelial (n = 10)

Pleomorphic adenoma

Lymphadenoma

- Sebaceous
- Nonsebaceous

Ductal papilloma

- Inverted ductal papilloma
- Intraductal papilloma
- Sialadenoma papilliferum

Myoepithelioma

Basal cell adenoma

Warthin tumor

Oncocytoma

Canalicular adenoma

Sebaceous adenoma

Cystadenoma

Table 1. WHO (2005) histological classification of epithelial tumors of the salivary glands, squamous cell carcinoma (SCC) and tumors like "carcinoma in pleomorphic adenoma".

100,000 patients) [25, 26]. Patients with AcCC have a median age of 52 years at the time of diagnosis and it occurs more in younger ages than other salivary gland tumors [27]. One-third of patients are under 40, one-third between 40 and 59 and one-third above 60 years of age [24]. AcCC more frequently occurs in whites (85%) than in blacks (7%) or other races (8%) [24, 28]. There are no known risk factors for AcCC; however, family history and radiation exposure have been proposed as potential risk factors [29].

The most common clinical feature of AcCC is a slow-growing swelling and its association with pain or fixation to neighboring structures is an indicator of poor prognosis [25]. Nodal metastasis is really uncommon at the time of diagnosis [26]. AcCC is less common in minor salivary glands and comprises only 9% according to SEER database [30]. AcCC of minor salivary glands mostly occur in buccal mucosa and upper lip in contrast to other types of minor salivary glands which mostly occur in palate [31, 32].

3.1.1. Diagnosis and preoperative assessment

Since AcCC often presents symptomless, preoperative assessment seems necessary to determine location of tumor, extent and malignancy indicators as in parotid surgery these factors show the risk of facial nerve injury [33]. Imaging is highly suggested when a glandular swelling is accompanied by impaired mobility or when involvement of deeper structures or nerves is suspected [34–37].

Imaging modalities include ultrasound (US), computed tomography (CT), magnetic resonance imaging (MRI) and positron emission tomography (PET) [33]. AcCC is appeared defined, lobular, hypoechoic, heterogeneous and poorly vascularized; while on CT, it is appeared regular and variably defined with heterogeneous enhancement [38].

MRI is preferred to CT for assessment of parotid, stylomastoid foramen and neural or perineural invasion [35, 37, 39, 40]. However, it is a rare condition; PET scan is indicated only when there is a high suspicion of distant metastatic disease. Also it is indicated postoperatively in case of AcCC with high-grade transformation [33, 41–43]. Ultrasound-guided fine needle aspiration cytology (FNAC) and ultrasound-guided core biopsy (USCB) are needling procedures for diagnosing AcCC [22, 44].

3.1.2. Management

The main treatment for AcCC is surgical resection, as AcCC do not show distant metastasis at the time of diagnosis and is usually an accessible tumor [25, 33]. For low-grade AcCC, surgery alone may be curative; while for known high-grade tumors in risk of positive margins, bone or nerve invasion and nodal metastasis a more aggressive approach is needed. A preoperatively paralyzed or involved facial nerve should be resected and repaired by interposition graft from greater auricular or sural nerve [22]. Elective neck dissection is not recommended; nevertheless patients with large or high-grade tumors may benefit from level II, III and IV neck dissections [26].

Radiotherapy is not necessary for low grade, low stage and adequately resected AcCCs [45]. As like other salivary gland cancers, criteria for radiotherapy include recurrent disease, advanced T-classification (T3/T4), positive margins, pathologically positive cervical lymph nodes, perineural invasion, high-grade and high proliferative tumors [24, 26, 28].

Role of chemotherapy is not exactly known in treatment of AcCCs; however, mTOR inhibitors may be beneficial [22].

3.2. Mucoepidermoid carcinoma

Defined as "a malignant glandular epithelial neoplasm characterised by mucous, intermediate and epidermoid cells, with columnar, clear cell and oncocytoid features" by World Health Organization (WHO), mucoepidermoid carcinoma (MEC) was first described by Masson and Berger [46–48]. MEC is considered as the most common primary salivary gland malignancy and patients have a mean age of 45 years old at the time of diagnosis [49, 50]. Children are rarely involved and gender differences are not marked [51, 52].

Parotid is the most commonly involved major salivary gland and MEC of minor salivary glands is usually found on the palate followed by buccal mucosa, tongue, lips and floor of mouth [51]. Another important location is retromolar area in which 18% of intra-oral MECs can be detected [53]. MEC may also be rose from salivary-type glands in sinonasal and laryngeal mucosa lachrymal and ceruminous glands, and even nodal glandular inclusions [54–57].

The most common clinical manifestation of MEC is a painless, variously fixed, rubbery or soft mass. Intra-oral tumors may appear as a blue-red tinged swelling which mimics a mucocele or vascular tumor because of their superficial location [51, 53]. The interval between initial symptoms and diagnosis differs depending on the site of origin [16]. Sublingual MEC is painful and patients are usually diagnosed earlier than parotid or submandibular tumors [16].

3.2.1. Preoperative assessment

Imaging is less necessary for diagnosing MECs unless they are located on the palate or retromolar area of mandible or involvement of deeper structures or cranial nerves is suspected [46]. CT scan is beneficiary for assessment of bone invasion by the tumor; while MRI is better for soft tissue. Ultrasound (US) may be satisfactory if small tumors are located in major salivary glands; for larger tumors or tumors outside these glands, a combination of CT and MRI is suggested. According to recent studies, positron emission tomography (PET) has been beneficial in loco-regionally advanced tumors [58]. Fine needle aspiration biopsy (FNAB) is another preoperative diagnostic modality which is dependent on expertise of pathologist and number of patients treated in the institute [59].

3.2.2. Management

Complete surgical removal of tumor is the treatment of choice in case of anatomically accessible MECs [32]. More treatment planning is needed when MECs are locally advanced, incompletely resected or with positive margins, invaded to bone or nerves, metastasized to lymph nodes or high grade [18, 60].

For low-grade tumors, surgery alone is curative; however, site and size of tumor influence the extent of surgery. For parotid, superficial parotidectomy is enough unless the tumor involves deep lobe [61]. Resection of facial nerve is recommended if there is preoperative facial nerve paralysis or weakness or there is evidence of perineural invasion in frozen section [46]. If submandibular or sublingual glands are involved, resection of the anterior mandible or mylohyoid muscle should be considered. Wide local excision is usually curative if minor salivary glands are involved with low-grade small MECs. Mandibulectomy, maxillectomy, mastoidectomy, infratemporal fossa, anterior craniofacial resection, soft or hard palate resection or resection of cranial nerves may be required in more extensive disease [62]. For tumors in tonsillar area, radical tonsillectomy and ipsilateral neck dissection is applied [32, 63]. Elective neck dissection should be done in high-grade MEC and avoided in low- or intermediate-grade tumors [32].

Radiotherapy is recommended for high-grade MECs and patients with perineural invasion, positive margins and T3–4 classification [64, 65]. For patients with increased risk of nodal metastasis, elective neck irradiation may be applicable [32, 66]. The role of chemotherapy is not approved in the treatment of MECs and some clinical trials are being conducted regarding this issue.

3.3. Adenoid cystic carcinoma (cylindroma)

Accounting for about 1% of all head and neck cancers and 10% of all salivary gland tumors, adenoid cystic carcinoma (AdCC) is a rare tumor with a yearly incidence of about 3–4.5 cases per million [67–70]. On the other hand, it is the most common malignancy of minor salivary gland tumors with a proportion ranging from 32 to 71% [67]. AdCC may involve other sites and glands such as lacrimal and ceruminous glands as well as nasal and paranasal sinuses, larynx and trachea [32, 67, 71–74]. AdCC is mostly found in the parotid, submandibular and minor salivary glands. Based on previous studies, AdCC was the most frequent histology of parotid carcinoma [23]. In the submandibular gland, the likelihood of AdCC is even greater as it accounts for 40% of salivary gland cancers [75, 76]. AdCC of minor salivary glands is most frequently found in the palate followed by paranasal sinuses and other parts of salivary glands [32, 77].

Although more prevalent in middle-aged and older patients in fifth and sixth decades of life, AdCC occurs in all age groups [12, 78–81]. Until now, there are no known risk factors for AdCC and smoking has not been proven to affect incidence [82].

The characteristic cribriform arrangement of tumor cells on microscopy and invasion to surrounding structures and nerves were first described in 1853 and 1854 by Robin, Lorain and Laboulbene [83].

AdCC is a really invasive tumor which is recognized by perineural invasion and multiple local recurrences. Although considered rarely, but regional lymph node metastasis may be hidden according to its occult and clinically undetectable nature and lack of pathological assessment of lymph nodes. Hematogenous metastasis is also common especially to lung, bone and liver [83, 84].

As one of the most biologically destructive and unpredictable tumors of the head and neck, the most common clinical manifestation of AdCC is a slowly growing mass followed by pain. AdCC symptoms vary according to the site of disease. The tumor usually presents with a mass in major salivary glands and may lead to facial nerve paralysis when located in parotid [69, 85]. When located in the palate, a mass is common; however, ulcer or even oroantral fistula may be detected. Dyspnea is the first symptom in larynx and nasal obstruction, epistaxis, eye symptoms and deep facial pain are presenting symptoms of nose and paranasal sinuses involvement [32, 86, 87].

3.3.1. Preoperative assessment

As other salivary gland malignancies, preoperative imaging of AdCC includes computed tomography (CT) and magnetic resonance imaging (MRI) which help with estimation of disease extent. CT scan is preferred for bone invasion assessment and MRI is more appropriate for evaluation of soft tissue extension or suspected neural invasion presenting as pain or facial nerve analysis [88]. Positron emission tomography (PET) scan in combination with CT is applied for excluding distant metastasis [89].

3.3.2. Management

Decision-making for treatment of AdCC depends on tumor location, stage at diagnosis and biologic behavior of tumor reflected in histologic grading [90]. Radical surgical resection of tumor, ensuring free margins, followed by postoperative radiotherapy is the gold-standard treatment for AdCC. Since AdCC has a high potential for infiltrating to neighboring tissue, mainly by perineural invasion, the free margin may not be reached. In anatomical sites with difficult access, incomplete resection has remained as a problem.

In case of parotid involvement, facial nerve should be preserved if it is not paralyzed preoperatively and not involved by tumor at the time of surgery. Radiotherapy after surgery is considered as an appropriate adjuvant therapy for possible residual tumors on nerve branches [45, 91, 92].

Neck dissection is only performed in patients with clinically positive lymph nodes; however, it is not common in AdCC especially for parotid malignancies [93]. The number of involved lymph nodes is higher in minor salivary glands AdCC. Lymph nodes could also be involved by direct extension of primary tumor when AdCC is located in parotid, submandibular gland and larynx [94, 95]. Despite combination therapy with surgery and radiotherapy, local recurrence happens [69]. Chemoradiotherapy may be considered using various agents in patients with adverse prognostic factors [96]. To the best of scientists' knowledge, patients with locally recurrent or metastatic AdCC may not experience cure by systemic treatment using cytotoxic chemotherapy or targeted molecular therapies [69]. So chemotherapy may be considered as a palliative treatment for patients with poorly-controlled disease or symptomatic metastasis [97].

3.4. Basal cell adenocarcinoma

Basal cell adenocarcinoma (BCAC) occurs equally in both genders and usually involves patients in fifth or sixth decades of their lives [98]. In the setting of syndromic disease, it may have multifocal lesions of multiple cylindromatosis and trichoepitheliomas (Brooke-Spiegler syndrome) [99]. Basal cell adenocarcinoma usually has an indolent behavior but may be locally aggressive and one-third of cases experience recurrence. It has been reported that BCACs have a regional and distant metastatic rates ranging from 8 to 12% and 2 to 4%, respectively [100, 101]. The main treatment strategy for basal cell adenocarcinoma is surgery with lymph node dissection, if required. High-stage tumors are treated with radiotherapy which may improve outcome [101].

3.5. Epithelial-myoepithelial carcinoma

As a biphasic salivary gland malignancy, epithelial-myoepithelial carcinoma (EMCA) may occur at any sites containing salivary or seromucinous glands [98]. It is mostly (60–80%) prevalent in parotid glands and involves people in sixth decade of life. Female-male ratio is 3:2 [102]. *RAS* mutation is detected in 20 to 25% of cases with predominancy of HRAS codon 61 mutations [103]. EMCA is typically a low-grade tumor and has an estimated 5-year disease-specific survival (DSS) of 90–95% and 10-year DSS of 80–90% [102, 104]. Often late, but about one-third of patients experience recurrence with a median disease-free survival (DFS) of 11 years. Regional and distant metastases are uncommon [104]. Factors like margin status, vascular invasion, necrosis, and high-grade features are among important prognostic factors [102]. EMCA is surgically treated with no sensible effect of radiotherapy [102, 104].

3.6. Mammary analogue secretory carcinoma, a new entity

Mammary analogue secretory carcinoma (MASC) is a newly defined salivary gland malignancy based on morphologic and molecular features [44, 105]. Previously, most of MASC were marked as acinic cell carcinoma or adenocarcinoma not otherwise specified [98]. Both genders are equally involved and MASC typically occurs in fifth to sixth decades of life.

There are limited data on management of MASC; it may have a higher rate of lymph node metastasis (up to 25%) than acinic cell carcinoma [106]. Nonetheless, surgery is the main treatment for MASC.

4. TNM classification and staging of major salivary gland tumors

The most common system for cancers in the major salivary glands is the TNM system of the American Joint Committee on Cancer (AJCC), available at (https://www.cancer.org/cancer/salivary-gland-cancer/detection-diagnosis-staging/staging.html).

T groups for major salivary gland cancers:

TX: The main (primary) tumor cannot be assessed; information not known.

T0: No evidence of a primary tumor. (For example, the cancer was first found in the lymph nodes, but the main tumor itself can't be found.)

T1: Tumor is 2 cm (about ¾ inch) across or smaller. It's not growing into nearby tissues.

T2: Tumor is larger than 2 cm but no larger than 4 cm (about 1½ inch) across. It is not growing into nearby tissues.

T3: Tumor is larger than 4 cm across and/or is growing into nearby soft tissues.

T4a: Tumor is any size and is growing into nearby structures such as the jaw bone, skin, ear canal, and/or facial nerve. This is known as *moderately advanced disease.*

T4b: Tumor is any size and is growing into nearby structures such as the base of the skull or other bones nearby, or it surrounds the carotid artery. This is known as *very advanced disease.*

N groups for major salivary gland cancers:

NX: Nearby (regional) lymph nodes cannot be assessed; information not known.

N0: No spread to regional lymph nodes.

N1: The cancer has spread to one lymph node on the same side of the head or neck as the primary tumor. The lymph node is no larger than 3 cm (about 1¼ inch) across.

N2: This group includes 3 subgroups:

- **N2a:** The cancer has spread to one lymph node on the same side as the primary tumor. The lymph node is larger than 3 cm but not larger than 6 cm (about 2½ inches) across.
- **N2b:** The cancer has spread to more than one lymph node on the same side as the primary tumor, but none of the lymph nodes are larger than 6 cm across.
- **N2c:** The cancer has spread to one or more lymph nodes, none larger than 6 cm across, either on the side opposite the primary tumor or on both sides of the neck.

N3: The cancer has spread to a lymph node that is larger than 6 cm across.

M groups for major salivary gland cancers:

M0: The cancer has not spread to tissues or organs far away from the salivary glands.

M1: The cancer has spread to tissues or organs far away from the salivary glands.

Stage grouping:

Stage I: T1, N0, M0: The tumor is no more than 2 cm across and is not growing into nearby tissues (T1). It has not spread to nearby lymph nodes (N0) or distant sites (M0).

Stage II: T2, N0, M0: The tumor is larger than 2 cm but is no larger than 4 cm across and is not growing into nearby tissues (T2). It has not spread to nearby lymph nodes (N0) or distant sites (M0).

Stage III: Either of the following:

T3, N0, M0: The tumor is larger than 4 cm across and/or is growing into nearby soft tissues (T3). It has not spread to nearby lymph nodes (N0) or to distant sites (M0).

or

T1 to T3, N1, M0: The tumor is any size and may have grown into nearby soft tissues (T1 to T3). The cancer has spread to one lymph node on the same side of the head or neck as the primary tumor, but the lymph node is no larger than 3 cm across (N1). The cancer has not spread to distant sites (M0).

Stage IVA: Either of the following:

T4a, N0 or N1, M0: The tumor is any size but has grown into nearby structures such as the jaw bone, skin, ear canal, and/or facial nerve (T4a). It may or may not have spread to one lymph node (no larger than 3 cm across) on the same side of the head or neck as the primary tumor (N0 or N1). The cancer has not spread to distant sites (M0).

or

T1 to T4a, N2, M0: The tumor is any size and may or may not have grown into nearby soft tissues or structures such as the jaw bone, skin, ear canal, and/or facial nerve (T1 to T4a). The cancer has spread to more than one lymph node, to a lymph node larger than 3 cm across, or to lymph nodes on the other or both sides of the neck. None of the lymph nodes are larger than 6 cm across (N2). The cancer has not spread to distant sites (M0).

Stage IVB: Either of the following:

T4b, Any N, M0: The tumor is any size and has grown into nearby structures such as the base of the skull or other bones nearby, or it surrounds the carotid artery (T4b). The cancer may or may not have spread to nearby lymph nodes (any N). It has not spread to distant sites (M0).

or

Any T, N3, M0: The tumor is any size and may or may not have grown into nearby soft tissues or other structures (any T). The cancer has spread to at least one lymph node that's larger than 6 cm across (N3). It has not spread to distant sites (M0).

Stage IVC: Any T, Any N, M1: The tumor is any size and may or may not have grown into nearby soft tissues or other structures (any T). The cancer may or may not have spread to nearby lymph nodes (any N). It has spread to distant sites (M1).

Author details

Mohammad Hossein Khosravi[1,2], Ali Bagherihagh[2,4], Masoumeh Saeedi[2,4], Payman Dabirmoghaddam[5], Ali Kouhi[2,3]* and Mohammad Hosein Amirzade-Iranaq[2,6]

*Address all correspondence to: alikouhi@gmail.com

1 Student Research Committee (SRC), Baqiyatallah University of Medical Sciences, Tehran, Iran

2 International Otorhinolaryngology Research Association (IORA), Universal Scientific Education and Research Network (USERN), Tehran, Iran

3 Department of Otolaryngology-Head and Neck Surgery, Otorhinolaryngology Research Center, Tehran University of Medical Sciences, Tehran, Iran

4 Department of Otorhinolaryngology-Head and Neck Surgery, Faculty of Medicine, Baqiatallah University of Medical Sciences, Tehran, Iran

5 Tehran University of Medical Sciences, Tehran, Iran

6 Student Research Committee, Shahid Sadoughi University of Medical Sciences, Yazd, Iran

References

[1] Holmberg KV, Hoffman MP. Anatomy, biogenesis and regeneration of salivary glands. Ligtenberg AJM, Veerman ECI (eds). In: Saliva: Secretion and Functions. Vol. 24. Karger Publishers, Basel; 2014. pp. 1-13

[2] Johns M. The salivary glands: Anatomy and embryology. Otolaryngologic Clinics of North America. 1977;**10**(2):261

[3] Cate-Ten A. Oral Histology: Development, Structure, and Function. Saint Louis, Missouri: Mosby; 1998

[4] Tucker AS, editor. Salivary gland development. Seminars in cell & developmental biology. Elsevier: 2007 Apr;**18**(2):237-44. DOI:10.1016/j.semcdb.2007.01.006

[5] Speight P, Barrett A. Salivary gland tumours. Oral diseases. 2002;**8**(5):229-240

[6] Mendenhall WM, Werning JW, Pfister DG. Treatment of head and neck cancer. In: DeVita VT Jr, Lawrence TS, Rosenberg SA, editors. Cancer: Principles and Practice of Oncology. 9th ed. Philadelphia: Lippincott Williams & Wilkins; 2011. pp. 729-780

[7] Ellis GL, Auclair PL. Tumors of the salivary glands. atlas of tumor pathology, 3rd series, fascicle 17. Washington DC: Armed Forces Institute of Pathology; 1996

[8] Wahlberg P, Anderson H, Biörklund A, Möller T, Perfekt R. Carcinoma of the parotid and submandibular glands—A study of survival in 2465 patients. Oral Oncology. 2002;**38**(7):706-713

[9] Del Signore AG, Megwalu UC. The rising incidence of major salivary gland cancer in the United States. Ear, Nose, & Throat Journal. 2017;**96**(3):E13

[10] Scanlon EF, Sener SF. Head and neck neoplasia following irradiation for benign conditions. Head & Neck Surgery. 1981;**4**(2):139-145

[11] Van der Laan B, Baris G, Gregor RT, Hilgers F, Balm A. Radiation-induced tumours of the head and neck. The Journal of Laryngology & Otology. 1995;**109**(04):346-349

[12] Spiro RH, Thaler HT, Hicks WF, Kher UA, Huvos AH, Strong EW. The importance of clinical staging of minor salivary gland carcinoma. The American Journal of Surgery. 1991;**162**(4):330-336

[13] Gooden E, Witterick IJ, Hacker D, Rosen IB, Freeman JL. Parotid gland tumours in 255 consecutive patients: Mount Sinai Hospital's quality assurance review. Journal of Otolaryngology. 2002;**31**(6)

[14] Theriault C, Fitzpatrick P. Malignant parotid tumors prognostic factors and optimum treatment. American Journal of Clinical Oncology. 1986;**9**(6):510-516

[15] Guzzo M, Andreola S, Sirizzotti G, Cantu G. Mucoepidermoid carcinoma of the salivary glands: Clinicopathologic review of 108 patients treated at the National Cancer Institute of Milan. Annals of Surgical Oncology. 2002;**9**(7):688-695

[16] Goode RK, Auclair PL, Ellis GL. Mucoepidermoid carcinoma of the major salivary glands. Cancer. 1998;**82**(7):1217-1224

[17] Parsons JT, Mendenhall WM, Stringer SP, Cassisi NJ, Million RR. Management of minor salivary gland carcinomas. International Journal of Radiation Oncology Biology Physics. 1996;**35**(3):443-454

[18] Terhaard CH, Lubsen H, Van der Tweel I, Hilgers F, Eijkenboom W, Marres H, et al. Salivary gland carcinoma: Independent prognostic factors for locoregional control, distant metastases, and overall survival: Results of the Dutch head and neck oncology cooperative group. Head & Neck. 2004;**26**(8):681-693

[19] Vander Poorten VL, Balm AJ, Hilgers FJ, Tan IB, Loftus-Coll BM, Keus RB, et al. The development of a prognostic score for patients with parotid carcinoma. Cancer. 1999; **85**(9):2057-2067

[20] Eveson JW, Auclair P, Gnepp DR, et al. Tumours of the Salivary Glands. World Health Organisation Classification of Tumours Pathology and Genetics of Head and Neck Tumours. Lyon: IARC Press; 2005. pp. 212-215

[21] Al-Mamgani A, van Rooij P, Verduijn GM, Meeuwis CA, Levendag PC. Long-term outcomes and quality of life of 186 patients with primary parotid carcinoma treated with surgery and radiotherapy at the Daniel den Hoed Cancer Center. International Journal of Radiation Oncology Biology Physics. 2012;**84**(1):189-195

[22] Vander Poorten V, Triantafyllou A, Thompson L, Bishop J, Hauben E, Hunt J, et al. Salivary acinic cell carcinoma: Reappraisal and update. European Archives of Oto-Rhino-Laryngology. 2016;**273**(11):3511-3531

[23] Vander Poorten VL, Hart AA, van der Laan BF, de Jong RJB, Manni JJ, Marres HA, et al. Prognostic index for patients with parotid carcinoma. Cancer. 2003;**97**(6):1453-1463

[24] Patel NR, Sanghvi S, Khan MN, Husain Q, Baredes S, Eloy JA. Demographic trends and disease-specific survival in salivary acinic cell carcinoma: An analysis of 1129 cases. The Laryngoscope. 2014;**124**(1):172-178

[25] Lewis JE, Olsen KD, Weiland LH. Acinic cell carcinoma. Clinicopathologic review. Cancer. 1991;**67**(1):172-179

[26] Neskey DM, Klein JD, Hicks S, Garden AS, Bell DM, El-Naggar AK, et al. Prognostic factors associated with decreased survival in patients with acinic cell carcinoma. JAMA Otolaryngology–Head & Neck Surgery. 2013;**139**(11):1195-1202

[27] Hoffman HT, Karnell LH, Robinson RA, Pinkston JA, Menck HR. National Cancer Data Base report on cancer of the head and neck: Acinic cell carcinoma. Head & Neck. 1999;21(4):297-309

[28] Gomez DR, Katabi N, Zhung J, Wolden SL, Zelefsky MJ, Kraus DH, et al. Clinical and pathologic prognostic features in acinic cell carcinoma of the parotid gland. Cancer. 2009;**115**(10):2128-2137

[29] Saku T, Hayashi Y, Takahara O, Matsuura H, Tokunaga M, Tokuoka S, et al. Salivary gland tumors among atomic bomb survivors, 1950-1987. Cancer. 1997;**79**(8):1465-1475

[30] Biron VL, Lentsch EJ, Gerry DR, Bewley AF. Factors influencing survival in acinic cell carcinoma: A retrospective survival analysis of 2061 patients. Head & Neck. 2015;**37**(6):870-877

[31] Omlie JE, Koutlas IG. Acinic cell carcinoma of minor salivary glands: A clinicopathologic study of 21 cases. Journal of Oral and Maxillofacial Surgery. 2010;**68**(9):2053-2057

[32] Poorten VV, Hunt J, Bradley PJ, Haigentz M, Rinaldo A, Mendenhall WM, et al. Recent trends in the management of minor salivary gland carcinoma. Head & Neck. 2014;**36**(3):444-455

[33] Vander Poorten V, Bradley PJ, Takes RP, Rinaldo A, Woolgar JA, Ferlito A. Diagnosis and management of parotid carcinoma with a special focus on recent advances in molecular biology. Head & Neck. 2012;**34**(3):429-440

[34] Cheung RL, Russell AC, Freeman J. Does routine preoperative imaging of parotid tumours affect surgical management decision making? Journal of Otolaryngology--Head & Neck Surgery. 2008;**37**(3)

[35] Eisele D, Kleinberg L, O'Malley B. Management of malignant salivary gland tumors. In: Harrison LB, Sessions RB, Hong KH, editors. Head and Neck Cancer: A Multidisciplinary Approach. 1st ed. Philadelphia-New York: Lippincott-Raven; 1999. 721-748

[36] Spiro R. Management of malignant tumors of the salivary glands. Oncology (Williston Park, NY). 1998;**12**(5):671-680; discussion 83

[37] Yousem DM, Kraut MA, Chalian AA. Major salivary gland imaging 1. Radiology. 2000;**216**(1):19-29

[38] Li J, Gong X, Xiong P, Xu Q, Liu Y, Chen Y, et al. Ultrasound and computed tomography features of primary acinic cell carcinoma in the parotid gland: A retrospective study. European Journal of Radiology. 2014;**83**(7):1152-1156

[39] Jungehuelsing M, Sittel C, Fischbach R, Wagner M, Stennert E. Limitations of magnetic resonance imaging in the evaluation of perineural tumor spread causing facial nerve paralysis. Archives of Otolaryngology–Head & Neck Surgery. 2000;**126**(4):506-510

[40] Lee Y, Wong K, King A, Ahuja A. Imaging of salivary gland tumours. European Journal of Radiology. 2008;**66**(3):419-436

[41] Johnykutty S, Miller CH, Hoda RS, Giampoli EJ. Fine-needle aspiration of dedifferentiated acinic cell carcinoma: Report of a case with cyto-histological correlation. Diagnostic Cytopathology. 2009;**37**(10):763-768

[42] Stanley RJ, Weiland LH, Olsen KD, Pearson BW. Dedifferentiated acinic cell (acinous) carcinoma of the parotid gland. Otolaryngology—Head and Neck Surgery. 1988;**98**(2):155-161

[43] Yoo IR, Jung C-K, Kim SH, Chung SK. F-18 FDG PET/CT findings of dedifferentiated acinic cell carcinoma. Clinical Nuclear Medicine. 2010;**35**(6):473-474

[44] Skálová A, Vanecek T, Sima R, Laco J, Weinreb I, Perez-Ordonez B, et al. Mammary analogue secretory carcinoma of salivary glands, containing the ETV6-NTRK3 fusion gene: A hitherto undescribed salivary gland tumor entity. The American Journal of Surgical Pathology. 2010;**34**(5):599-608

[45] Vander Poorten VL, Balm AJ, Hilgers FJ. Management of cancer of the parotid gland. Current Opinion in Otolaryngology & Head and Neck Surgery. 2002;**10**(2):134-144

[46] Coca-Pelaz A, Rodrigo JP, Triantafyllou A, Hunt JL, Rinaldo A, Strojan P, et al. Salivary mucoepidermoid carcinoma revisited. European Archives of Oto-Rhino-Laryngology. 2015;**272**(4):799-819

[47] Goode RK, El-Naggar AK. Mucoepidermoid carcinoma. In: Barnes L, Eveson JW, Reichart P, Sidransky D, editors. World Health Organization Classification of Tumours. Pathology and Genetics of Head and Neck Tumours. Lyon: IARC Press; 2005. pp. 219-220

[48] Masson P, Berger L. Epitheliomas a double metaplasie de la parotide. Bulletin De l'Association Francaise Pour L'Etude Du Cancer. 1924;**13**:366-373

[49] Ellis GL, Auclair PL. Tumors of the Salivary Glands. Atlas of Tumor Pathology, 3rd Series, Fascicle 17. Washington, DC: Armed Forces Institute of Pathology; 1996. pp. 39-57, 155-175, 452-454

[50] Spiro RH. Salivary neoplasms: Overview of a 35-year experience with 2,807 patients. Head & Neck Surgery. 1986;**8**(3):177-184

[51] Eversole L. Mucoepidermoid carcinoma: Review of 815 reported cases. Journal of Oral Surgery (American Dental Association: 1965). 1970;**28**(7):490

[52] Yoshida EJ, García J, Eisele DW, Chen AM. Salivary gland malignancies in children. International Journal of Pediatric Otorhinolaryngology. 2014;**78**(2):174-178

[53] Melrose RJ, Abrams AM, Howell FV. Mucoepidermoid tumors of the intraoral minor salivary glands: A clinicopathologic study of 54 cases. Journal of Oral Pathology & Medicine. 1973;**2**(6):314-325

[54] Crain N, Nelson BL, Barnes EL, Thompson LD. Ceruminous gland carcinomas: A clinicopathologic and immunophenotypic study of 17 cases. Head and Neck Pathology. 2009;**3**(1):1-17

[55] Ferlito A, Recher G, Bottin R. Mucoepidermoid carcinoma of the larynx. A clinicopathological study of 11 cases with review of the literature. ORL; Journal for Oto-Rhino-Laryngology and Its Related Specialties. 1981;**43**:280-299

[56] Paulino AF, Huvos AG. Epithelial tumors of the lacrimal glands: A clinicopathologic study. Annals of Diagnostic Pathology. 1999;**3**(4):199-204

[57] Wolfish EB, Nelson BL, Thompson LD. Sinonasal tract mucoepidermoid carcinoma: A clinicopathologic and immunophenotypic study of 19 cases combined with a comprehensive review of the literature. Head and Neck Pathology. 2012;**6**(2):191-207

[58] Sharma P, Jain TK, Singh H, Suman SK, Faizi NA, Kumar R, et al. Utility of 18F-FDG PET-CT in staging and restaging of patients with malignant salivary gland tumours: A single-institutional experience. Nuclear Medicine Communications. 2013;**34**(3):211-219

[59] Adelstein DJ, Koyfman SA, El-Naggar AK, Hanna EY, editors. Biology and management of salivary gland cancers. Seminars in Radiation Oncology. 2012: Elsevier

[60] Garden AS, El-Naggar AK, Morrison WH, Callender DL, Ang KK, Peters LJ. Postoperative radiotherapy for malignant tumors of the parotid gland. International Journal of Radiation Oncology Biology Physics. 1997;**37**(1):79-85

[61] Chen AM, Lau VH, Farwell DG, Luu Q, Donald PJ. Mucoepidermoid carcinoma of the parotid gland treated by surgery and postoperative radiation therapy: Clinicopathologic correlates of outcome. The Laryngoscope. 2013;**123**(12):3049-3055

[62] Byrd SA, Spector ME, Carey TE, Bradford CR, McHugh JB. Predictors of recurrence and survival for head and neck mucoepidermoid carcinoma. Otolaryngology--Head and Neck Surgery. 2013;**149**(3):402-408

[63] Jarvis S, Giangrande V, Brennan P. Mucoepidermoid carcinoma of the tonsil: A very rare presentation. Acta Otorhinolaryngologica Italica. 2013;**33**(4):286

[64] Chen AM, Granchi PJ, Garcia J, Bucci MK, Fu KK, Eisele DW. Local-regional recurrence after surgery without postoperative irradiation for carcinomas of the major salivary glands: Implications for adjuvant therapy. International Journal of Radiation Oncology Biology Physics. 2007;**67**(4):982-987

[65] Ghosh-Laskar S, Murthy V, Wadasadawala T, Agarwal J, Budrukkar A, Patil N, et al. Mucoepidermoid carcinoma of the parotid gland: Factors affecting outcome. Head & Neck. 2011;**33**(4):497-503

[66] Chen AM, Garcia J, Lee NY, Bucci MK, Eisele DW. Patterns of nodal relapse after surgery and postoperative radiation therapy for carcinomas of the major and minor salivary glands: What is the role of elective neck irradiation? International Journal of Radiation Oncology Biology Physics. 2007;**67**(4):988-994

[67] Bjørndal K, Krogdahl A, Therkildsen MH, Overgaard J, Johansen J, Kristensen CA, et al. Salivary gland carcinoma in Denmark 1990-2005: A national study of incidence, site and histology. Results of the Danish Head and Neck Cancer Group (DAHANCA). Oral oncology. 2011;**47**(7):677-682

[68] Bradley PJ. Adenoid cystic carcinoma of the head and neck: A review. Current Opinion in Otolaryngology & Head and Neck Surgery. 2004;**12**(2):127-132

[69] Coca-Pelaz A, Rodrigo JP, Bradley PJ, Vander Poorten V, Triantafyllou A, Hunt JL, et al. Adenoid cystic carcinoma of the head and neck–An update. Oral Oncology. 2015;**51**(7):652-661

[70] Dodd R, Slevin NJ. Salivary gland adenoid cystic carcinoma: A review of chemotherapy and molecular therapies. Oral Oncology. 2006;**42**(8):759-769

[71] Argyris PP, Pambuccian SE, Cayci Z, Singh C, Tosios KI, Koutlas IG. Lacrimal gland adenoid cystic carcinoma with high-grade transformation to myoepithelial carcinoma: Report of a case and review of literature. Head and Neck Pathology. 2013;**7**(1):85-92

[72] Azar T, Abdul-Karim FW, Tucker HM. Adenoid cystic carcinoma of the trachea. The Laryngoscope. 1998;**108**(9):1297-1300

[73] Gu F-M, Chi F-L, Dai C-F, Chen B, Li H-W. Surgical outcomes of 43 cases with adenoid cystic carcinoma of the external auditory canal. American Journal of Otolaryngology. 2013;**34**(5):394-398

[74] Saraydaroglu O, Coskun H, Kasap M. Unique presentation of adenoid cystic carcinoma in postcricoid region: A case report and review of the literature. Head and Neck Pathology. 2011;**5**(4):413-415

[75] Batsakis JG. Carcinomas of the submandibular and sublingual glands. Annals of Otology, Rhinology & Laryngology 1986**95**:211-212

[76] Vander Poorten VL, Balm AJ, Hilgers FJ, Tan IB, Loftus-Coll BM, Keus RB, et al. Prognostic factors for long term results of the treatment of patients with malignant submandibular gland tumors. Cancer. 1999;**85**(10):2255-2264

[77] van Weert S, Bloemena E, van der Waal I, de Bree R, Rietveld DH, Kuik JD, et al. Adenoid cystic carcinoma of the head and neck: A single-center analysis of 105 consecutive cases over a 30-year period. Oral Oncology. 2013;**49**(8):824-829

[78] Nascimento AG, Amaral ALP, Prado LAF, Kligerman J, Silveira TRP. Adenoid cystic carcinoma of salivary glands. A study of 61 cases with clinicopathologic correlation. Cancer. 1986;**57**(2):312-319

[79] Sequeiros SG, Rodrigo TJ, Llorente PJ, Suárez NC. Prognostic factors in adenoid cystic carcinoma of salivary glands. Acta Otorrinolaringologica Espanola. 2005;**56**(8):361-367

[80] Spiro RH, Huvos AG, Strong EW. Adenoid cystic carcinoma of salivary origin: A clinicopathologic study of 242 cases. The American Journal of Surgery. 1974;**128**(4):512-520

[81] Vander Poorten VL, Balm AJ, Hilgers FJ, Tan IB, Keus RB, Hart AA. Stage as major long term outcome predictor in minor salivary gland carcinoma. Cancer. 2000;**89**(6):1195-1204

[82] Zvrko E, Golubović M. Laryngeal adenoid cystic carcinoma. ACTA Otorhinolaryngologica Italica. 2009;**29**(5):279

[83] Stell PM. Adenoid cystic carcinoma. Clinical Otolaryngology and Allied Sciences. 1986;**11**:267-291

[84] Kokemueller H, Eckardt A, Brachvogel P, Hausamen J-E. Adenoid cystic carcinoma of the head and neck—A 20 years experience. International Journal of Oral and Maxillofacial Surgery. 2004;**33**(1):25-31

[85] Franchi A, Gallo O, Bocciolini C, Franchi L, Paglierani M, Santucci M. Reduced E-cadherin expression correlates with unfavorable prognosis in adenoid cystic carcinoma of salivary glands of the oral cavity. American Journal of Clinical Pathology. 1999;**111**(1):43-50

[86] Biswas KD, Saha J, Sen I, Biswas G, Sinha R, Saha D, et al. Unusual presentations of adenoid cystic carcinoma in extra-salivary gland subsites in head and neck region: A case series. Indian Journal of Otolaryngology and Head & Neck Surgery. 2014;**66**(1):286-290

[87] Husain Q, Kanumuri VV, Svider PF, Radvansky BM, Boghani Z, Liu JK, et al. Sinonasal adenoid cystic carcinoma: Systematic review of survival and treatment strategies. Otolaryngology--Head and Neck Surgery. 2013;**148**(1):29-39

[88] Matsuzaki H, Yanagi Y, Hara M, Katase N, Asaumi J, Hisatomi M, et al. Minor salivary gland tumors in the oral cavity: Diagnostic value of dynamic contrast-enhanced MRI. European Journal of Radiology. 2012;**81**(10):2684-2691

[89] Jeong H-S, Chung MK, Son Y-I, Choi JY, Kim HJ, Ko YH, et al. Role of 18F-FDG PET/CT in management of high-grade salivary gland malignancies. Journal of Nuclear Medicine. 2007;**48**(8):1237-1244

[90] Shen C, Xu T, Huang C, Hu C, He S. Treatment outcomes and prognostic features in adenoid cystic carcinoma originated from the head and neck. Oral Oncology. 2012;**48**(5): 445-449

[91] Renehan AG, Gleave E, Slevin NJ, McGurk M. Clinico-pathological and treatment-related factors influencing survival in parotid cancer. British Journal of Cancer. 1999;**80**(8):1296

[92] Spiro RH, Armstrong J, Harrison L, Geller NL, Lin S-Y, Strong EW. Carcinoma of major salivary glands: Recent trends. Archives of Otolaryngology–Head & Neck Surgery. 1989;**115**(3):316-321

[93] Ferlito A, Shaha AR, Rinaldo A, Mondin V. Management of clinically negative cervical lymph nodes in patients with malignant neoplasms of the parotid gland. ORL. 2001;**63**(3):123-126

[94] Ferlito A, Barnes L, Myers EN. Neck dissection for laryngeal adenoid cystic carcinoma: Is it indicated? Annals of Otology, Rhinology & Laryngology. 1990;**99**(4):277-280

[95] Spiro RH. Distant metastasis in adenoid cystic carcinoma of salivary origin. The American Journal of Surgery. 1997;**174**(5):495-498

[96] Pederson AW, Salama JK, Haraf DJ, Witt ME, Stenson KM, Portugal L, et al. Adjuvant chemoradiotherapy for locoregionally advanced and high-risk salivary gland malignancies. Head & Neck Oncology. 2011;**3**(1):31

[97] Dillon PM, Chakraborty S, Moskaluk CA, Joshi PJ, Thomas CY. Adenoid cystic carcinoma: A review of recent advances, molecular targets, and clinical trials. Head & Neck. 2016;**38**(4):620-627

[98] Seethala RR. Salivary gland tumors: Current concepts and controversies. Surgical Pathology Clinics. 2017;**10**(1):155-176

[99] Kazakov DV, Schaller J, Vanecek T, Kacerovska D, Michal M. Brooke-Spiegler syndrome: Report of a case with a novel mutation in the CYLD gene and different types of somatic mutations in benign and malignant tumors. Journal of Cutaneous Pathology. 2010;**37**(8):886-890

[100] Muller S, Barnes L. Basal cell adenocarcinoma of the salivary glands: Report of seven cases and review of the literature. Cancer. 1996;**78**(12):2471-2477

[101] Zhan KY, Lentsch EJ. Basal cell adenocarcinoma of the major salivary glands: A population-level study of 509 cases. The Laryngoscope. 2016;**126**(5):1086-1090

[102] Seethala RR, Barnes EL, Hunt JL. Epithelial-myoepithelial carcinoma: A review of the clinicopathologic spectrum and immunophenotypic characteristics in 61 tumors of the salivary glands and upper aerodigestive tract. The American Journal of Surgical Pathology. 2007;**31**(1):44-57

[103] Chiosea SI, Miller M, Seethala RR. HRAS mutations in epithelial–myoepithelial carcinoma. Head and Neck Pathology. 2014;**8**(2):146-150

[104] Vázquez A, Patel TD, D'Aguillo CM, Abdou RY, Farver W, Baredes S, et al. Epithelial-myoepithelial carcinoma of the salivary glands: An Analysis of 246 Cases. Otolaryngology--Head and Neck Surgery. 2015;**153**(4):569-574

[105] Chiosea SI, Griffith C, Assaad A, Seethala RR. The profile of acinic cell carcinoma after recognition of mammary analog secretory carcinoma. The American Journal of Surgical Pathology. 2012;**36**(3):343-350

[106] Chiosea SI, Griffith C, Assaad A, Seethala RR. Clinicopathological characterization of mammary analogue secretory carcinoma of salivary glands. Histopathology. 2012;**61**(3):387-394

4

The Role of Cancer Stem Cells in Head and Neck Squamous Cell Carcinoma and its Clinical Implications

Kaveh Karimnejad, Nathan Lindquist and Reigh-Yi Lin

Abstract

Worldwide, more than 550, 000 new cases of head and neck squamous cell carcinoma (HNSCC) are estimated to occur annually, making it the sixth most common human malignancy. Since their discovery in 2007, cancer stem cells (CSCs) in HNSCC have garnered increased interest secondary to their properties of tumorigenicity, differenti- ation, proliferation, and self-renewal. CSCs are intrinsically more resistant to tradi- tional treatments such as radiation and chemotherapy, contributing to potential metastasis and recurrence of HNSCC. This chapter focuses first on normal head and neck stem cells, providing background for the discussion of a number of topics pertaining to the study of HNSCC CSCs including molecular biomarkers and clinical implications. Continued research to elucidate the properties of CSCs will undoubt- edly expand our knowledge surrounding the pathogenesis, metastasis, and relapse of HNSCC. Ultimately, a better understanding of CSC biomarkers, signaling pathways, and mechanisms of resistance will improve therapies and patient outcomes through targeted interventions.

Keywords: Head and neck squamous cell carcinoma, Stem cells, Cancer stem cells, Chemoresistance, Metastasis

1. Introduction

In the United States, over 53, 000 new cases of head and neck squamous cell carcinoma (HNSCC) are estimated to occur each year, with roughly 11, 000 deaths annually [1]. Across the globe, HNSCC has an annual incidence of over 550, 000 cases, making it the sixth most common cancer worldwide. HNSCC accounts for 90% of the malignancies in the head and neck region, affecting the nasal vestibule, nasal cavity, paranasal sinuses, nasopharynx, lips, oral cavity, oropharynx, pharynx, hypopharynx, and larynx. The foundation of treatment for head and neck cancer has been surgery and radiation therapy, while chemotherapy may also be employed as an adjunctive treatment. Advancements in surgical technique, radiation strategies and technologies, as well as chemotherapeutic drugs have led to improvements in patient's overall quality of life. However, the prognosis for HNSCC has improved only marginally over the past thirty years, with the five-year survival rate remaining at 50% [2-4]. Even after standard therapy, patients with HNSCC exhibit relatively high rates of local recurrence, regional cervical lymph node recurrence, and to a lesser degree distant metastasis, all of which contribute to significant morbidity and mortality [5]. Often, these recurrences and metastases are more resistant to traditional treatment modalities such as chemoradiation. Unfortunately, primary site recurrence occurs in 10-30% of all patients [6].

Traditional approaches to understanding and treating HNSCC are based on the stochastic model of cancer, where all tumor cells are identical (Figure 1). More recently, the cancer stem cell (CSC) hypothesis has gained increasing traction in explaining tumorigenesis [7]. This theory proposes that cancer maintains a hierarchical order of cells, with only a small subpopulation of CSCs capable of tumor initiation, propagation, and regeneration [8]. Conventional therapies that target rapidly cycling cells are less effective in killing CSCs. CSCs also display increased intrinsic resistance to chemotherapy and radiation therapy. As a result, CSCs are likely to contribute to cancer relapse.

This review aims to provide a succinct yet thorough overview of our current basis for the CSC hypothesis as it pertains to HNSCC. We will start with a brief discussion of the normal epithelium of the head and neck region as well as our current understanding of normal endogenous stem cells of the head and neck region. Evidence for the CSC hypothesis of

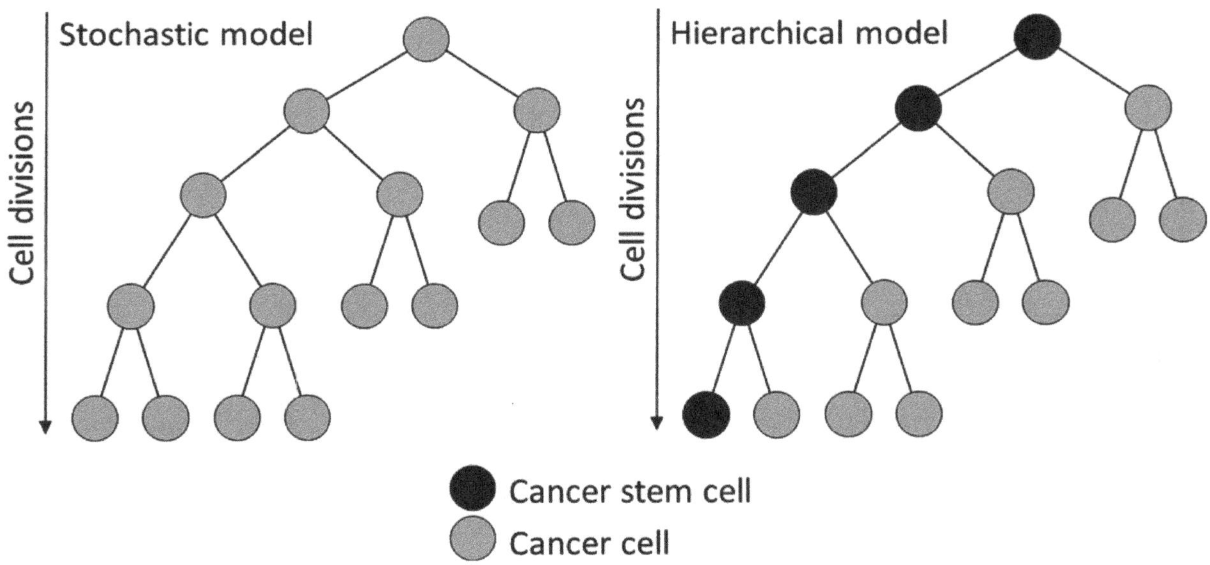

Figure 1. In the stochastic model, all tumor cells have equal abilities to propagate, initiate tumors, and seed metastases. The heterogeneity of tumors in this model is derived from spontaneous phenotypic shifts. The emerging cancer stem cell hypothesis dictates the hierarchical model, in which asymmetric division results in specific and well-defined populations of cancer stem cells and other cancer cells that do not initiate tumors or seed metastases. These cells may consist of populations with decreased proliferative ability (i.e., transit-amplifying cells) or post-mitotic differentiated cells with no further proliferative ability or activity.

HNSCC will include a discussion of the prospective markers for CSCs in HNSCC, as well as a closer look at the cellular regulation of these CSCs and the clinical implications of these cancer- initiating and propagating cells.

2. Head and neck stem cells in normal tissues

Stem cells are unique in their ability to maintain self-renewal, differentiate into multiple lineage types in the same tissue, and display a high degree of proliferative potential [9]. The somatic stem cell microenvironment or cellular "niche" is vital in maintaining the delicate distinction between self-renewal and uncontrolled proliferation of stem cells [10]. Stem cells and the extracellular matrix secrete factors to maintain the microenvironment, while inhibitory signals from this local microenvironment provide necessary control of proliferation and differentiation to sustain this important subpopulation of cells [11, 12]. Importantly, these quiescent, undifferentiated somatic stem cells also depend on the niche for the transient stimulatory signals necessary for cell division and tissue regeneration [13]. Unlike most of the gastrointestinal tract, which contains a simple epithelial layer to allow for increased absorption, the oral cavity, pharynx, and esophagus are covered by a stratified epithelium that is more similar in structure to other tissues such as skin [14]. The stratified epithelium is composed of multiple layers of cell types oriented in order of increasing differentiation from basal to superficial.

In the normal squamous stratified epithelium, stem cells are located in the basal layer. To replenish the more superficial layers, these stem cells divide asymmetrically to self-renew and produce cells to undergo subsequent differentiation and amplification [11]. Cell division in stratified squamous epithelium results in differentiation, superficial cellular movement, stratification, and ultimately, tissue turnover. In the stratified squamous epithelium, for example, a layer of small, cuboidal, basal stem cells are responsible for cell division and regeneration [15]. Moving superficially, these committed cells further differentiate to increase keratin filament production, flatten, and decrease the size and volume of the nucleus and organelles. The most superficial (corneal or superficial) layers of the oral mucosa demonstrate cell flattening, mem- brane thickening, decreased desmosomes, and eventual sloughing of cells into the oral cavity [16]. The hierarchical normal oral epithelium is renewed approximately every 14–24 days [17]. Increasingly, endogenous oral cavity stem cells are theorized to precede CSCs, as these are the only cells with life span sufficient to accumulate the genetic mutations necessary for malignant transformation [18].

3. Head and neck stem cell markers

In contrast to other tissues or organ systems, relatively few markers have been identified or characterized for normal endogenous stem cells of the head and neck region. To date, most of our knowledge of normal head and neck stem cells is based largely on work on oral epithelial stem cells (OESCs) and corollaries from the skin and hair follicle, which also maintain a squamous stratified epithelium.

In the 1960s, the first experiments to identify potential stem cells in the oral mucosa utilized pulse-chase experiments with tritiated-thymidine ($_3$H-TdR) to elucidate cell turnover rates in the skin and oral mucosa and identify label-retaining cells in the basal layer [19]. Of the few candidate cell surface markers for OESCs, most are also expressed in other normal oral epithelial basal cells, meaning that much of the research involving OESC markers has involved purification rather than isolation of these cells [20]. Such work is often accomplished based on sorting for cell markers and performing subsequent *in vitro* experiments to test the self-renewal and proliferative properties of these subpopulations. So far, notable candidate oral stem cell markers include keratins K5, 14, 15, and 19, β1- and α6-integrins, integrin $\alpha_6\beta_4$, melanoma chondroitin sulfate proteoglycan (MCSP), $p75_{NGFR}$, B-cell-specific Moloney murine leukemia virus integration site 1 (BMI1), and the p63 transcription factor (Table 1) [20-37].

Aida *et al.* performed telomere analysis of different cell types in normal lingual epithelium to calculate normalized telomere:centromere ratios (NTCRs). Overall, the basal cell group demonstrated the largest NTCR, with a smaller subgroup of these cells maintaining an exceptionally large NTCR, suggesting the presence of stem cells. In general, stem cells are thought to maintain relatively longer telomeres due to a lower telomere turnover rate as well as the potential for telomere upregulation. In addition, samples from older patients contained relatively shorter telomeres, confirming a measurable age-related progression. Finally, immunohistochemistry confirmed the presence of p27, p63, and K19 in the basal layer with relatively scant staining for Ki-67, a well-known marker of cell proliferation [22].

In one study, the magnetic separation of oral human keratinocytes yielded a fraction of α6β +CD71 cells that could regenerate a stratified oral epithelial equivalent *in vitro*. Unlike either of the α6β +CD71+ or or $\alpha_6\beta$ keratinocyte groups, $\alpha_6\beta_+CD71_-$ cells also expressed the candidate stem cell markers p63 and Keratin 19 and were negative for two recognized markers of differentiation: cytokeratin 10 or involucrin [23].

Tao *et al.* demonstrate a method of enriching a subpopulation containing both potential stem cells and transit amplifying cells through integrin-β1 adherence to collagen IV. While their subsequent study of p63 expression could not confirm specificity for stem cells in the basal layer, the ΔNp63α and ΔNp63β isoforms may be more specific markers for undifferentiated or immature cells [21].

Through cell lineage mapping, Hogan and coworkers noted a $K14_+K5_+Trp63_+Sox2_+$ subpopulation of long-term stem or progenitor cells located outside the taste buds that are capable of differentiating into both mature taste bud receptor cells as well as keratinocytes. The authors suggest that a similar model may apply to the taste buds of the circumvallate papillae and soft palate, and that their work may prove a model system for future study of these endogenous stem cells [24]. This same group isolated a population of undifferentiated tongue basal cells using Krt5-eGFP transgenic mice that demonstrated self-renewal and differentiation to stratified keratinized epithelial cells *in vitro*.

Candidate Normal Stem Cell Marker	Site(s) Studied	Function and Significance in Stem Cell Biology	References
Keratin 5	Mouse tongue and soft palate	ntermediate filament protein expressed by basal epithelial cells, only small fraction may actually replicate	[24,29,31]
Keratin 14	Mouse tongue and oral mucosa	Intermediate filament protein expressed by basal epithelial cells, only small fraction of these cells may actually replicate	[24,29,32]
Keratin 15	Human hard palate	Intermediate filament protein, marker of stem cells in hair follicle bulge, expressed in deep tips of palatal epithelial papillae	[33]
Keratin 19	Human hard palate and gingiva	Intermediate filament protein, stem cell marker for cells of hair follicle	[22,23,34,35]
β1-integrin	Cultured human epidermal, buccal, and gingival cells	Important in adhesion to extracellular matrix proteins, increased in cells with higher colony-forming efficiency	[21,36]
α6β4-integrin	Human hard palate and gingiva	Important in adhesion to basement membrane, expressed on α6β4 CD71 basal cells capable of oral epithelium regeneration	[23,33,34]
MCSP	Human hard palate	Cellular surface proteoglycan associated with migration and invasion of melanoma cells, important for maintenance of patterned distribution and clustering of epidermal stem cells	[20,33,37]
p75NGFR	Human esophageal, buccal, gingival, and laryngeal epithelium	Low-affinity neurotrophin receptor in TNF receptor superfamily important in proliferation, cell migration, and tissue regeneration	[25-28]
p63	Rat palate and oral mucosa, human tongue, gingival and buccal epithelium	Transcription factor with multiple isoforms responsible for epidermal stem cell maintenance and regulation	[21,22,24,34]
BMI1	Mouse lingual epithelium	Protein involved with epithelial cell maintenance, proliferation, and tissue regeneration	[29]

Table 1. The function and significance of candidate normal stem cell markers in the head and neck region.

The low-affinity neurotrophin receptor $p75_{NGFR}$ is a member of the tumor necrosis factor receptor superfamily and has effects in cell survival, apoptosis, and intercellular signaling [25]. It has been put forth as a possible stem cell marker for neural crest, mesenchymal, esophageal, oral mucosa [25], and most recently laryngeal epithelium [25, 26]. In addition, $p75_{NGFR}$-positive basal keratinocytes are able to migrate and initiate regeneration of damaged buccal epithelium [27]. Furthermore, expression of $p75_{NGFR}$ has been shown to be closely related to CSCs in esophageal squamous cell carcinoma as well as laryngeal squamous cell carcinoma [26, 28].

Recent interest in lingual epithelial stem cells has provided some evidence that keratins K5 and K14 may not be specific stem cell markers in this system. Ueno and coworkers utilized immunostaining to reveal that only a small fraction of these keratins K14/K5-positive cells were actually replicating to supply epithelial cells [29]. Rather, this group identified a group of BMI1-positive stem cells that maintain the epithelial cells and can regenerate after irradia- tion-induced tissue injury. Curiously, these potential stem cells were located in the second or third epithelial layer of the interpapillary pit of the filiform papillae. Increasingly, BMI1 is viewed as a candidate marker for CSCs of the head and neck, with the potential for prognostic value based on the location of this intracellular oncoprotein [30].

MCSP, melanoma-associated chondroitin sulfate proteoglycan; NGFR, nerve growth factor receptor; TNF, tumor necrosis factor; BMI1, B-cell-specific Moloney murine leukemia virus integration site 1

4. Origin of head and neck cancer stem cells

In most instances, HNSCC is caused by the accumulation of multiple genetic mutations based on genetic predisposition, which is induced by environmental factors such as tobacco and alcohol abuse or persistent human papilloma virus infection [38]. However, the alterations of multiple molecular and cellular pathways that lead to the development and recurrence of HNSCC are still not well understood. Recently, recurrence and therapeutic resistance of HNSCC has been attributed to a subpopulation of self-sustaining, tumor-initiating CSCs. CSCs are defined by several exclusive features that allow propagation as well as tumor formation and maintenance. These features are: (1) differentiation, giving rise to heterogeneous progeny; (2) self-renewal, which maintains a pool of stem cells which can expand; and (3) homeostatic control, which accounts for tissue specificity [4].

Multiple possible origins for CSCs have been proposed wherein a population of self-renewing cells are formed, leading to tumorigenesis (Figure 2) [39]. In one such scenario, normal stem cells undergo mutations that diminish restraint on replication, thereby creating CSCs that are unresponsive to environmental or intrinsic controls on self-renewal. Another potential source of CSCs are the more differentiated progenitor cells, also known as transit-amplifying cells, which maintain a more limited role in self-renewal yet are far more numerous than stem cells. A third motif of CSC generation explains that well-differentiated, mature cells undergo mutations to dedifferentiate and obtain greater self-renewal potential [5]. There is evidence that these dedifferentiated HNSCC cells may undergo epithelial-mesenchymal transition and invasion, leading to the development of cells with CSC- or mesenchymal characteristics [40].

5. Initial clues to the concept of head and neck cancer stem cells

The first "leukemia-initiating" CSCs were identified in 1994 by Dick and co-workers through their work with acute myeloid leukemia [41]. In 2003, Al-Hajj *et al.* reported the first CSCs in a solid tumor by separating a tumorigenic subpopulation of breast cancer cells based on the surface cell markers $CD44_{+}/CD24_{-/low}$ [42]. In 2007, a landmark study by Prince *et al.* described a subpopulation of $CD44_{+}$ tumor-initiating cells isolated from HNSCC, although the cell surface markers CD44s and CD44v6 were subsequently described in a majority of normal head and neck tissues as well as HNSCC [43, 44]. Other subpopulations of tumor-initiating cells have since been identified in HNSCC that also fulfill the criteria for CSCs. Furthermore, several of the putative markers of these CSC subpopulations have been linked to cancer recurrence and therapeutic resistance, augmenting the evidence for the CSC hypothesis in HNSCC. Recent interest in the identification of new and improved biomarkers for HNSCC CSCs has spiked due to the prospect of using these tools to improve treatment approaches and overall mortality in this deadly disease.

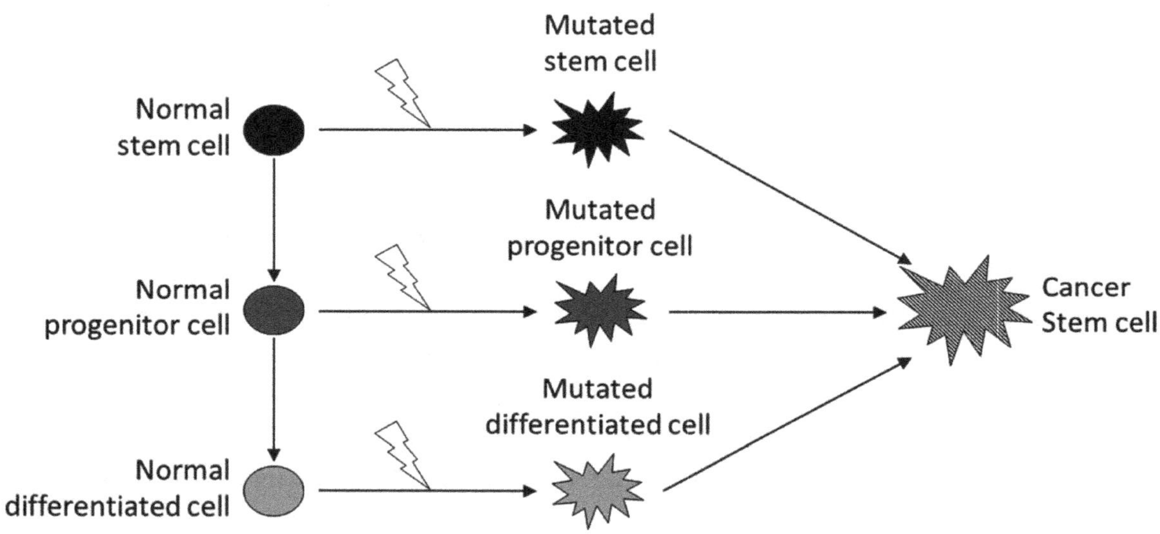

Figure 2. Potential origins for cancer stem cells include normal stem cells, progenitor cells, or fully differentiated cells. To give rise to cancer stem cells, the progenitor and fully differentiated cells acquire mutations to reactivate genes responsible for increased proliferative activity, cell-division, and dedifferentiation.

6. Cancer stem cell assays

The isolation and identification of CSCs is a hefty experimental challenge, as there is no established protocol to verify putative CSCs. Current experimental goals aim to satisfy the CSC criteria of both self-renewal as well as the capacity to develop heterogeneous cell lineages capable of forming tumors identical to the original [45]. Isolation strategies attempt to exploit the unique properties of CSCs that distinguish them from their differentiated progeny. Such capacities include the efflux of vital dyes by multidrug transporters, enzymatic activity, sphere-forming capacity in low attachment conditions, and the expression of cell surface antigens [46]. There are currently four main strategies for isolation of CSCs: (1) detection of side-population phenotypes by Hoechst 33342 exclusion, (2) sphere-formation assays, (3) assessment of aldehyde dehydrogenase (ALDH) activity, and (4) identification of CSC-specific cell surface markers [45]. To date, the most common modality in identifying HNSCC CSCs relies upon the expression of membrane cell surface antigens present in stem-like cells. As a result, most potential CSC populations are detected by immunohistochemistry or flow cytometry. Many of these antigens were originally put forth as potential targets as a result of their expression in normal stem cells [47, 48]. Herein, we present a review of the most promising putative HNSCC CSC markers: CD44, CD133, and ALDH. We also include a discussion of CD24 and CD10.

Putative Cancer Stem Cell Markers in HNSCC Sites Studied	Biological Function	Significance in HNSCC Stem Cell Biology	References
CD44	Surface glycoprotein involved in cell migration and adhesion	Showed the ability to regenerate tumor *in vivo* but also abundantly expressed in normal squamous epithelia of the head and neck. Associated with Snail (chemoresistance and radioresistance) as well as high coexpression of BMI1 (important for self-renewal and tumorigenesis)	[43,44,49,50,55]
CD133 (Prominin 1)	Transmembrane glycoprotein localized on membrane protrusions and microvilli	Correlated with lymph node metastases and decreased overall survival	[51,52,54,55]
ALDH	Intracellular enzyme most commonly found in the liver. ALDH detoxifies intracellular aldehydes through oxidation	Tumor cells expressing relatively high levels of ALDH have increased tumorigenicity, stem-cell-related genes, drug-resistant genes, and EMT-related genes. Associated with high co-expression of Snail protein, which is an EMT regulator and key factor in self- renewal and tumorigenicity	[47,56,65]

Putative Cancer Stem Cell Markers in HNSCC Sites Studied	Biological Function	Significance in HNSCC Stem Cell Biology	References
CD24	Mucin adhesion molecule for P-selectin and L1 expressed by pre-B lymphocytes and neutrophils during cell development	Associated with increased proliferation and invasion *in vitro* and tumorigenicity *in vivo*, correlates with increased resistance to chemotherapeutic agents	[47,60,62]
CD10	Zinc-dependent metalloendoprotease that cleaves signaling peptides and is found in a wide range of normal tissues	Described as a potential marker for therapeutic resistance and tumor recurrence in HNSCC	[64]

Table 2. The function, significance, and associations of putative cancer stem cell markers in HNSCC.

7. Putative head and neck cancer stem cell markers

7.1. CD44

CD44 is a surface glycoprotein involved in cell migration and adhesion. Prince *et al.* demonstrated the ability of a subpopulation of $CD44_+$ HNSCC cells to regenerate a tumor *in vivo* after transplantation of as few as $5x10_3$ cells into an immunocompromised mouse model [44]. $CD44_+$ cells have been shown to express a high level of BMI1, a prospective normal stem cell bio- marker that also plays a key role in self-renewal and tumorigenesis in malignancy [49, 50]. While CD44 was the first CSC marker established for HNSCC, its role has since come into question. In contrast to earlier studies involving CD44, recent studies have demonstrated the abundant expression of CD44 in most HNSCC tumor cells. In one such study, CD44 was present in 80-100% of tumor cells [43]. However, according to the *hierarchical model*, only a small subset of cells within malignant tissue that are able to generate tumors should stain positive for CSC markers. Furthermore, high percentages of $CD44_+$ cells have been identified in normal squamous epithelia of the head and neck, with up to 60–95% of normal head and neck epithelial cells demonstrating CD44 positivity. Although the role of CD44 in HNSCC has raised some questions, this protein may still prove a valuable role in the identification of CSCs when used in combination with other markers. In the 2009 study by Chen *et al.*, not only did knockdown of Snail expression in $CD44_+ALDH_+$ cells decrease tumor invasion and colony formation, but it also significantly increased sensitivity to chemotherapy and radiotherapy. Specifically, following seven days of Snail siRNA treatment, the $CD44_+ALDH_+$ CSCs exhibited increased sensitivity to cisplatin and etoposide, and radiotherapy. These findings illustrate the potential utility of CSCs as unique cell targets for both chemotherapy and radiation therapy.

7.2. CD133

First described in 1997, CD133 (Prominin 1) is a transmembrane glycoprotein expressed in several normal stem cell populations and malignancies [51]. CD133 is localized to cellular membrane protrusions and microvilli [52]. It is expressed in several solid malignancies including brain, colon, liver, and lung, and has been purported as a unique, specific marker for sarcomas [38]. In 2007, Zhou *et al.* demonstrated the presence of a $CD133_{+}$ subpopulation in 3.5% of the native cells from a HEp-2 laryngeal cancer cell line. These $CD133_{+}$ cells continued to proliferate and expand the tumor cell population in sphere formation assays. In cell culture assays, the majority of terminal cells did not express CD133, a finding consistent with the criteria for CSC self-renewal as well as the capacity to give rise to phenotypically unique tumor daughter cells [53]. More recent studies have supported these findings, suggesting the utility of CD133 as a clinically relevant prognostic marker in HNSCC. Canis *et al.* demonstrated an inversely proportional correlation between CD133 expression in primary tumors and overall survival in addition to a positive correlation between CD133 expression and the presence of lymph node metastases [54]. In addition, Yu *et al.* describe an oral cavity squamous cell carcinoma-derived side population of cells with high expression of CD133 and ALDH showed high tumorigenic capacity [55]. Cell viability assays revealed that these side populations of cells were more chemoresistant to cisplatin, fluorouracil, or doxorubicin treatment when compared to the major population of the same cell line. The researchers hypothesized that CD133 may be crucial to modulation of chemosensitivity. They subsequently performed lentiviral-mediated transduction in the side population of cells, which resulted in significant decrease in expression of CD133 mRNA and protein. The silencing of CD133 decreased the percentage of the side population in the cancer cell lines and decreased *in vivo* tumor growth. Furthermore, cisplatin treatment of the CD133 knockdown population diminished cell invasion and clonogenicity, demonstrating the enhanced sensitivity to chemotherapy by targeting CD133. These findings support the role of HNSCC CSCs as novel therapeutic targets in the development of chemotherapeutic drugs.

7.3. ALDH

ALDH is an intracellular enzyme most commonly found in the liver [47]. ALDH detoxifies intracellular aldehydes through oxidation and may play a role in the differentiation of stem cells by oxidizing retinol into retinoic acid. With regard to cancer, high ALDH activity has been linked to subsets of multiple myeloma and acute myeloid leukemia [56]. Prior to its identification with HNSCC, ALDH was labeled a putative CSC marker in both breast and colon cancer. Ginestier *et al.* successfully used high ALDH activity to identify a tumorigenic breast cancer cell fraction capable of self-renewal and generating heterogeneous tumors. In their study, expression of ALDH as detected by immunohistochemistry correlated with a poorer prognosis for breast carcinomas [57].

Expression of ALDH1 in inflammatory breast cancer has been put forth as an independent predictor of early metastasis and decreased survival [58]. In 2009, Chen *et al.* published the first study demonstrating that cells of $ALDH1_{+}$ lineage have CSC properties and play a role in self- renewal in HNSCC [3]. In a study by Clay *et al.*, HNSCC cells were categorized and isolated based on either high or low ALDH activity and subsequently implanted into immunocompromised mice. Cells with relatively high levels of ALDH represented a small percentage of cells (1% to 7.8%), but gave rise to tumors from as few as 500 cells in 53% of implantations. In contrast, only 8% of similar implantations with cells expressing low levels of ALDH formed tumor. As a result, ALDH appears to be a relatively selective marker for HNSCC CSCs [56]. In a similar study, 87% of implantations with 1000 ALDH$_+$CD44$_+$ HNSCC cells generated tumors, compared to only 13% of ALDH$_-$CD44$_-$ cell implantations, despite utilizing ten times more cells: 10, 000 [59]. ALDH$_+$ cells have also been shown to exhibit higher expression levels of stem cell-related, drug-resistance-associated, and epithelial-mesenchymal-transformation-related (EMT) genes such as Snail [3]. In fact, Snail protein overexpression transformed ALDH$_-$ cells to ALDH$_+$ cells, resulting in increased invasion and tumorigenic properties [65]. Given this association with Snail and EMT, as well as the ability to recapitulate tumors in high percentages after *in vivo* implantation in multiple studies, ALDH may be the most well-established HNSCC CSC marker to date.

7.4. CD24 and CD10

CD24 is a mucin adhesion molecule for P-selectin and L1 expressed by pre-B lymphocytes and neutrophils during cell development [47, 60]. CD24 expression has been shown to increase tumor cell proliferation and further shown to regulate multiple cell properties which contribute to tumor growth and metastasis [60]. It has been correlated with increased spread of breast cancer and has been further identified as a putative CSC marker in pancreatic, ovarian, and colorectal cancers [61, 62]. CD24 has also been associated with tumorigenesis, tumor progression, and malignant transformation of stomach and gallbladder cancers [63]. In a study by Han *et al.* CD24$_+$CD44$_+$ HNSCC cells were demonstrated to be more proliferative and invasive *in vitro* and more tumorigenic *in vivo.* After implantation in immunodeficient mice, CD24$_+$CD44$_+$ *cells* formed larger tumors than the CD24$_-$CD44$_+$ group. CD24$_+$CD44$_+$ cells were also correlated with slightly increased resistance to chemotherapeutic agents [62]. CD24 is one of the primary surface antigens involved in solid tumors and its role has been established in various human epithelial neoplasias. However, the paucity of research concerning HNSCC precludes its inclu- sion as a CSC biomarker at the present time.

CD10 is a zinc-dependent metalloendoprotease that cleaves signaling peptides and is found in a wide range of normal tissues. It has been described as a potential marker for therapeutic resistance and tumor recurrence in HNSCC [64]. As the field of CSCs remains in its infancy, further investigation regarding the roles of CD24 and CD10 will better elucidate the role of these proteins in HNSCC.

8. Clinical relevance of head and neck cancer stem cells

Today, few studies have evaluated patient HNSCC tumors or tissues and the correlation with clinical data and outcomes. One barrier to the establishment of clinically significant CSC markers in the head and neck region is secondary to the convention of amassing malignancies from various upper aerodigestive sites with distinctly diverse embryological and biological characteristics [47]. As a result, there is little definitive data with regard to clinical implications of CSCs within HNSCC, the primary exception being prognostic value. Furthermore, no single biomarker for CSC cells in HNSCC has proven absolute in distinguishing this vital subpopulation. The continued study of current prospective CSC markers in HNSCC, combined with the investigation of putative CSC biomarkers from other malignancies, will undoubtedly augment our knowledge and improve our understanding of the pathogenesis of HNSCC. In addition, further knowledge regarding the biomarkers and regulation of normal, native stem cells in the head and neck region will serve as a strong foundation for oncological research. Ultimately, CSCs may prove to be useful diagnostic and prognostic markers for HNSCC, guiding therapy and treatment through personalized approaches and interventions.

Author details

Kaveh Karimnejad[#], Nathan Lindquist[#], Reigh-Yi Lin[*]

*Address all correspondence to: rlin7@slu.edu

Department of Otolaryngology – Head and Neck Surgery, Saint Louis University School of Medicine, Saint Louis, Missouri, USA

[#] These authors contribute equally to this work.

References

[1] Siegel R, Naishadham D, Jemal A. Cancer statistics, 2013. *CA*: A cancer journal for clinicians. 2013;63(1):11–30.

[2] Anderson RT, Keysar SB, Bowles DW, Glogowska MJ, Astling DP, Morton JJ, et al. The dual pathway inhibitor rigosertib is effective in direct patient tumor xenografts of head and neck squamous cell carcinomas. *Mol Canc Therapeut*. 2013;12(10):1994–2005.

[3] Chen Z. The cancer stem cell concept in progression of head and neck cancer. *J Oncol*. 2009;2009:8.

[4] Bhaijee F, Pepper DJ, Pitman KT, Bell D. Cancer stem cells in head and neck squamous cell carcinoma: a review of current knowledge and future applications. *Head Neck*. 2012;34(6):894–9.

[5] Shah A, Patel S, Pathak J, Swain N, Kumar S. The evolving concepts of cancer stem cells in head and neck squamous cell carcinoma. *Scientific World J*. 2014;2014:8.

[6] Wolf GT. Surgical margins in the genomic era: The Hayes Martin Lecture, 2012. *Arch Otolaryngol Head Neck Surg*. 2012;138(11):1001–13.

[7] Wicha MS, Liu S, Dontu G. Cancer stem cells: an old idea – a paradigm shift. *Canc Res*. 2006;66(4):1883–90; discussion 95–6.

[8] Reya T, Morrison SJ, Clarke MF, Weissman IL. Stem cells, cancer, and cancer stem cells. *Nature*. 2001;414(6859):105–11.

[9] Jordan CT, Guzman ML, Noble M. Cancer Stem Cells. *N Eng J Med*. 2006;355(12): 1253–61.

[10] Li L, Neaves WB. Normal stem cells and cancer stem cells: the niche matters. *Canc Res*. 2006;66(9):4553–7.

[11] Mannelli G, Gallo O. Cancer stem cells hypothesis and stem cells in head and neck cancers. *Canc Treat Rev*. 2012;38(5):515–39.

[12] Scadden DT. The stem-cell niche as an entity of action. *Nature*. 2006;441(7097):1075–9.

[13] Fuchs E, Tumbar T, Guasch G. Socializing with the neighbors: stem cells and their niche. *Cell*. 2004;116(6):769–78.

[14] Squier CA, Kremer MJ. Biology of oral mucosa and esophagus. *J Natl Canc Instit Mono- graphs*. 2001(29):7–15.

[15] Nguyen LV, Vanner R, Dirks P, Eaves CJ. Cancer stem cells: an evolving concept. *Nature Rev Canc*. 2012;12(2):133–43.

[16] Winning TA, Townsend GC. Oral mucosal embryology and histology. *Clinics Dermatol*. 2000;18(5):499–511.

[17] Richard V, Pillai MR. The stem cell code in oral epithelial tumorigenesis: 'the cancer stem cell shift hypothesis'. *Biochim Biophys Acta*. 2010;1806(2):146–62.

[18] Costea DE, Tsinkalovsky O, Vintermyr OK, Johannessen AC, Mackenzie IC. Cancer stem cells – new and potentially important targets for the therapy of oral squamous cell carcinoma. *Oral Dis*. 2006;12(5):443–54.

[19] Cutright DE, Bauer H. Cell renewal in the oral mucosa and skin of the rat. I. Turnover time. *Oral Surg Oral Med Oral Pathol*. 1967;23(2):249–59.

[20] Jones KB, Klein OD. Oral epithelial stem cells in tissue maintenance and disease: the first steps in a long journey. *Int J Oral Sci*. 2013;5(3):121–9.

[21] Tao Q, Qiao B, Lv B, Zheng C, Chen Z, Huang H. p63 and its isoforms as markers of rat oral mucosa epidermal stem cells in vitro. *Cell Biochem Funct*. 2009;27(8):535–41.

[22] Aida J, Izumiyama-Shimomura N, Nakamura K, Ishikawa N, Poon SS, Kammori M, et al. Basal cells have longest telomeres measured by tissue Q-FISH method in lingual epithe- lium. *Exper Gerontol*. 2008;43(9):833–9.

[23] Calenic B, Ishkitiev N, Yaegaki K, Imai T, Costache M, Tovaru M, et al. Characterization of oral keratinocyte stem cells and prospects of its differentiation to oral epithelial equiv- alents. Romanian journal of morphology and embryology = *Rev Roumaine Morphol Embryolog*. 2010;51(4):641–5.

[24] Okubo T, Clark C, Hogan BL. Cell lineage mapping of taste bud cells and keratinocytes in the mouse tongue and soft palate. *Stem Cells* (Dayton, Ohio). 2009;27(2):442–50.

[25] Nakamura T, Endo K, Kinoshita S. Identification of human oral keratinocyte stem/pro- genitor cells by neurotrophin receptor p75 and the role of neurotrophin/p75 signaling. *Stem Cells* (Dayton, Ohio). 2007;25(3):628–38.

[26] Li X, Shen Y, Di B, Li J, Geng J, Lu X, et al. Biological and clinical significance of p75NTR expression in laryngeal squamous epithelia and laryngocarcinoma. *Acta Oto-laryngol*. 2012;132(3):314–24.

[27] Ishii A, Muramatsu T, Lee JM, Higa K, Shinozaki N, Jung HS, et al. Expression of p75 (NGFR), a proliferative and basal cell Marker, in the buccal mucosa epithelium during re- epithelialization. *Acta Histochem Cytochem*. 2014;47(4):145–53.

[28] Huang SD, Yuan Y, Liu XH, Gong DJ, Bai CG, Wang F, et al. Self-renewal and chemother- apy resistance of p75NTR positive cells in esophageal squamous cell carcinomas. *BMC Canc*. 2009;9:9.

[29] Tanaka T, Komai Y, Tokuyama Y, Yanai H, Ohe S, Okazaki K, et al. Identification of stem cells that maintain and regenerate lingual keratinized epithelial cells. *Natur Cell Biol*. 2013;15(5):511–8.

[30] Allegra E, Trapasso S, Pisani D, Puzzo L. The role of BMI1 as a biomarker of cancer stem cells in head and neck cancer: a review. *Oncology*. 2014;86(4):199–205.

[31] Luo X, Okubo T, Randell S, Hogan BL. Culture of endodermal stem/progenitor cells of the mouse tongue. In vitro cellular & developmental biology. *Animal*. 2009;45(1–2):44–54.

[32] Raimondi AR, Molinolo A, Gutkind JS. Rapamycin prevents early onset of tumorigenesis in an oral-specific K-ras and p53 two-hit carcinogenesis model. *Canc Res*. 2009;69 (10):4159–66.

[33] Mackenzie IC. Stem cells in oral mucosal epithelia. *Oral Biosci Med*. 2005;2(2):95–103.

[34] Calenic B, Ishkitiev N, Yaegaki K, Imai T, Kumazawa Y, Nasu M, et al. Magnetic separa- tion and characterization of keratinocyte stem cells from human gingiva. *J Periodontal Res*. 2010;45(6):703–8.

[35] Michel M, Torok N, Godbout MJ, Lussier M, Gaudreau P, Royal A, et al. Keratin 19 as a biochemical marker of skin stem cells in vivo and in vitro: keratin 19 expressing

cells are differentially localized in function of anatomic sites, and their number varies with donor age and culture stage. *J Cell Sci*. 1996;109 (Pt 5):1017–28.

[36] Jones PH, Watt FM. Separation of human epidermal stem cells from transit amplifying cells on the basis of differences in integrin function and expression. *Cell*. 1993;73 (4):713–24.

[37] Legg J, Jensen UB, Broad S, Leigh I, Watt FM. Role of melanoma chondroitin sulphate proteoglycan in patterning stem cells in human interfollicular epidermis. *Development* (Cambridge, England). 2003;130(24):6049–63.

[38] Albers AE, Chen C, Koberle B, Qian X, Klussmann JP, Wollenberg B, et al. Stem cells in squamous head and neck cancer. *Critic Rev Oncol/Hematol*. 2012;81(3):224–40.

[39] Clarke MF, Fuller M. Stem cells and cancer: two faces of eve. *Cell*. 2006;124(6):1111–5.

[40] Chen C, Wei Y, Hummel M, Hoffmann TK, Gross M, Kaufmann AM, et al. Evidence for epithelial-mesenchymal transition in cancer stem cells of head and neck squamous cell carcinoma. *PLoS One*. 2011;6(1):e16466.

[41] Lapidot T, Sirard C, Vormoor J, Murdoch B, Hoang T, Caceres-Cortes J, et al. A cell initiating human acute myeloid leukaemia after transplantation into SCID mice. *Nature*. 1994;367(6464):645–8.

[42] Al-Hajj M, Wicha MS, Benito-Hernandez A, Morrison SJ, Clarke MF. Prospective identi- fication of tumorigenic breast cancer cells. *Proc Natl Acad Sci*. 2003;100(7): 3983–8.

[43] Mack B, Gires O. CD44s and CD44v6 expression in head and neck epithelia. *PLoS One*. 2008;3(10):e3360.

[44] Prince ME, Sivanandan R, Kaczorowski A, Wolf GT, Kaplan MJ, Dalerba P, et al. Identi- fication of a subpopulation of cells with cancer stem cell properties in head and neck squamous cell carcinoma. *Proc Natl Acad Sci*. 2007;104(3):973–8.

[45] Tirino V, Desiderio V, Paino F, De Rosa A, Papaccio F, La Noce M, et al. Cancer stem cells in solid tumors: an overview and new approaches for their isolation and characterization. *FASEB J* : official publication of the Federation of American Societies for Experimental Biology. 2013;27(1):13–24.

[46] Krishnamurthy S, Nör JE. Head and neck cancer stem cells. *J Dental Res*. 2012;91 (4): 334–40.

[47] Allegra E, Trapasso S. Cancer stem cells in head and neck cancer. *OncoTargets Ther*. 2012;5:375–83.

[48] Monroe MM, Anderson EC, Clayburgh DR, Wong MH. Cancer stem cells in head and neck squamous cell carcinoma. *J Oncol*. 2011;2011:762780.

[49] Lessard J, Sauvageau G. Bmi-1 determines the proliferative capacity of normal and leukaemic stem cells. *Nature*. 2003;423(6937):255–60.

[50] Park IK, Morrison SJ, Clarke MF. Bmi1, stem cells, and senescence regulation. *J Clin Invest*. 2004;113(2):175–9.

[51] Yin AH, Miraglia S, Zanjani ED, Almeida-Porada G, Ogawa M, Leary AG, et al. AC133, a novel marker for human hematopoietic stem and progenitor cells. *Blood*. 1997;90 (12):5002–12.

[52] Corbeil D, Marzesco AM, Wilsch-Brauninger M, Huttner WB. The intriguing links between prominin-1 (CD133), cholesterol-based membrane microdomains, remodeling of apical plasma membrane protrusions, extracellular membrane particles, and (neuro) epithelial cell differentiation. *FEBS Lett*. 2010;584(9):1659–64.

[53] Zhou L, Wei X, Cheng L, Tian J, Jiang JJ. CD133, one of the markers of cancer stem cells in Hep-2 cell line. *Laryngoscope*. 2007;117(3):455–60.

[54] Canis M, Lechner A, Mack B, Zengel P, Laubender RP, Koehler U, et al. CD133 is a predictor of poor survival in head and neck squamous cell carcinomas. *Canc Biomarkers*: section A of Disease Markers. 2012;12(2):97–105.

[55] Yu CC, Hu FW, Ph DC, Chou MY. Targeting CD133 in the enhancement of chemosen- sitivity in oral squamous cell carcinomas-derived side population cancer stem cells. *Head Neck*. 2014.

[56] Clay MR, Tabor M, Owen JH, Carey TE, Bradford CR, Wolf GT, et al. Single-marker identification of head and neck squamous cell carcinoma cancer stem cells with aldehyde dehydrogenase. *Head Neck*. 2010;32(9):1195–201.

[57] Ginestier C, Hur MH, Charafe-Jauffret E, Monville F, Dutcher J, Brown M, et al. ALDH1 is a marker of normal and malignant human mammary stem cells and a predictor of poor clinical outcome. *Cell Stem Cell*. 2007;1(5):555–67.

[58] Charafe-Jauffret E, Ginestier C, Iovino F, Tarpin C, Diebel M, Esterni B, et al. Aldehyde dehydrogenase 1-positive cancer stem cells mediate metastasis and poor clinical outcome in inflammatory breast cancer. Clin Canc Res: an official journal of the American Associ- ation for Cancer Research. 2010;16(1):45–55.

[59] Krishnamurthy S, Dong Z, Vodopyanov D, Imai A, Helman JI, Prince ME, et al. Endothe- lial cell-initiated signaling promotes the survival and self-renewal of cancer stem cells. *Canc Res*. 2010;70(23):9969–78.

[60] Baumann P, Cremers N, Kroese F, Orend G, Chiquet-Ehrismann R, Uede T, et al. CD24 expression causes the acquisition of multiple cellular properties associated with tumor growth and metastasis. *Canc Res*. 2005;65(23):10783–93.

[61] Aigner S, Ramos CL, Hafezi-Moghadam A, Lawrence MB, Friederichs J, Altevogt P, et al. CD24 mediates rolling of breast carcinoma cells on P-selectin. *FASEB J*: official

publica- tion of the Federation of American Societies for Experimental Biology. 1998;12 (12):1241–51.

[62] Han J, Fujisawa T, Husain SR, Puri RK. Identification and characterization of cancer stem cells in human head and neck squamous cell carcinoma. *BMC Canc*. 2014;14:173.

[63] Lim SC, Oh SH. The role of CD24 in various human epithelial neoplasias. *Pathol Res Pract*. 2005;201(7):479–86.

[64] Fukusumi T, Ishii H, Konno M, Yasui, Nakahara S, Takenaka Y, et al. CD10 as a novel marker of therapeutic resistance and cancer stem cells in head and neck squamous cell carcinoma. *Brit J Canc*. 2014;111(3):506–14.

[65] Chen YC, Chen YW, Hsu HS, Tseng LM, Huang PI, Lu KH, et al. Aldehyde dehydroge- nase 1 is a putative marker for cancer stem cells in head and neck squamous cancer. *Biochem Biophys Res Commun*. 2009;385(3):307–13.

5

Oral Side Effects of Head and Neck Irradiation

Vlaho Brailo, Vanja Vučićević Boras,
Danica Vidović Juras, Ana Andabak Rogulj,
Božana Lončar Brzak and Ivan Alajbeg

Abstract

Head and neck irradiation is the standard treatment of advanced oral/oropharyngeal cancer. The treatment has severe side effects such as mucositis, xerostomia, irradiation caries, trismus, and osteoradionecrosis. Side effects can lead to treatment discontinuation, infection, increased drug consumption, and increased duration of hospital admission and can have negative impact on the quality of life and overall survival. Furthermore, some of them (mucositis and xerostomia) affect almost every (>90%) patient. Since nearly two-thirds of oral/oropharyngeal cancers are diagnosed in advanced stage, one might conclude that the great majority of patients will be affected. However, these side effects can be prevented or at least reduced by proper oral/dental care. Therefore, every patient planned for head and neck irradiation should undergo dental evaluation before beginning of the treatment.

Keywords: oral cancer, radiotherapy, mucositis, xerostomia, osteoradionecrosis, radiation caries

1. Introduction

Head and neck irradiation is the standard treatment of advanced oral/oropharyngeal cancer. Most often, radiotherapy (RT) is delivered after surgery, alone or in combination with chemotherapy to assure better locoregional control. Indication for postoperative radio-/chemoradiotherapy includes: T3 or T4 tumor, close (<5 mm) or positive surgical margin, positive cervical lymph nodes with or without extracapsular spread, lymphovascular and/or perineural invasion. RT can be delivered as a primary treatment in cases of unresectable disease, compromised patient's health, unfavorable cosmetic, or functional outcome of anticipated surgery and recurrent disease with multiple previous surgeries [1].

Head and neck cancer patients usually receive the total dose of 60–70 Gy divided into 2 Gy daily fractions (5 days a week) over 6–7 weeks. Along with therapeutic action on tumor cells, ionizing radiation causes damage to surrounding healthy tissues located in the radiation field. Radiation induced damage to surrounding healthy tissues is responsible for complications that arise during and after radiotherapy. There are several reasons why these complications are very frequent in the oral cavity:

- fast turnover rate of oral mucosal cells
- rich and complex oral microflora
- mucosal microtrauma during mastication [2]

Most orofacial complications are dose-dependent and side effects occur when doses greater than 45 Gy are delivered. Apart from the total dose, intensity of oral side effects depends on the fraction size and scheduling, field size/affected tissue volume, and concomitant use of chemotherapy. In order to minimize the irradiation damage to surrounding tissue, novel techniques such as 3D (three-dimensional) conformal radiotherapy and intensity-modulated radiotherapy (IMRT) are introduced. These techniques allow more precise design of radiation field enabling delivery of high doses to the target tissue while reducing doses to surrounding structures [3].

Radiation-related oral side effects can be acute or chronic. Acute side effects begin during the RT and last several weeks after the therapy cessation. Acute side effects include

- oral mucositis
- taste disorder
- xerostomia

Chronic oral side effects begin several weeks, months, or even years after the RT. Chronic side effects are as follows:

- trismus
- radiation-induced dental caries
- osteoradionecrosis [4]

Patients undergoing RT demand a multidisciplinary approach in order to reduce the intensity of radiation-induced oral side effects and understand the role of dentist and themselves in their prevention and therapy.

2. Acute side effects of head and neck irradiation

2.1. Oral mucositis

Oral mucositis (OM) is the most common complication of head and neck irradiation affecting 80–90% of the patients. Oral mucositis is defined as reactive inflammation of oral mucosa due to radiation-induced damage of cellular DNA and subsequent cellular death of basal keratinocytes. Mucositis manifests as ulcerative inflammation of the oral mucosa (**Figure 1**) which can cause severe pain, deteriorated oral function, increased drug consumption, and can lead to temporary treatment interruption with consequent reduction in therapeutic effect [4].

Pathogenesis of oral mucositis can be divided into five stages: initiation, upregulation/activation, signal amplification, ulceration, and healing. First step, initiation is characterized by radiation-induced DNA damage and generation of reactive oxygen species (ROS). In the next step, ROS activate nuclear factor-κB (NF-κB) transcription factor, which further upregulates genes responsible for the synthesis of pro-inflammatory cytokines like interleukin 6 (IL-6) and tumor necrosis factor alpha (TNF-α). As the RT continues, generated pro-inflammatory cytokines further amplify inflammatory mucosal damage by providing positive feedback on NF-κB activation. In the next stage, patients develop ulcerations which are colonized by oral microorganisms that further promote epithelial damage. Last stage characterized by healing of the ulcers occurs when radiation-induced DNA damage stops [5].

First clinical sign of oral mucositis is whitish appearance of oral mucosa which begins at the end of the first week of irradiation. In the third week, patients usually develop ulcerations covered with fibrinous pseudomembranes that are prone to secondary infection. Mucositis persists throughout the radiotherapy with a peak at the end of irradiation and lasts for 2–4 weeks after treatment cessation. Intensity of mucositis is strongly dependent on the total dose, fraction size, field size, number and frequency of fraction delivery, and type of ionizing irradiation [4, 5].

Even though there are numerous scales for the assessment/classification of mucositis available, most commonly used scoring system is the one established by the World Health Organization [6–9]. The scoring system is very simple to apply and based on patient's ability to eat solid food. According to WHO, oral mucositis can be divided into four stages as follows [9]:

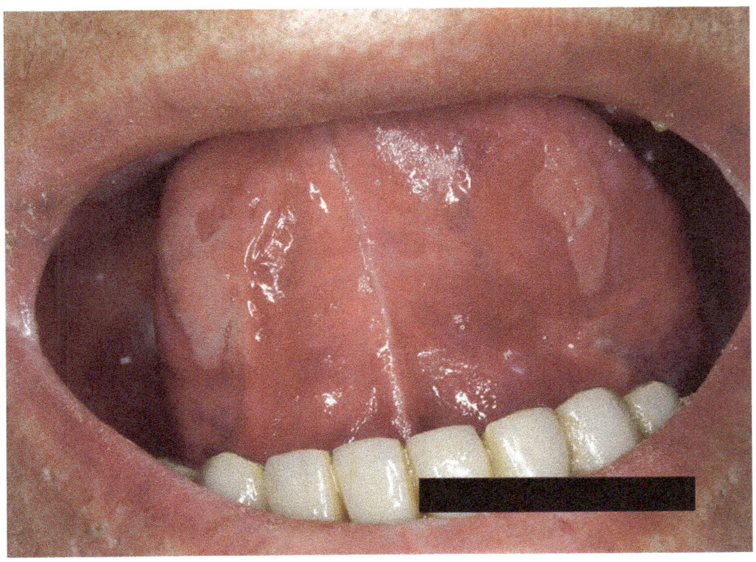

Figure 1. Oral mucositis.

- stage 0 = no pain
- stage 1 = erythema and mild edema
- stage 2 = erythema and ulcers, patient is able to eat solid food
- stage 3 = erythema and ulcers, patient is unable to eat solid food
- stage 4 = peroral alimentation is not possible

There is still no effective agent that could prevent the development of oral mucositis in patients undergoing head and neck irradiation [10]. The treatment of oral mucositis therefore remains symptomatic, aimed at relieving pain, preventing infection of oral lesions, and maintaining normal functioning of oral cavity.

2.2. Xerostomia

Xerostomia is one of the most frequent and debilitating side effects of head and neck RT. It develops acutely (early in the course of irradiation), but frequently remains chronic (permanent) complication (**Figure 2**). Lack of saliva affects the health of the entire oral cavity and favors the occurrence of other oral complications, which impair patient's quality of life, such as development of dental caries, oral infections, dysgeusia, dysphagia, oral discomfort, and pain [11]. Major salivary glands produce 70–80% of the total salivary flow. Parotid gland predominantly produces stimulated, watery saliva, and its serous acinar cells are more radiosensitive than mucous cells of submandibular and sublingual glands [12]. It seems that the extent of parotid irradiation is a major contributing factor for the development of xerostomia, as well as a total dose of received irradiation [3]. Xerostomia often remains permanent if radiation dose is greater than 40 Gy. Head and neck tumors are usually treated with a total dose greater than 60 Gy, during 6 weeks, which can lead to decrease in salivary production by 80% [2].

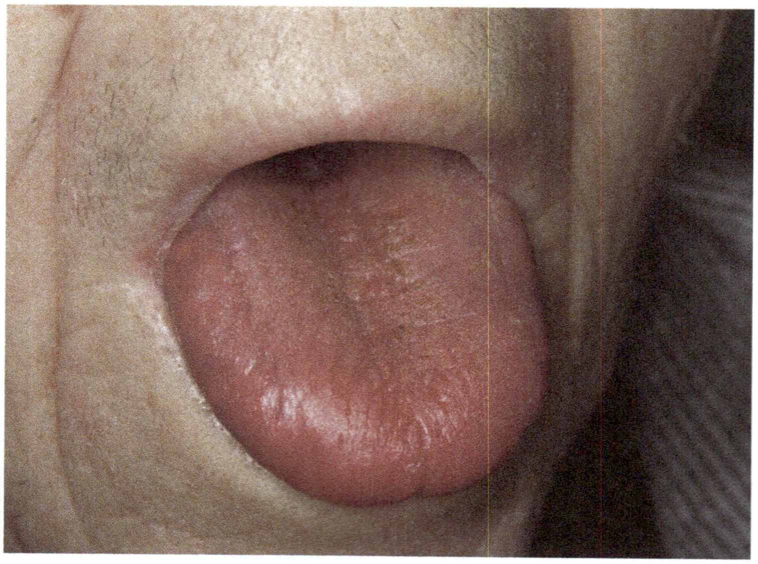

Figure 2. Xerostomia.

Together with quantitative effect on salivary flow, RT also changes the composition of saliva. Concentration of different ions and proteins in saliva rises, while the bicarbonate concentration decreases, causing a low salivary pH and a low buffering capacity [13, 14]. Quantitative and qualitative changes in saliva seriously impair patient's quality of life. Sparing salivary glands during irradiation, if possible, can reduce the long-term reduction in salivary flow [11].

2.3. Taste disorder

During the RT, majority of patients experience complete or partial taste loss. According to a recent literature review, taste disorder affects 66.5% of patients undergoing RT alone and 76% of patients undergoing combined chemoradiotherapy [15].

Taste disorder is a result of two factors: (i) a direct radiation effect on the taste buds and (ii) changes in salivary flow and composition. Taste buds are very sensitive to irradiation and demonstrate signs of degeneration and atrophy at doses of 10 Gy [4]. Decreased salivary flow disrupts transport of flavor molecules to taste buds while changed ionic composition of saliva further impairs taste perception. Most patients report their taste disorder as mild. Impact of taste disorder on the quality of life is difficult to assess because patients often report taste disorder along with other, more severe side effects of head and neck irradiation like xerostomia, sticky saliva, and difficulty swallowing [15].

In majority of cases, taste gradually returns to normal or near-normal levels within 1 year after RT. Because of this transitory aspect, there is usually no need for treatment. However, in around 15% of patients, taste disorder can last longer. There have been cases of patients whose taste disorder lasted 5–7 years after RT. To date, no universally recommended preventive or management strategies are available [15].

3. Chronic side effects of head and neck irradiation

3.1. Radiation-induced dental caries

The primary cause of radiation-induced dental caries is change in quality and quantity of saliva, due to radiation-induced salivary gland damage. After RT, salivary viscosity is increased and its buffering capacity and pH are reduced. Salivary pH becomes cariogenic, decreasing from 7.0 to 5.0 and making minerals of enamel and dentin dissolve easily [16]. A defensive role of saliva is impaired, which leads to changes in oral flora of these patients. Within 3 months of completing RT, oral flora becomes more acidogenic and cariogenic because of increased concentration of *Streptococcus mutans*, *Lactobacillus*, and *Candida* species [17, 18]. If the teeth are located in the irradiation field, irradiation also has a direct destructive effect on dental hard tissue, causing decreased circulation through pulp, secondary fibrosis, and degeneration of the odontoblast processes. As shown from the literature, the effect of irradiation on tooth structure is dose-dependent. Doses lower than 30 Gy cause minimal tooth damage, doses 30–60 Gy increase risk of tooth breakdown two to three times while doses greater than 60 Gy increase risk of tooth damage 10 times [19]. Radiation-induced caries characteristically has a quick progress and affects smooth tooth surfaces where caries in nonradiated patients seldom occurs. The affected teeth become discolored and demineralized, with erosions in the cervical region, which makes them fracture easily (**Figure 3**). Despite advanced clinical presentation, the lesions are painless [16]. The risk of occurrence of radiation caries is lifelong so patients should be instructed to maintain adequate oral hygiene and to come to regular dental check-ups every 1–3 months.

3.2. Osteoradionecrosis

Osteoradionecrosis (ORN) is the most serious complication of head and neck RT, which affects the bone in irradiated area. RT alters collagen synthesis and induces inflammation and obliteration of the blood vessels that provide blood supply to the bone. Irradiated bone becomes hypovascularized and hypoxic, with impaired healing capacity [20]. The process is irreversible and progressive, and the risk of osteonecrosis is lifelong. The most commonly used definition of ORN implies exposed bone without healing for 3 months, without recurrence of the tumor [2], although there is no universally accepted definition in the literature. Due to the disagreement about the definition, there are no accurate data about the prevalence and incidence of ORN in the jaws. The reported relative frequency of ORN is between 0 and 7.1%, but patients with tumors localized in the oral cavity have higher relative frequency of ORN, up to 13.6% [21]. Results from one literature review report a weighed ORN prevalence of 7.4% for conventional radiotherapy, 5.1% for IMRT, 6.8% for chemoradiotherapy, and 5.3% for brachytherapy [22]. The literature shows that two-thirds of ORN in the orofacial region appear after a traumatic event, such as tooth extractions, ill-fitting dentures, biopsies, or periodontal dental procedures, while one-third can appear spontaneously. The most frequently affected bone in the head and neck region is the mandible [21, 22].

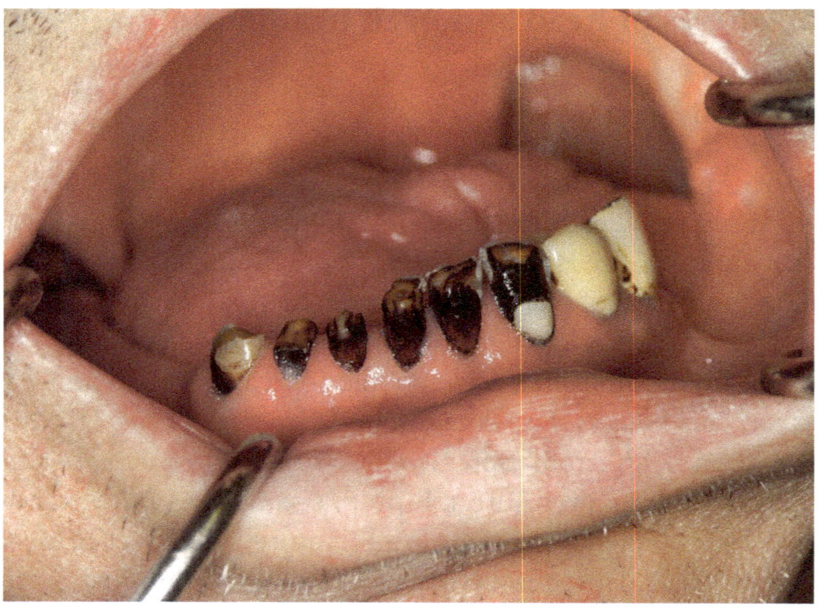

Figure 3. Radiation caries.

Risk factors for the development of ORN include therapeutic dose and mode of irradiation or combined chemotherapy and radiotherapy. Doses greater than 60 Gy, use of brachytherapy, or combined chemo- and radiotherapy increases the risk of development of ORN, while hyperfractioned RT or moderately accelerated fractioned RT, even in greater doses, decrease the risk of its occurrence [23]. Other risk factors include poor oral hygiene, malnutrition, chronic trauma from ill-fitting dentures, or acute trauma from surgical procedures in the jaw, especially in posterior mandible [24].

ORN manifests as an area of exposed bone in the oral cavity (**Figure 4**). Symptoms of ORN include pain, dysgeusia, dysesthesia, halitosis, or food impaction in the area of exposed bone, although in early stages it can be asymptomatic. Untreated, it can lead to fistulas and pathological fractures of the bone (**Figure 5**) [20–24]. Still, there is no universally accepted classification system for ORN, which makes comparison of different studies difficult [25].

3.3. Trismus

Trismus can occur if temporomandibular joint and masticatory muscles are located in irradiated area during head and neck cancer therapy. Irradiation causes spasm and fibrosis of masticatory muscles, which limits mouth opening [26, 27]. Trismus is often defined as reduced mouth opening with interincisal space less than 35 mm, but there is no universally accepted definition in the literature which is the reason for a wide range of reported prevalence of trismus after head and neck RT, ranging from 5 to 38% of patients [28, 29]. Trismus is often underreported as RT side effect, although it seriously impairs quality of life, resulting with difficulties in patient's social life, affecting speech, food intake, and oral hygiene maintaining and even leading to depression [30]. Risk factors for the occurrence of the trismus are similar as for other late oral side effects of RT and include the total dose of radiation, fractionation

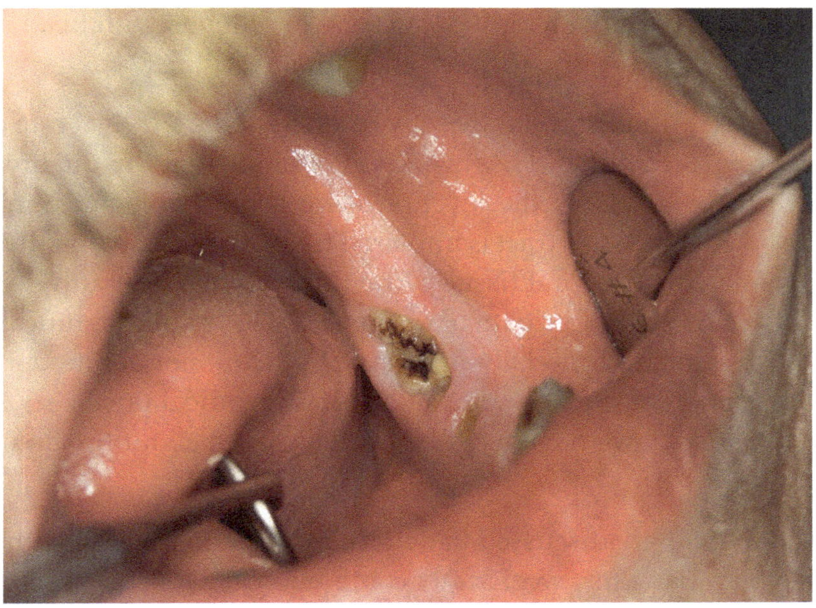

Figure 4. Osteoradionecrosis.

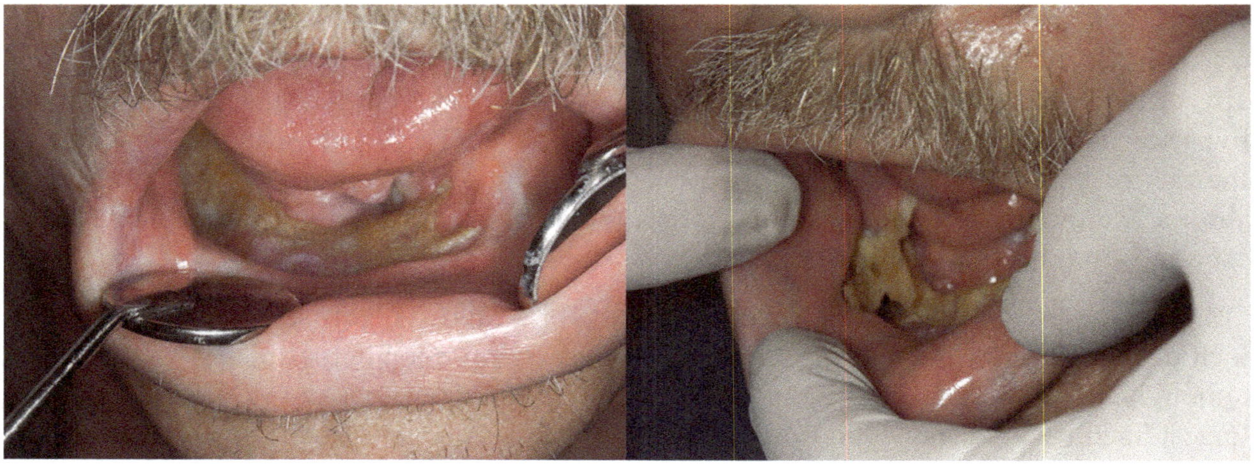

Figure 5. Osteoradionecrosis progressing to pathological fracture of the mandible (*Courtesy of Prof. Alajbeg*).

regimen (mode of irradiation), treatment modality (conventional RT vs. intensity-modulated radiotherapy (IMRT)), overall duration of RT, tumor location, and poor physical condition [26, 27, 31, 32]. Some results show that a total dose of RT greater than 55 Gy increases the incidence of trismus up to 47%, while treatment modality as conventional RT compared to IMRT decreases the mean incidence of trismus from 25.4 to 5% [27, 33]. Patients receiving RT to head and neck area should be instructed in rehabilitative exercises during and after RT to prevent the trismus development.

4. Dentist's role in head and neck cancer team

As early as 1995, experts of the health system of the United Kingdom concluded that health policy in addition to acting on the length of survival of patients with head and neck tumors (PwHNTs) must take all measures to increase their quality of life [34].

Over decades, modern treatment modalities have increased the survival rate of these patients, owing to the great efforts invested. However, it is obvious that the quality of life to which PwHNTs are destined is far below the level of being comfortable and functional [35]. The function of the upper aerodigestive tract is impaired following the treatment in PwHNT, especially of structures related to the oral tissues. The function of the mouth is a very important aspect of the quality of life of cancer patients in general [36]. While significant developments occur in the field of treatment, especially in terms of procurement of modern equipment for RT, as well as in education of radiation oncologists and medical physicists, which improves the survival rate of patients, we have to ask ourselves: what about the quality of life of our PwHNT following RT?

Oral toxicities related to RT are discussed in detail elsewhere in the text. Although oral mucositis does not last longer than a few weeks after completion of RT, its most serious consequence is interruption of RT [37]. The practice in which oncologists would temporarily interrupt radiation in case of severe form of mucositis "until the PwHNT gets his oral situation improved" might still exist. This practice reduces the cure rate by 1–2% per each day of interruption [38]. Therefore, the dentists must take all measures to help PwHNT withstand the uninterrupted treatment, no matter how uncomfortable it gets.

Although it might require a lot of effort in continuous communication with oncology surgeons and oncologists, our profession must strive to provide arguments against interruption of radiation. Dentists need to convince oncologists that good preparation of PwHNT and close monitoring during RT at 2-week intervals can effectively prevent the need for interruption of RT, and this practice should be ever so rarer. Centers that include collaborative dentist would not normally interrupt radiation in cases of severe mucositis.

As discussed elsewhere in the chapter, there are also lifelong complications of head and neck RT, which ultimately can cause pathological fractures of the jaw and, indirectly, death. It is a cascade process with connected temporal occurrences. Briefly described, it begins with the destruction of acini of the salivary glands by radiation. The teeth, as there is no saliva, cannot defend demineralization, which leads to the inevitable radiation caries. The destruction of tooth leads toward the need for extraction, which is a high-risk procedure in the irradiated bone, because of RT-induced hypovascularity, ultimately leading toward ORN [39]. ORN can be so extensive that it may cause pathological fracture of the mandible (**Figure 5**). This "domino effect" could be prevented if dental profession is included into multidisciplinary approach.

Good protocols for an interdisciplinary approach to PwHNT clearly emphasize that the dentist is a part of the oncology team [40]. Unfortunately, is not usually so. There are exceptions in most developed countries, but it really is not a part of standard of care, especially in developing countries such as Croatia. The causes of such inappropriate practices lay on both sides of the bridge: medical doctor (head and neck surgeon) generally is not aware of the true significance and is not easily bothered to spend his limited energy on oral complications. A dentist, on the other hand, often has "better things to do" than to deal with a handful of neglected people of low socioeconomic status, who seem hopelessly ill. It could be due to personal ignorance on the subject, and due to a fear to treat PwHNT. And so, our task is twofold: as representatives of the profession called "oral medicine" to build a bridge between our fellow dentists and fellow medical doctors, and to strive to persuade them how important it is to cooperate. In addition, we have to introduce an educational intervention among fellow dentists to foster their engagement in this important activity. What we still do not know is how to motivate fellow dentists to enthusiastically participate in the care of PwHNT. Until then, only few institutions in Croatia, such as ours, will remain one of the few places that provide this type of care.

Dentists' activities are directed to adherence to guidelines for oral care, which improve the quality of life in PwHNT, especially those who are treated with RT. Those include the reduction of the inevitable side effects of treatment, as well as the prevention of long-term complications of treatment.

Oral care needs to be based on the good practices from developed countries. The US National Comprehensive Cancer Network ("National Comprehensive Cancer Network," NCCN) brings together 26 of the top cancer centers in the United States and publishes guidelines for good clinical practice of treating head and neck tumors [41]. According to their guidelines, it is clearly stated that patients should be referred to dental evaluation before the treatment of any head and neck cancer site: lip cancer, oral cavity, oropharynx, hypopharynx, nasopharynx, glottic, and supraglottic larynx, paranasal sinuses (pp. 11–59). With the obligatory oral and dental evaluation and treatment before cancer treatment, NCCN guidelines emphasize the necessary oral evaluation and care during and after radiotherapy, stating that dental evaluation is recommended for oral cavity and all sites exposed to significant radiotherapy (p. 83) [41]. As a mandatory postulate, the NCCN approach describes the integration of treatment, stating that it is critically important that a multidisciplinary evaluation and treatment are prospectively coordinated and integrated by all disciplines involved in the care before starting any treatment (p. 84) [41].

Timing of RT as the part of multimodal treatment is important. It is well established that time elapsed between surgery and RT inversely affects the prognosis [42]. There are, however, papers questioning this concept, but today it is considered the best to start RT 6 weeks following the surgery [43]. This leaves enough time for dental treatment to be completed before the RT.

However, it is not unusual that dentists sees PwHNT scheduled for RT, who comes at their first dental appointment only several days before the actual start of RT. If a dentist extracts their teeth, he would be causing further postponing of RT, which may be disastrous for the patient. Today, thanks to better planning in health care, waiting for RT is not so long anymore (at least in the institutions we work with), but the PwHNTs also come to point of oral care soon after discharge after surgery, which is early enough so that all dental procedures can be performed at a normal pace prior to the RT. This minimizes the risk of toxicities, eliminating the need for extractions after radiation. During and after RT, specific procedures are followed, as discussed elsewhere in the chapter.

Guidelines of the British Society for Disability and Oral Health, by Kumar et al., offer an elaborate approach to pathways of oral care in PwHNT [44]. Their basic postulate, without which we will certainly fail, is that clear pathway of care is necessary if we want to prevent or minimize oral complications. Regardless of how simple this may look, the lack of "clear pathway of care" was what caused the previous absence of this specific care. It requires strong dedication, exceptional effort, time, and preparedness for countless disappointments along the journey our profession takes in order to foster this type of oral care.

One should be aware that most of PwHNTs are not easy to motivate for compliance to oral care. It is very difficult to explain PwHNT how important the preventative effect of fluoridation is, when combined with good oral hygiene. A typical PwHNT has a history of consuming large amounts of alcohol and tobacco products, and is not easily motivated to suddenly start adhering to very strict oral hygiene measures. However, the efforts lead to success in a considerable number of patients.

Dentists should be aware of obstacles inherent in most health systems. One of them is was that primary care dentists usually are unprepared and uninterested to participate in oral care.

The probable reason is the lack of specific knowledge and skills. These patients should be continuously motivated, closely followed up, and helped to obtain good adherence to our recommendations. If their primary care dentist is not collaborating with specialists, PwHNT most certainly will not comply.

Specialists should write very extensive medical histories, explaining the primary care dentist what and why certain dental procedures must be done in their offices and the therapeutic rationale behind these procedures. These are written dental recommendations with an educational component. Secondary and tertiary care professionals who coordinate oral care should always clearly emphasize that they would be available for telephone or other types of consultation. Furthermore, it has been noted that the advice on oral and dental complications of head and neck RT treatment communicated by head and neck surgeon had much more impact on patients than if that same advice was communicated by the responsible dentist. It is therefore of utmost importance that head and neck surgeon possesses basic knowledge of the subject matter and that is willing to firmly insist that PwHNT complies with oral health measures. Regardless of how disappointing this might be for oral care professionals, this discovery is very important and should help guiding efforts to change oral behavior in our PwHNT. Head and neck surgeons who assume a role of "oral health advocates" can help dentists to significantly increase patients' compliance. We have observed that if surgeons also motivate patients for good oral care, a significant increase in compliance with the recommendations will be achieved [45]. The ideal would be that the oral assessment is introduced as a legal requirement before the radiation of the head and neck. Listed experiences should be of practical help to readers who plan to start this service [46].

5. Dental management prior radiation therapy for head and neck cancers

Prior to the head and neck RT, all patients without exception should be referred for oral/dental care. There are no generally accepted evidence-based clinical guidelines for dentists how to prepare patients for RT; however, it is rational to follow effective strategies from the relevant literature [47].

The main purposes of pretreatment dental evaluation are as follows:

- to prevent or minimize acute and chronic oral side effects associated with RT
- to facilitate submission of RT and radiation-induced sequelae

(1) The task of the dentist, as a member of the oncology team preparing the patients for head and neck RT, is to perform the following procedures:

(a) treatment of oral and dental diseases

(b) implementation of preventive procedures

(c) education of the patients

5.1. Treatment of oral and dental diseases

Since treating diseased oral tissues prior to RT prevents or minimizes the development of many radiation-induced complications, a thorough oral examination before RT is essential. The fact that some patients are edentulous does not mean that for them dental management before, during, and after radiotherapy is not or is less important.

In order to reveal the presence of periapical lesions, impacted teeth, general bone conditions, and tumor rarefications, a panoramic radiograph is performed [48]. Dental caries with or without root canal infection, necrotic pulps, periodontitis, periodontal abscesses, diseases of oral mucosa are additionally assessed trough clinical dental evaluation. Oral status is evaluated and recorded: present teeth, clinical and radiographic findings (carious lesions, oral mucosa status, periodontal status, salivary gland functional assessment, interincisal opening), presence of orthodontic devices, and denture use.

Prophylactic dental clearance includes restorative treatments, periodontal scaling, fluoride therapy, and dental extractions. The following teeth need to be extracted [49]:

- Teeth with advanced caries lesions with questionable pulpal status or pulpal involvement
- Teeth with extensive periapical lesions
- Teeth with signs of severe periodontal disease (advanced bone loss and mobility or furcation involvement)
- Residual root tips not fully covered with bone or showing radiolucency
- Impacted or incompletely erupted teeth, particularly third molars that are not fully covered by alveolar bone or that are in contact with the oral environment

Three weeks before radiation therapy begins, all dental treatments should be completed. In the case there is less than 10 days to the beginning of the RT, teeth extractions are delayed for the "window" period after radiation (within 5–6 months after completion of RT) [50].

5.2. Implementation of preventive procedures

The elimination of all potential causes of local trauma is mandatory. It is known that ORN can develop also in edentulous patients [45] and therefore the adjustment of ill-fitting dentures is necessary. It is important to remove sharp edges and protruding teeth fillings. Orthodontic braces should be removed before the beginning of the RT.

5.3. Education of the patients

Besides teeth preservation and elimination of potential trauma, it is necessary that dentist educates the patient prior to RT. The dentist should explain the expected and possible RT-induced complications. Patients must be aware that the salivary glands may be affected by irradiation, which can result in severe decrease of salivary function [51]. Radiation-induced xerostomia is an important chronic side effect of RT that can lead to many oral diseases and patients should be warned on the rapid occurrence of dental caries [52]. Untreated on time, it results in the extraction of teeth and the possible development of ORN. During preirradiation, dental management dentist should strongly emphasize to the patients that postirradiation caries and following oral diseases are avoidable through the regular and meticulous dental hygiene, daily fluoridation, and regular dental checkups.

Regrettably, in addition to poor oral health, before RT in many head and neck squamous cell carcinoma patients, even from developed countries and regardless of their dental status, poor oral hygiene is common [45]. Patients should therefore receive optimal mouth care before RT begins. During the preirradiation treatment, it is important that the dentist provides patients with instructions for oral hygiene during and after radiation therapy.

It is useful to provide the patient with the Fact Sheets created by the Oral Care Study Group of the Multinational Association of Supportive Care in Cancer (MASCC) and the International Society of Oral Oncology (ISOO) [53]. These are available online, multilingual, and written in plain language and the notable parts of the Fact Sheets are provided below along with their original section numbers.

1.3.1. Oral care advices that dentist should give to the patient before RT include instructions about [53]

1.3.1.1. proper toothbrushing: "Use a soft toothbrush. Brush before bed. Gently brush tongue. Brush within 30 minutes of eating."

1.3.1.2. dental floss use: "Floss at least once daily with waxed floss."

1.3.1.3. rinsing: "Rinse, swish and spit rinse several times after brushing or flossing. Ensure medicated rinses are done 20 minutes apart.

HOW TO MAKE YOUR MOUTH RINSE 1. Mix 1 teaspoon of baking soda and 1 teaspoon of salt with 4 cups of water. 2. Put the mouthwash in a container with a lid. 3. The mouthwash should be kept at room temperature. 4. Discard at the end of each day and make a new batch.

HOW TO USE YOUR MOUTH RINSE Shake well before using. • Rinse and gargle with one tablespoon (15 mL) and then spit out. • Repeat 2 or 3 times at each use. • Use mouthwash every 2 hours during the day."

1.3.1.4. oral moisturizing: "Moisturize nasal passages through the night with a steam vaporizer in your room. Moisturize with mouth rinse and water based lubricants often. Avoid petroleum jelly and glycerin products."

1.3.1.5. lip care: "Use water-soluble, wax-based, or oil-based lubricants. • Apply after cleaning, at bedtime and as needed. Do not apply petroleum Jelly."

1.3.3.6. fluoridation

> "INSTRUCTIONS FOR USE OF FLUORIDE TRAYS 1. Brush and floss before wearing trays. 2. Fill the grooves of the trays 1/3 full with gel. 3. Insert tray and spit out any excess gel. 4. Leave the tray in for 5 minutes. • Use at bedtime for longer lasting results. • Brush trays and air dry after each use. • Do not use hot water to clean trays (hot water will distort the tray). • Do not eat, drink or rinse for 30 minutes after tray use."

Besides explaining how to perform fluoridation, dentist should emphasize the importance of fluoridation in preventing post-radiation dental caries.

1.3.1.7. Denture care instructions

"• Keep your dentures out as much as possible. • Remove dentures, plates and prostheses before brushing. • Brush and rinse dentures after meals and before bed. • Soak dentures in cleansing solution for at least 8 hours. • If you are on antifungal therapy, soak in anti-fungal solution." [53]

Edentulous patient should also be instructed to remove dentures during RT. [48]

As a member of oncology team, the dentist should also explain to the patients:

1.3.2. The necessity of avoiding the consumption of cigarettes and alcohol

1.3.3. The necessity of regular dental visits during and after RT.

Dental consultation should always be in order prior to RT. During the first pre irradiation dental visit, patient should become aware that the dentist plays very important role in the management of head and neck cancer. They should realize that dental treatment before, during, and after head and neck RT is mandatory part of the more successful oncological therapy, which reduces the morbidity and mortality associated with RT.

6. Oral care during head and neck radiotherapy

Oral care during head and neck RT is directed to the treatment of acute complications—oral mucositis, xerostomia and taste alterations.

6.1. Oral mucositis

Most pronounced symptom of oral mucositis is pain associated with dysphagia, odynophagia, and difficulty speaking. Symptoms usually begin in the third week of RT. Sometimes pain can be so intense that it can prevent oral food intake resulting in the need for parenteral nutrition, and in some cases discontinuation of RT. During this period, regular checkups at dental office every 7–10 days are recommended [54]. Up to now, a lot of treatment modalities for OM have been tested, but most of them with varying success.

The treatment of OM is symptomatic, and it mainly consists of pain management and infection control. For the pain management, mouthwash containing topical anesthetic agent such as lidocaine is usually prescribed. Tetracaine, amethocaine, dyclonine, and benzocaine are also used for pain relief. The use of topical anesthetics allows patients to do regular daily activities such as eating and tooth brushing. Most of the studies, aimed at pain relief, reported less frequent interruption of RT, when topical anesthetic is used [55–57]. Administration of systemic analgesics, including opioids, is used in most patients with moderate or severe OM [58]. Except topical anesthetic, mouthwash can contain ant-inflammatory and antimicrobial agents. A nonsteroidal anti-inflammatory drug, benzydamine hydrochloride, is effective in reducing the intensity and duration of mucosal damage [10, 59]. Plaque control and oral hygiene is very important in controlling OM. Even though chlorhexidine (CHX) is not recommended in the prevention or management of oral mucositis, its administration may provide indirect benefits like plaque control and gingivitis prevention, as well as oral candidosis prevention [10]. In the case of oral candidosis, local antifungal drugs such as miconazole or nystatin are prescribed [54]. Cytoprotective drug amifostine and biological response modifiers (interleukin 1, interleukin 11, and transforming growth factor β) have also been introduced for management of OM, but with varying success and are not recommended [10]. From all of the above mentioned, it can be concluded that there is still no effective therapy for the prevention and treatment of OM. However, it is important to emphasize that dentist can significantly contribute to the implementation of RT in its entirety, without interrupting it.

6.2. Taste disorder

The prevalence of taste alterations in patients receiving RT is 66.5%, and approximately 15% of them continue to experience this problem after cessation of the treatment [15]. Taste disorder has a negative impact on quality of life and may cause malnutrition, weight loss, and in severe cases, significant morbidity. However, it is important to note that this problem is reversible, and in most of the patients spontaneous return of taste occurs within a year and therefore no specific treatment is necessary [15]. Additionally, up to now no efficient agent for treating or preventing RT related taste disorder exists [15]. Zinc gluconate, amifostine, and dietary counseling have been studied for that purpose. Studies that tested administration of zinc gluconate reported variable results [60, 61]. Zinc gluconate is therefore not recommended for taste disorder prevention in head and neck cancer patients, even though it was found to be beneficial in a noncancer idiopathic dysgeusia [15]. It has been shown that use of amifostine only modestly helps in reducing the severity of taste disorder, without affecting the incidence [62, 63]. Because of conflicting results of the studies which examined the use of amifostine in the prevention and/or management of taste disorder, recommendation is not to use it in head and neck cancer patients [15]. Use of dietary and educational counseling on the incidence and severity of dysgeusia in cancer patients has shown a minor impact on early-onset taste disorder (30% vs. 40%), but with a greater effect on long-term taste disorder (5% vs. 25%) [64].

6.3. Xerostomia

It is well known that salivary gland hypofunction and xerostomia are significant morbidities during and following head and neck RT, resulting in decrease of salivary flow rates. Treatment goals for salivary gland hypofunction are stimulation of residual salivary gland tissue, relief of oral dryness, prevention of tooth demineralization, caries, and oral infection [11]. Pilocarpine, cevimeline, bethanechol HCl, and amifostine have been tested for the prevention of salivary gland hypofunction in cancer patient undergoing RT. Due to conflicting results their use is not recommended [11]. On the other hand, recent systematic review suggested that both pilocarpine and cevimeline can reduce xerostomia symptoms and increase salivary flow compared to placebo *after* RT but "some aspects of the relevant effect size, duration of the benefit, and clinical meaningfulness remain unclear" [65].

Intensity-modulated radiation therapy (IMRT) can reduce the radiation dose to salivary glands, thus helping in decrease of salivary gland hypofunction and symptoms of xerostomia [66, 67]. Surgical transfer of submandibular gland to the submental space can contribute to preservation of salivary gland function and reducing xerostomia symptoms. However, this method applies only to patients with clinically negative cervical lymph nodes [11]. Despite their short-term effect, it has been shown that use of saliva substitutes is more effective in the treatment of dry mouth than placebo. The saliva substitutes are mainly based on carboxymethylcellulose,

Oral care during head and neck radiotherapy
• regular checkups every 7–10 days during RT
• for the pain management prescribe topical anesthetics and/or analgesics
• use a soft toothbrush with a fluoride toothpaste for brushing after meals and before bed. Floss at least once a day (use xylocaine anesthetic rinse prior to brushing and flossing)
• if brushing is too painful, use a clean moist gauze or foam swab soaked in baking soda mouth rinse
• rinse the mouth with a baking soda and salt solution (mix 1 teaspoon of baking soda and 1 teaspoon of sat with four cups of water) several times a day. Avoid salt during mucositis
• management of dry mouth (sip water frequently, use saliva substitutes, use sugar-free candies, and gums)
• keep dentures out of the mouth as much as possible; soak it in cleansing solution for at least 8 hours
• exercises for the jaw muscles at least three times a day to avoid trismus
• avoid spicy or acidic foods, tobacco, and alcohol

Table 1. Oral care during head and neck radiotherapy (modified from Refs. [68–70]).

hydroxypropylmethylcellulose, hydroxyethylcellulose, and plyglycerylmethacrylate. Some of them contain electrolytes and fluoride for preventing teeth demineralization. Artificial saliva substitutes come in the form of gel, spray, and solution. Because its lubricating effect lasts longer, saliva substitute gel is recommended, especially during the night or other periods of severe oral dryness [11].

Points to remember for the oral care during head and neck RT are presented in **Table 1** [68–70].

7. Oral care after head and neck radiotherapy

After completion of RT, frequent follow-up appointments at dental office and good oral hygiene are of utmost importance. Initially, follow-up appointments are carried out once a month, and subsequently their dynamics is determined individually. Xerostomia and salivary gland dysfunction as acute complication of RT continues in the posttreatment period, thereby becoming chronic, which greatly increases the risk of dental caries and its sequelae. Radiation caries is extremely progressive and highly destructive type of caries, which certainly increases the risk of ORN by increasing risk for tooth extraction. Therefore, every effort should be focused on caries prevention. In order to avoid difficulties in maintaining oral hygiene and the implementation of necessary dental procedure, early signs of trismus should be recognized.

7.1. Radiation caries

Radiation caries is primarily a consequence of salivary hypofunction, saliva composition changes, and increase in acidogenic bacteria number. Furthermore, direct damage on the hard dental tissues frequently occurs from RT. For caries prevention good preoperative dental treatment, frequent dental evaluation and treatment after RT, consistent home care that includes brushing after meals and before bed, daily flossing, plaque control, self-applied fluoride products, and restricted intake of cariogenic foods are required [54].

It is considered that the fluoride therapy is the best option for the prevention and treatment of radiation caries. The use of fluoride products significantly reduces caries activity in postRT patients. High concentrated fluorides (≥5000 ppm) directly applied on tooth surfaces or with custom-made carriers should be maintained every day. Literature data have demonstrated no significant difference on caries activity related to the type of fluoride gel or fluoride delivery system [71].

Chlorhexidine (CHX) as a bisguanide with bactericidal activity reduces plaque accumulation and helps in reducing mainly Gram-positive and bit less Gram-negative bacteria. It is interesting that use of CHX has shown decrease in oral *Streptococcus mutans*, with no influence on oral lactobacillus counts [72, 73]. Generally, CHX is recommended for maintaining oral health, although potential side effects such as tooth staining, taste changes, and increased calculus deposits should be taken into account. CHX mouthwashes should be administered daily after tooth brushing [71].

In cases where radiation caries is not possible to prevent, restoration with a proper dental material is required. Lack of salivary buffering, reduction of normal plaque pH, and formation of the hydrofluoric acid in patients with xerostomia lead to erosion of glass ionomer restorations [74]. Hence, conventional glass ionomer restorations are not recommended in patients who have been treated with RT. For the dental restoration in patients who have been treated with RT, the use of resin-modified glass ionomer, composite resin, and amalgam restorations are recommended [71].

7.2. Trismus

Reduced mouth opening is a result of the damaging effects of RT on the masticatory muscles. It is very important to identify early signs of trismus considering the fact that early treatment can significantly affect its prevention. For the prevention as well as for the treatment of reduced mouth opening, passive and active physiotherapy from the commencement of RT can be performed. Active physiotherapy is carried out with the muscles placed around the joint, while passive motion includes use of various devices [33]. Passive physiotherapy implies the use of tongue depressors, a hand operated device "Therabite Jaw Motion Rehabilitation System,", and forced mouth opening with finger pressure several times a day [75]. Except of the aforementioned therapeutic options, pentoxifylline and botulinum toxins have shown efficacy in reducing radiation-induced trismus [76, 77]. However, the latter needs to be confirmed by randomized controlled studies. Whenever possible, sophisticated multiple-field techniques should be used to reduce the dose of radiation to the mastication muscles and temporomandibular joint [2].

7.3. Osteoradionecrosis

Head and neck cancer patients undergoing RT are at lifelong risk of developing ORN. Therefore, dental extractions after RT should be avoided if possible. Furthermore, every local trauma must be avoided, and endodontic therapy, instead of extractions, should be the treatment of choice. Otherwise, if there is a need for extractions in postradiation period, they should be performed during first 5–6 months after RT with minimal trauma and primary closure [25]. Obliteration of the blood vessels and hypovascularity of the bone that occurs after RT is not an overnight process and it takes 5–6 months to develop [20, 50]. This "window" period should therefore be used for necessary extractions if possible. Literature results on the incidence of ORN after tooth extraction support this as significantly lower incidence of ORN was reported when extractions were performed within 1 year postRT compared to extractions performed 2–5 years postRT (7.5% vs. 22.6%) [78]. Use of antibiotic prophylaxis for the prevention of ORN is widespread in the literature, but there is no consensus on the type and dose of application. Their administration is empirical [23]. Hyperbaric oxygen therapy (HBO) is not strongly recommended for the prevention of ORN prior dental extractions, due to unclear clinical efficacy and cost-effectiveness. No specific and universally accepted guideline for the administration of HBO therapy exists [22]. Most of the protocols propose 20–30 dives before and 10 dives after dental extraction at 2.0–2.5 atmosphere pressure [22, 23]. Despite that, recent Cochrane systematic review concluded that HBO therapy "appears to reduce the chance of ORN following tooth extraction in an irradiated field" and that "the application of HBOT to selected participants and tissues may be justified" [79].

Management of ORN includes conservative treatment, surgical debridement with the use of adjunctive antibiotics and reconstructive surgery. Conservative treatment should be the first line therapy for ORN because surgical procedure may enhance the necrotic process [23]. Treatment consists of local wound care and good oral hygiene using 0.2% chlorhexidine mouthwashes and course of systemic antibiotics in acute episodes [80, 81]. If a conservative

Oral care after head and neck radiotherapy
• regular checkups every 4–8 weeks for the first 6 months (afterwards based on the patient's needs)
• avoid invasive surgical procedures including dental extractions (if necessary, the use of antibiotics and HBO therapy before and after surgery should be considered)
• daily fluoride application (using a tray or brush-on method), flossing and meticulous oral hygiene (use a soft toothbrush and 0.02% CHX mouthwash) must be performed
• management of dry mouth (sip water frequently, use saliva substitutes, sugar-free candies, and gums)
• exercises for the jaw muscles at least three times a day (minimum first 6 months postRT)
• a new removable denture can be made 3–6 months postRT (avoid any tissue irritation/trauma)

Table 2. Oral care after head and neck radiotherapy (modified from Refs. [68–70]).

approach does not achieve wound healing, surgical removal of necrotic bone is indicated. Indications for reconstructive surgery include advanced cases with oral and/or cutaneous fistula, radiographically visible osteolysis, and pathologic fracture [81, 82]. The use of antioxidant agent pentoxifylline and tocopherol (vitamin E) for the treatment of ORN has shown promising results but more clinical trials are needed to confirm their efficacy [82].

Points to remember for the oral care after head and neck RT are presented in **Table 2** [68–70].

8. Conclusion

Efforts of dental professionals will have a significant clinical and financial impact on the treatment of PwHNT. The dentist must be a member of the oncology team and must have knowledge on the specific complications of head and neck RT. Dentist should make a plan of treatment and prevention before the start of RT. Surgeons, radiation oncologists, and medical oncologists can find valuable partners in dental profession, with the aim of improving patients' overall quality of life. Such care can greatly prevent and reduce side effects of treatment, resulting in a significant reduction in the cost of treatment, and some of those aspects facilitate implementation of radiation therapy without interruption, which increases the chances of cure.

Author details

Vlaho Brailo[1,2*], Vanja Vučićević Boras[1,2], Danica Vidović Juras[1,2], Ana Andabak Rogulj[1], Božana Lončar Brzak[1] and Ivan Alajbeg[1,2]

*Address all correspondence to: brailo@sfzg.hr

1 Department of Oral Medicine, School of Dental Medicine, University of Zagreb, Zagreb, Croatia

2 Oral Medicine Unit, Dental Clinic, University Clinical Hospital Zagreb, Zagreb, Croatia

References

[1] Huang SH, O'Sullivan B. Oral cancer: Current role of radiotherapy and chemotherapy. Medicina Oral, Patologia Oral Y Cirugia Bucal. 2013;**18**(2):e233-e240

[2] Sciubba JJ, Goldenberg D. Oral complications of radiotherapy. Lancet Oncology. 2006;**7**:175-183

[3] Dirix P1, Nuyts S. Evidence-based organ-sparing radiotherapy in head and neck cancer. Lancet Oncology. 2010;**11**(1):85-91

[4] Vissink A, Jansma J, Spijkervet FK, Burlage FR, Coppes RP. Oral sequelae of head and neck radiotherapy. Critical Reviews in Oral Biology & Medicine Journal. 2003;**14**(3):199-212

[5] Villa A, Sonis ST. Mucositis: pathobiology and management. Current Opinion in Oncology. 2015;**27**(3):159-164

[6] Potting CM, Blijlevens NA, Donnelly JP, Feuth T, Van Achterberg T. A scoring system for the assessment of oral mucositis in daily nursing practice. European Journal of Cancer Care (England). 2006;**15**(3):228-234

[7] Sonis ST, Eilers JP, Epstein JB, LeVeque FG, Liggett Jr. WH, Mulagha MT, et al. Validation of a new scoring system for the assessment of clinical trial research of oral mucositis induced by radiation or chemotherapy. Mucositis Study Group. Cancer. 1999;**85**(10):2103-2113

[8] Schubert MM, Williams BE, Lloid ME, Donaldson G, Chapko MK. Clinical assessment scale for the rating of oral mucosal changes associated with bone marrow transplantation. Development of an oral mucositis index. Cancer. 1992;**69**(10):2469-2477

[9] World Health Organization. Handbook for Reporting Results of Cancer Treatment. Geneva, Switzerland: World Health Organization; 1997. pp. 15-22

[10] Lalla RV, Bowen J, Barasch A, Elting L, Epstein J, Keefe DM, et al. MASCC/ISOO clinical practice guidelines for the management of mucositis secondary to cancer therapy. Cancer. 2014;**120**(10):1453-1461

[11] Jensen SB, Pedersen AM, Vissink A, Andersen E, Brown CG, Davies AN, et al. A systematic review of salivary gland hypofunction and xerostomia induced by cancer therapies: Management strategies and economic impact. Support Care Cancer. 2010;**18**(8):1061-1079

[12] Vissink A, Burlage FR, Spijkervet FK, Jansma J, Coppes RP. Prevention and treatment of the consequences of head and neck radiotherapy. Critical Reviews in Oral Biology and Medicine. 2003;**14**(3):213-225

[13] Chambers MS, Garden AS, Kies MS, Martin JW. Radiation-induced xerostomia in patients with head and neck cancer: pathogenesis, impact on quality of life, and management, Head Neck. 2004;**26**(9):796-807

[14] Dirix P, Nuyts S, Van den Bogaert W. Radiation-induced xerostomia in patients with head and neck cancer: A literature review. Cancer. 2006;**107**(11):2525-2534

[15] Hovan AJ, Williams PM, Stevenson-Moore P, Wahlin YB, Ohrn KE, Elting LS, et al. A systematic review of dysgeusia induced by cancer therapies. Support Care Cancer. 2010;**18**(8):1081-1087

[16] Kielbassa A, Hinkelbein W, Hellwig E, Meyer-Lückel H. Radiation-related damage to dentition. Lancet Oncology. 2006;**7**:326-335

[17] Epstein J, Chin E, Jacobson J, Rishiraj B, Le N. The relationships among fluoride, cariogenic oral flora, and salivary flow rate during radiation therapy. Oral Surgery, Oral Medicine, Oral Pathology, Oral Radiology, and Endodontology. 1998;**86**:286-292

[18] Keene H, Daly T, Brown L, Dreizen S, Drane J, Horton I, et al. Dental caries and *Streptococcus mutans* prevalence in cancer patients with irradiation-induced xerostomia: 1-13 years after radiotherapy. Caries Research. 1981;**15**:416-427

[19] Walker M, Wichman B, Cheng A, Coster J, Williams K. Impact of radiotherapy dose on dentition breakdown in head and neck cancer patients. Practical Radiation Oncology. 2011;**1**:142-148

[20] Silvestre-Rangil J, Silvestre F. Clinico-therapeutic management of osteoradionecrosis: A literature review and update. Medicina Oral, Patologia Oral Y Cirugia Bucal. 2011;**16**(7):e900-e904

[21] Nabil S, Samman N. Risk factors for osteoradionecrosis after head and neck radiation: A systematic review. Oral Surgery, Oral Medicine, Oral Pathology and Oral Radiology. 2012;**113**:54-69

[22] Peterson D, Doerr W, Hovan A, Pinto A, Saunders D, Elting L, et al. Osteoradionecrosis in cancer patients: The evidence base for treatment-dependent frequency, current management strategies, and future studies. Support Care Cancer. 2010;**18**(8):1089-1098

[23] Lyons A, Ghazali N. Osteoradionecrosis of the jaws: Current understanding of its pathophysiology and treatment. British Journal of Oral and Maxillofacial Surgery. 2008;**46**:653-660

[24] Jacobson A, Buchbinder D, Hu K, Urken M. Paradigm shifts in the management of osteoradionecrosis of the mandible. Oral Oncology. 2010;**46**(11):795-801

[25] Chrcanovic BR, Reher P, Sousa AA, Harris M. Osteoradionecrosis of the jaws—A current overview—Part 1: Physiopathology and risk and predisposing factors. Journal of Maxillofacial and Oral Surgery. 2010;**14**(1):3-16

[26] Teguh D, Levendag P, Voet P, van der Est H, Noever I, de Kruijf W, et al. Trismus in patients with oropharyngeal cancer: Relationship with dose in structures of mastication apparatus. Head Neck. 2008;**30**(5):622-630

[27] Louise Kent M, Brennan M, Noll J, Fox P, Burri S, Hunter J, et al. Radiation-induced trismus in head and neck cancer patients. Support Care Cancer. 2008;**16**(3):305-309

[28] Scott B, Butterworth C, Lowe D, Rogers S. Factors associated with restricted mouth opening and its relationship to health-related quality of life in patients attending a maxillofacial oncology clinic. Oral Oncology. 2008;**44**:430-438

[29] Dijkstra P, Kalk W, Roodenburg J. Trismus in head and neck oncology: A systematic review. Oral Oncology. 2004;**40**(9):879-889

[30] Lee R, Slevin N, Musgrove B, Swindell R, Molassiotis A. Prediction of post-treatment trismus in head and neck cancer patients. British Journal of Oral and Maxillofacial Surgery. 2012;**50**(4):328-332

[31] van der Molen L, Heemsbergen W, de Jong R, van Rossum M, Smeele L, Rasch C, et al. Dysphagia and trismus after concomitant chemo-intensity-modulated radiation therapy (chemo-IMRT) in advanced head and neck cancer; dose-effect relationships for swallowing and mastication structures. Radiotherapy & Oncology. 2013;**106**:364-369

[32] Chen Y, Zhao C, Wang J, Ma H, Lai S, Liu Y, et al. Intensity-modulated radiation therapy reduces radiation-induced trismus in patients with nasopharyngeal carcinoma: A prospective study with>5 years of follow-up. Cancer. 2011;**117**:2910-2916

[33] Bensadoun R, Riesenbeck D, Lockhart P, Elting L, Spijkervet F, Brennan M, et al. A systematic review of trismus induced by cancer therapies in head and neck cancer patients. Support Care Cancer. 2010;**18**(8):1033-1038

[34] Calman, K., Hine, D. A Policy Framework for Commissioning Cancer Services: A Report by the Expert Advisory Group on Cancer to the Chief Medical Officers of England and Wales. Department of Health; April 1995

[35] Vaughan ED. An analysis of morbidity following major head and neck surgery with particular reference to mouth function. Journal of Maxillofacial Surgery. 1982;**10**: 129-134

[36] Sonis ST, Sonis AT, Lieberman A. Oral complications in patients receiving treatment for malignancies other than of the head and neck. The Journal of the American Dental Association. 1978;**97**:468-472

[37] Maxymiw WG, Wood RE. The role of dentistry in head and neck radiation therapy. Journal of the Canadian Dental Association. 1989;**55**(3):193-198

[38] Russo G, Haddad R, Posner M, Machtay M. Radiation treatment breaks and ulcerative mucositis in head and neck cancer. Oncologist. 2008;**13**(8):886-898

[39] Thorn JJ, Hansen HS, Specht L, Bastholt L. Osteoradionecrosis of the jaws: Clinical characteristics and relation to the field of irradiation. Journal of Oral and Maxillofacial Surgery. 2000;**58**(10):1088-1093

[40] HAZU. Kliničke smjernice u dijagnostici i liječenju tumora glave i vrata. http://info.hazu.hr/upload/file/Kal_11/simpozij%20pozivnica%2004-2011.pdf [Internet] 2011. [Cited: 21 March 2017]

[41] NCCN. NCCN Guidelines. Head and Neck Cancer. version 02.2013. 2013. [Internet] 2011. Available from: http://oralcancerfoundation.org/treatment/pdf/head-and-neck.pdf. [Accessed: March 21st, 2017]

[42] Kajanti M, Holsti LR, Holsti P. Radical surgery and postoperative split-course radiotherapy in squamous cell carcinoma of the mobile tongue: Factors influencing local control and the time to recurrence. Radiotherapy & Oncology. 1991;**22**(3):174-179

[43] Amar A, Chedid HM, Curioni OA, Dedivitis RA, Rapoport A, Cernea CR, Brandão LG. Delayed postoperative radiation therapy in local control of squamous cell carcinoma of the tongue and floor of the mouth. Einstein (Sao Paulo). 2014;**12**(4):477-479

[44] Kumar N, Brooke A, Burke M, et al. The Royal College of Surgeons of England/The British Society for Disability and Oral Health. The Oral Management of Oncology Patients Requiring Radiotherapy, Chemotherapy and/or Bone Marrow Transplantation-Clinical Guidelines. Updated 2012 (Update of the 1997 Guideline by Shaw J, Kumar N,

Duggal M et al.). [Internet] 2011. Available from: https://www.rcseng.ac.uk/dental-faculties/fds/publications-guidelines/clinical-guidelines/. [Accessed: 21 March 2017]

[45] Alajbeg I, Pastorčić Grgić M, Gršić K, Andabak-Rogulj A, Stubljar B, Tomičević T. Strategies for prevention and treatment of head and neck radiotherapy complications—Our experiences. Book of Abstracts of the 1st International Congress on head and neck tumors; 19—22 October 2011; Zagreb, Hrvatska

[46] Alajbeg I. Stomatologist—A member of the oncology team for chemo-radiotherapy of head and neck. In: Topić B, editor. Proceedings of the Symposium "Interdisciplinary diagnosis and treatment of premalignant and malignant lesions of oral mucosa" (Sarajevo, Oct. 3, 2015). Vol. 47. Academy of Sciences and Arts of Bosnia and Hezegovina, Department of Medical Sciences; 2016. pp. 151-161

[47] Barker GJ, Epstein JB, Williams KB, Gorsky M, Raber-Durlacher JE. Current practice and knowledge of oral care for cancer patients: A survey of supportive health care providers. Support Care Cancer. 2005;**13**:32-41

[48] Bonan PR, Lopes MA, Pires FR, Almeida OP. Dental management of low socioeconomic level patients before radiotherapy of the head and neck with special emphasis on the prevention of osteoradionecrosis. The Brazilian Dental Journal. 2006;**17**:36-42

[49] Jawad H, Hodson NA, Nixon PJ. A review of dental treatment of head and neck cancer patients, before, during and after radiotherapy: Part 1. The Brazilian Dental Journal. 2015;**218**(2):65-68

[50] Bagheri SC. Clinical Review of Oral and Maxillofacial Surgery: A Case-based Approach. 2nd ed. St. Louis: Mosby, Inc.; 2014. p. 221

[51] Cotrim AP, Sowers A, Mitchell JB, Baum BJ. Prevention of irradiation-induced salivary hypofunction by microvessel protection in mouse salivary glands. Molecular Therapy. 2007;**15**:2101-2106

[52] Tschoppe P, Meyer-Lueckel H, Toll R, Kielbassa AM. In vitro analysis of an new saliva substitute (Saliva natura) on enamel and dentin [Article in German]. Laryngorhinootologie. 2007;**86**:723-727

[53] MASCC/ISOO Oral Care Study Group, International Society of Oral Oncology (ISOO). How to Care for Yourself before Head and Neck Radiation Begins [Internet]. 2014. Available from: http://www.mascc.org/assets/StudyGroups/oralcare/en_head_neck_beforeradiation.pdf. [Accessed: 1 March 2017]

[54] Little JW, Falace DA, Miller CS, Rhodus NL. Cancer and oral care of the patient. In: Dental Management of the Medically Compromised Patient. James W. Little, 7th ed. St. Louis: Mosby Elsevier; 2008. pp. 433-461

[55] Alterio D, Jereczek-Fossa BA, Zuccotti GF, et al. Tetracaine oral gel in patients treated with radiotherapy for head-and-neck cancer: Final results of a phase II study. International Journal of Radiation Oncology, Biology, Physics. 2006;**64**(2):392-395

[56] Logan RM. Oral mucositis—Current concepts and management. Annals of the Royal Australasian College of Dental Surgeons. 2006;**16**:54-57

[57] Carnel SB, Blakeslee DB, Oswald SG, Barnes M. Treatment of radiation- and chemotherapy-induced stomatitis. Otolaryngology–Head and Neck Surgery. 1990;**102**(4):326-330

[58] Saadeh CE. Chemotherapy- and radiotherapy-induced oral mucositis: Review of preventive strategies and treatment. Pharmacotherapy. 2005;**25**:540-554

[59] Epstein JB, Silverman Jr S, Paggiarino DA, Crockett S, Schubert MM, Senzer NN, et al. Benzydamine HCl for prophylaxis of radiation-induced oral mucositis: Results from a multicenter, randomized, double-blind, placebo-controlled clinical trial. Cancer. 2001;**92**:875-885

[60] Halyard M. Taste and smell alterations in cancer patients—Real problems with few solutions. Journal of Supportive Care in Cancer. 2009;**7**(2):68-69

[61] Heckmann SM, Hujoel P, Habiger S, et al. Zinc gluconate in the treatment of dysgeusia—A randomized clinical trial. Journal of Dental Research. 2005;**84**(1):35-38

[62] Komaki R, Lee JS, Milas L, et al. Effects of amifostine on acute toxicity from concurrent chemotherapy and radiotherapy for inoperable non-small-cell lung cancer: Report of a randomized comparative trial. International Journal of Radiation Oncology, Biology, Physics. 2004;**58**(5):1369-1377

[63] Büntzel J, Schuth J, Küttner K, Glatzel M. Radiochemotherapy with amifostine cytoprotection for head and neck cancer. Support Care Cancer. 1998;**6**(2):155-160

[64] Ravasco P, Monteiro-Grillo I, Marques Vidal P, Camilo ME. Impact of nutrition on outcome: A prospective randomized controlled trial in patients with head and neck cancer undergoing radiotherapy. Head Neck. 2005;**27**:659-668

[65] Mercadante V, Al Hamad A, Lodi G, Porter S, Fedele S. Interventions for the management of radiotherapy-induced xerostomia and hyposalivation: A systematic review and meta-analysis. Oral Oncology. 2017;**66**:64-74

[66] Hsiung CY, Ting HM, Huang HY, Lee CH, Huang EY, Hsu HC. Parotid-sparing intensity-modulated radiotherapy (IMRT) for nasopharyngeal carcinoma: Preserved parotid function after IMRT on quantitative salivary scintigraphy, and comparison with historical data after conventional radiotherapy. International Journal of Radiation Oncology, Biology, Physics. 2006;**66**:454-461

[67] Graff P, Lapeyre M, Desandes E, Ortholan C, Bensadoun RJ, Alfonsi M. Impact of intensity-modulated radiotherapy on health-related quality of life for head and neck cancer patients: Matched-pair comparison with conventional radiotherapy. International Journal of Radiation Oncology, Biology, Physics. 2007;**67**:1309-1317

[68] Keefe DM, Schubert MM, Elting LS, et al. Updated clinical practice guidelines for the prevention and treatment of mucositis. Cancer. 2007;**109**(5):820-831

[69] Shiboski CH, Hodgson TA, Ship JA, Schiødt M. Management of salivary hypofunction during and after radiotherapy. Oral Surgery, Oral Medicine, Oral Pathology and Oral Radiology. 2007;**103**(suppl 1):S66.e1-S66.e19

[70] National Cancer Institute. PDQ® Cancer Information Summaries. Oral Complications of Chemotherapy and Head/Neck Radiation [Internet]. Available from: http://www.cancer.gov/cancertopics/pdq/supportivecare/oralcomplications/healthprofessional

[71] Hong CH, Napeñas JJ, Hodgson BD, et al. Dental Disease Section, Oral Care Study Group, Multi-national Association of Supportive Care in Cancer (MASCC)/International Society of Oral Oncology (ISOO). A systematic review of dental disease in patients undergoing cancer therapy. Support Care Cancer. 2010;**18**(8):1007-1021

[72] Meurman JH, Laine P, Murtomaa H, et al. Effect of antiseptic mouthwashes on some clinical and microbiological findings in the mouths of lymphoma patients receiving cytostatic drugs. Journal of Clinical Periodontology. 1991;**18**:587-591

[73] Joyston-Bechal S, Hayes K, Davenport ES, Hardie JM. Caries incidence, mutans streptococci and lactobacilli in irradiated patients during a 12-month preventive programme using chlorhexidine and fluoride. Caries Research. 1992;**26**:384-390

[74] McComb D, Erickson RL, Maxymiw WG, Wood RE. A clinical comparison of glass ionomer, resin-modified glass ionomer and resin composite restorations in the treatment of cervical caries in xerostomic head and neck radiation patients. Operative Dentistry. 2002;**27**:430-437

[75] Melchers LJ, Van Weert E, Beurskens CH, et al. Exercise adherence in patients with trismus due to head and neck oncology: A qualitative study into the use of the Therabite. International Journal of Oral and Maxillofacial Surgery. 2009;**38**:947-954

[76] Chua DT, Lo C, Yuen J, Foo YC. A pilot study of pentoxifylline in the treatment of radiation-induced trismus. American Journal of Clinical Oncology. 2001;**24**:366-369

[77] Hartl DM, Cohen M, Juliéron M, Marandas P, Janot F, Bourhis J. Botulinum toxin for radiation-induced facial pain and trismus. Otolaryngology–Head and Neck Surgery. 2008;**138**:459-163

[78] Nabil S, Samman N. Incidence and prevention of osteoradionecrosis after dental extraction in irradiated patients: A systematic review. International Journal of Oral and Maxillofacial Surgery. 2011;**40**(3):229-243

[79] Bennett MH1, Feldmeier J, Hampson NB, Smee R, Milross C. Hyperbaric oxygen therapy for late radiation tissue injury. The Cochrane Database of Systematic Reviews. 2016;**4**:CD005005

[80] Costa DA, Costa TP, Netto EC, Joaquim N, Ventura I, Pratas AC, et al. New perspectives on the conservative management of osteoradionecrosis of the mandible: A literature review. Head Neck. 2016;**38**(11):1708-1716

[81] Nadella KR, Kodali RM, Guttikonda LK, Jonnalagadda A. Osteoradionecrosis of the jaws: Clinico-therapeutic management: A literature review and update. Journal of Maxillofacial and Oral Surgery. 2015;**14**(4):891-901

[82] Rice N, Polyzois I, Ekanayake K, Omer O, Stassen LF. The management of osteoradionecrosis of the jaws—A review. Surgeon. 2015;**13**(2):101-109

6

Human Papillomavirus in Head and Neck Cancer

Makbule Tambas, Musa Altun and Deniz Tural

Abstract

Throughout the last three decades, there has been a notable shift in the epidemiology of head and neck cancer (HNC) worldwide. A rapidly spreading subtype of HNCs is caused by human papillomavirus (HPV) infection. HPV-related cancers are now considered to constitute 30–65% of all HNC cases and 50–80% of oropharyngeal cancers. HPV-positive oropharyngeal cancers have a unique demographic profile and tumor biology characteristics. HPV-associated patients predominantly consist of younger men with better performance status and fewer comorbid diseases. They have better dentition, higher numbers of oral sex partners, and use less amount of tobacco or alcohol, higher amount of marijuana compared with HPV-negative patients. In addition, patients with HPV-positive tumors have a 60–80% reduced mortality rates, a finding that was confirmed by multiple trials and led to several ongoing deintensification studies. This chapter describes epidemiologic features of HPV-positive HNC, risk factors for HPV infection and HPV-associated oropharyngeal cancer, HPV detection methods, mechanisms of carcinogenesis and improved treatment response, and the impact of HPV status on clinical outcome as well as deintensification approaches and potential of vaccination.

Keywords: head and neck cancer, human papillomavirus, epidemiology, carcinogenesis, treatment

1. Introduction

Head and neck cancer (HNC) involves a wide field of tumors that originate from the skull base to the clavicles including the orbits, paranasal sinuses, nasopharynx, oropharynx, hypopharynx, oral cavity, and larynx. Worldwide, the incidence of HNC accounts for more than half a million each year, 5% of all cancer cases, with being the fifth most common cancer in the world [1, 2]. The distribution of HNC varies around world, such that it is 3–4% of all cancer diagnosed in North America and the Europe, whereas HNC consists of 30% of all cancer cases in men in India [3]. Yet, around 300,000 people die from HNC that can be seen in the global picture of the disease [4].

The well-known risk factors for HNC comprise tobacco, alcohol, poor oral health, human papillomavirus (HPV) infection (for oropharyngeal cancer), and Epstein-Barr virus (EBV) infection (for nasopharyngeal carcinoma) [5, 6]. Traditionally, HNC was related to tobacco use and alcohol exposure, and the synergistic increased risk with the combination of them [7]. HNCs are most common among 50–60 year-old individuals who are heavy smokers and alcohol users with lower socioeconomic status [8]. Additionally, the squamous cell carcinoma constitutes more than 90% of histological subtype of HNC [1].

2. Epidemiology

2.1. Changing trends in epidemiology of HPV-associated HNCs

Throughout the last three decades, there has been a notable shift in the epidemiology of HNC worldwide. The decrease in tobacco consumption has resulted in an entire reduction in the incidence of HNC during the past 30 years [9]. Since smoking maintains as the primary risk factor for the oral cavity, larynx, and hypopharynx, this declining trend is marked for these sites. However, up to 25% of all HNCs recently diagnosed are not related to tobacco use. A rapidly spreading subtype of HNCs is caused by HPV infection [10].

First suggested in 1983 by Syrjanen, HPV was reported as an initiative factor of HNC owing to its oncogenic potential, the parallel clinical characteristics in oral and genital damages, epithelia similarities, and HPV affinity for epithelial cells [11]. The evidence for a significant correlation was insufficient, until recently. In the 2000s, several reports, mainly from Sweden, established that a remarkable ratio of tonsillar cancers included HPV DNA. The increases by 2.8- and 2.9-fold were detected in the incidence of tonsillar cancer and ratio (23–68%) of HPV-positive tonsillar cancer between 1970 and 2002, in Sweden, in 2006 [12]. Immediately after this, in 2007, an arising HPV epidemic correlating with oropharyngeal SCC was reported in the United States [13]. The striking increases up to sevenfold in both HPV-positive tonsillar and base of tongue were demonstrated during the periods of 1970–2007 and 1998–2006 in 2009 and 2010 from Sweden, respectively [14, 15]. Following Dalianis group definition of "epidemic of viral-induced carcinoma," due to observation that most of the tonsillar carcinomas were HPV-associated in 2009 [14], a retrospective analysis of clinical trial material detected that HPV-related oropharyngeal cancer rate was 64% in the USA [16]. Similar retrospective analyses on oropharyngeal tumor samples revealed an increase in HPV incidence from 23, 28 to 57% from 1970s, 1980s to 1990s, respectively. Also, a constant trend in the increase was detected for recent term (68, 77, 93% incidence rates during 2000–2002, 2003–2005, 2006–2007, respectively [14]. Similarly, HPV association rate in oropharyngeal cases was increased from 16% to 73%, from 1984–1989 to 2000–2004 in the United States [17]. Furthermore, during the same periods, reports delivering similar striking rises in both oropharyngeal and HPV-positive oropharyngeal cancers have accumulated from several Western countries [3, 12–15, 17–23].

The oropharynx is distinctively sensitive to HPV, and as high as 70% of oropharyngeal cancers in the USA are HPV-related oropharyngeal squamous cell carcinomas [24]. The past 30-year Surveillance, Epidemiology, and End Results (SEER) population-based data were analyzed by Chaturvedi et al, and they evaluated the incidence trends of HPV-related and -unrelated HNC. They demonstrated a significant decline (1.85% annual reduction) in the incidence of HNC in HPV-unrelated fields (hypopharynx, oral cavity, larynx) and a remarkable rise (0.8% annual increase) in the incidence of HNC in HPV-associated oropharyngeal regions during the same period [9]. In addition, the incidence of hypopharyngeal, oral cavity, and laryngeal carcinomas notably reduced due to smoking and alcohol consumption declining in many countries [25]. On the contrary, the oropharyngeal carcinoma incidence has been reported to be increased in many countries including the UK [26], Canada [27], Australia [28], Norway [29], Denmark [30], and the Netherlands [20] over the last two decades, besides Sweden [12] and the USA [9]. HPV-related cancers are now considered to constitute 30–65% of all HNC cases and 50–80% of oropharyngeal cancers [9, 16]. HPV-positive HNC, which has distinctive epidemiologic and prognostic features [5–14] has become an expanding public health issue, is expected to be the main factor for HNC development in the forthcoming period [17].

Currently, the highest HPV-positive HNC incidence rates have been reported in Sweden and the USA. The genital HPV infection prevalence, sexual habits, and smoking and alcohol use may affect the population-specific HPV-positive HNC incidences. The focus of HPV-related malignancies has been shifted from anogenital cancers developing predominantly in women to oropharyngeal cancers developing mainly in men due to the fact that men were reported to have >70% HPV-positive oropharyngeal cancer cases [9, 12, 15, 16, 20–22]. By 2020, the number of HPV-mediated oropharyngeal patients per year is reflected to outnumber HPV-related cervical cancer cases in the USA [17]. The HPV-mediated oropharyngeal cancer has become an epidemic of our era [31].

2.2. HPV positivity in non-oropharyngeal sites of HNC

HPV detection rates were currently reported to be between 12.6% and 90.9% in oropharyngeal carcinoma [32]. One-quarter to one-half of unknown primaries originates from oropharyngeal region [33, 34] and the HPV presence in cervical lymph node metastases is a strong marker of oropharyngeal subsite for unknown primary regions [33, 35]. Although the association between oropharyngeal carcinoma (predominantly soft palate, the tonsils, base of tongue) and HPV is well known, the role of HPV in other head and neck subsites etiology is not well established. The presence of HPV DNA was not demonstrated in laryngeal, nasopharyngeal, hypopharyngeal, and oral cavity cancers in older studies, whereas recently published studies using more advanced methodologies and analyzed HPV gene expression products (e.g., p16) reported that HPV existed in non-oropharyngeal sites in small proportions which explains the increased incidence of oropharyngeal carcinoma compared with other HNCs [1, 36–38].

The prevalence of HPV-mediated HNCs was found as 25.9% in a systematic review of 60 published studies using PCR-based methods while it was higher in oropharyngeal carcinoma (35.6%) than both oral (23.5%) and laryngeal (24.0%) carcinoma. HPV-16 and the second most common high-risk type HPV-18 were detected in 86.7% and only 2.8% of the HPV-positive oropharyngeal carcinoma [39]. In addition, in a meta-analysis of 39 publications with 3649 HNC patients which investigated HPV in European population, the prevalence of HPV was found to be 40.0%, while it was most dominant in tonsillar cancer (66.4%) and lowest in pharyngeal (15.3%) and tongue (25.7%) cancers [36].

Unlike oropharyngeal cancers, HPV etiologic role in other HNC sites remains unclear. Concerning other head and neck subsites, HPV may play a role in the supraglottic larynx cancer [40], which might constitute the high-risk HPV infection rate established in laryngeal cancer, since its marginal field is adjacent with the oropharynx [28, 29, 41, 42]. Overall, contemporary studies using gold standard methods (type-specific HPV E6/E7 mRNA) from the United States detected the presence of HPV in less than 5% of non-oropharyngeal HNCs [17, 43]. Nevertheless, the estimate for the HPV infection-mediated non-oropharyngeal HNCs varies widely in the literature. While the estimated prevalence of HPV is 24% in the larynx, 31% in the nasopharynx, oral cavity 6–20%, and 21% in the sinonasal tract [44, 45], the studies mainly from the USA based on *in situ* hybridization (ISH) assays and E6/E7 mRNA detection suggest that the HPV association was found in 3% of oral cavity, 7% of larynx, and 0% of hypopharynx cancers [43]. Many factors including the border of anatomic classification of head and neck subsites and HPV detection methods contribute to this instability. The identification of certain markers of HPV-induced carcinogenesis and the correct rule out of the oropharynx as tumor origin site are substantial forthcoming issues in HPV-related non-oropharyngeal HNC estimation [43]. In addition, another topic which remains to be clarified is whether HPV tumor status in non-oropharyngeal sites may be implicated as a strong independent prognostic indicator such as in oropharyngeal cancers [16, 46–48].

2.3. The characteristics of HPV-positive HNC cancer patients

The demographic and risk features of HPV-positive and HPV-negative HNC patients differ remarkably. First, HPV(+) patients are younger than HPV(−) ones [49]. The HPV-related cancers develop in those aged 40–55 [50] who are 4–10 years younger than HPV-negative patients [16, 51]. This age difference might explain the increase in oropharyngeal cancer incidence in younger individuals in developed countries [17, 52]. Given that HPV-associated patients are younger at diagnosis, they have better performance status [16, 47, 50] with fewer comorbid diseases [16, 51, 53].

Second, although HNC is generally more common in men than women, a notably larger rate of HPV-positive oropharyngeal cancer is diagnosed in men than HPV-negative ones [17]. This is convenient with the data that oral HPV16 infection is five times more common in men compared with women in the USA [54].

Third, HPV-HNC has been found to develop more frequently in white than black patients. HPV-positivity rate is 29–34% in whites compared to only 0–4% in blacks [55, 56], while HPV-positive versus -negative rumors occurring in whites are 92–97% and 75–78%, respectively [16, 46, 55]. Thus, in contrast to blacks, the incidence of oropharyngeal cancer has increased in whites which is probably caused by higher HPV-HNC rates in whites compared with blacks in the USA [57]. Furthermore, the socioeconomic status differs in HPV-positive patients from

HPV-negative ones. HPV-positive patients have higher income and are more educated with higher rates of being married [51, 54].

The HPV-positive HNC patients have better dentition, higher numbers of oral sex partners, and use less amount of tobacco or alcohol, higher amount of marijuana compared with HPV-negative patients. In addition, these risk factors have a powerful dose effect, revealing the distinguishing risk profile for HPV-positive patients [17]. Furthermore, these patients without environmental risk factors have persistent infection with high-risk HPVs [17].

3. Risk factors for HPV infection and HPV(+) oropharyngeal cancers

HPV-16 which is detected in about 90% of the HPV(+) oropharyngeal cancers is the most common among several high-risk HPV types. Currently, HPV-16 is the only HPV type which is accepted as cancer inducing in the HNC [58, 59]. In addition, there are other high-risk HPV types with a less significant function and different manner than HPV-16 [37]. Among these, HPV-58, HPV-35, HPV-33, and HPV- 45 were detected in 10–15% of HPV(+) oropharyngeal cancer [38, 60, 61]. At present, HPV 16 constitutes 15- to 230-fold increased risk for oropharyngeal cancer [50, 62]. HPV has been confirmed to induce and promote the development of oropharyngeal cancer [63].

With the identification of HPV as a powerful and independent risk factor for HNC, data are accumulating concerning the oral HPV infection epidemiology. The prevalence of oral HPV infection has been estimated as 7% in population-based studies in the United States and significantly correlated with male gender, older age, current smoking, and various sexual habits (e.g., the number of oral sexual partners during lifetime) [54]. HPV infection which may be contaminated by any type of sexual contact has become the most frequent disease that transmits sexually in the world [64]. The estimated number of individuals who are currently infected and expected to be infected each year is 20 million and 6.2 million in the United States alone [65]. Even though the orally infected rate among the population aged between 14 and 69 (10% of men, 4% of women) is 7%, the cancer-causing HPV subtypes consist of only 1% of these infections [54].

HPV-infected persons are unaware of the infection, since there are no correlated signs or symptoms. No effective treatment has been developed for active HPV infection, currently. Fortunately, the virus will be cleared in most of the infected persons within 2 years. It remains unknown how to identify those in whom the infection will become chronic and progress to HPV-HNC in time. Since the most of carcinogenesis occurs deep in the crypts of the tonsils where simple "Pap smear equivalents" are inaccessible in contrast to anus or cervix, an efficient screening test for early detection of HPV-related oropharyngeal cancer does not exist, yet [31].

Marijuana smoking has been shown to be an independent risk factor for HPV-mediated HNC, while the duration, intensity, and total years of marijuana use increase the risk. Marijuana use is suggested to cause oropharyngeal cancer development since the cannabinoids bind to the

CB2 receptor of immune modulatory cells found in the tonsillar tissue which results in reduced immune response, lower resistance to viral infections, and antitumor functions [66].

It has been shown that HPV is less frequent in ex-, current-smokers, and tobacco chewers than nonsmokers and nonchewers [67]. Interestingly, in contrast to HPV(−) HNC, HPV(+) HNC decreases with increasing lifetime tobacco consumption [50]. On the one hand, rates of past and current tobacco use in HPV-oropharyngeal squamous cell carcinoma (OSCC) are reported to be 65% as opposed to 74% in HPV-negative OSCCs [6]. On the other hand, oral HPV infection presence is separately correlated with current smoking, but not lifetime smoking history [54]. Similarly, heavy alcohol consumption is less common in HPV(+) HNC patients compared with HPV-negative HNC ones [50]. Although heavy alcohol use (>21 drinks per week) is related to increased incidence of both HPV(+) and HPV(−) HNC, it is not correlated with oral HPV infection with the adjustment for sexual habits [54]. The complex role of alcohol remains to be identified.

Other significant factors in the increasing incidence of HPV infection and HPV(+) HNC are the changes in sexual behaviors, early sex debut, and number of oral-vaginal partners [68]. In addition, oral-oral contact and HPV transmission at birth may also lead to oral HPV infection [69, 70]. HPV transmits mainly through sexual contact directly with vaginal or anal intercourse, oral sex, or any mucosal contact. Also, oral HPV infection is more correlated with a genital HPV infection status, compared with oral sex activity in young males, suggesting autoinoculation as a potential HPV transmission route [71]. The first sexual encounter at younger ages, increasing number of sexual partners as well as more oral sex are reported by Americans [72, 73]. Additionally, the lifetime prevalence of oral sex was reported to be increased from 50% in 1970 to 90% in 2006 in a French study [73]. Furthermore, HPV exposure increases the HNC development risk, and HPV-16 seropositivity leads to cancer development 9 years earlier [74].

4. Diagnosis and histopathology

4.1. Clinical and pathologic presentation

An asymptomatic neck mass is the presentation of the disease in up to 90% of HPV(+) oropharyngeal cancer patients [75]. The neck nodes are generally in cystic structure which results in nondiagnostic aspiration materials. The diagnosis may be delayed due to no suspicious history because of being a nonsmoker, insufficient examination, and non-diagnostic aspirates of cystic lymph nodes. Ultrasound-guided fine-needle aspirates taken from cystic neck nodes may increase the chance of early diagnosis [76]. The utility of HPV detection in theses aspirates using p16 immunohistochemistry (IHC) and ISH has been shown [77]. In cases of unknown primary, a palatine and/or lingual tonsillectomy is superior to random biopsies.

HPV(+) oropharyngeal carcinoma exhibits a nonkeratinizing, basaloid, well-differentiated histology with diffuse nuclear and cytoplasmic p16 staining [66]. The HPV-positive tumor pathologic properties differ from HPV-negative ones showing lobular growth, having infiltrating lymphocytes, but not surface dysplasia or keratinization [66]. In addition, HPV-positive tumors present frequently with smaller primary tumors but advanced nodal metastasis [46, 50]. Despite being not pathognomonic, major histopathological features of HPV-mediated tumors are the presence of classic koilocytes, perinuclear cytoplasmic halos, nuclear dysplasia with the addition of presence of dyskeratosis, atypical immature metaplasia, macrocytes, and binucleation as minor properties [78].

4.2. HPV detection tests/methods

The detection of cyclin-dependent kinase inhibitor 2A (p16Ink4A or p16) by IHC is recognized as a standard test for HPV positivity in a tumor in many clinics and during clinical trial enrollment. The HPV-16 E7 protein downregulates Rb and frees E2F, its regulatory partner which upregulates p16. IHC detection of p16 is a fast, cheap, and easily available method and is the standard method for HPV status assessment in clinics [79].With a false-negative rate of 4%, p16 IHC is a reliable marker in HPV infection, given that strong nuclear and cytoplasmic staining is extremely predictive for HPV(+) HNC [80]. By contrast, in cases with intermediate p16 expression levels, ISH or reverse transcription-polymerase chain reaction (RT-PCR) is required [80]. The inability of PCR-based assays to distinguish integrated DNA from episomal viral DNA decreases the test specificity remarkably in contrast to ISH in which sensitivity is lower compared to PCR [81]. Furthermore, the RNA ISH E6/E7 microRNA probes enable the direct scanning of viral transcripts which means accurate HPV detection [82]. It may be used as a HPV confirmation test in p16-positive samples, due to the fact that p16 is also overexpressed in non-virally induced situations. Given the different survival rates of the p16(+)/HPV(−) subgroups, considering personalized approaches, these patients should be evaluated as a distinct subcategory that is why using both ISH and p16 is recommended for HPV assessment [83]. In a recent study, which used both three methods, the sensitivity of p16 was detected as 100%, whereas its specificity was 74% in oral cancer and 93% in oropharyngeal cancer [84]. Cancer Care Ontario recommends routine HPV test in oropharyngeal cancer, in metastatic cervical nodes from an unknown head and neck primary and the use of p16 IHC as an initial test for its high sensitivity in patients with HNC [31].

Antibodies against HPV in the serum can be used to measure the cumulative exposure to HPV infection [85]. HPV16 E6 or E7 antibodies were detected in 65% of HPV(+) oropharyngeal cancer patients which indicates that they are useful tools as HPV markers in the unavailability of appropriate cytologic or histologic materials [67]. The detection of HPV antibodies in saliva instead of serum may lead to common false negative results, since antibodies in oral sampling are fewer compared with those in serum [85].

Currently, several methods including The Roche linear array HPV genotyping test, the Hybrid Capture 2, and a PCR bead-based multiplex method present for HPV typing [86–88]. Nevertheless, since E6 and E7 mRNA by RT-PCR demonstrate functional HPV expression, it is widely accepted as the gold standard [89]. The correlation between the steps of HPV infection to cell, detection targets, and methods is shown in **Table 1**.

Step	HPV infection	Detection target	Suitable methods
1	HPV endocytosis HPV episome HPV DNA integration	DNA detection	PCR ISH
2	E6 mRNA E7 mRNA	RNA detection	PCR ISH
3	Protein E6 Protein E7	Oncoprotein detection	Monoclonal antibodies
4	Rb:E2F P16	P16 overexpression detection	Monoclonal antibodies

Table 1. Correlation between the steps of HPV infection to cell, detection targets and methods.

5. Carcinogenesis

Currently, HPVs consist of over 81 different subtypes of HPVs classified on the basis of their L1 protein, separated based on cutaneous and mucosal site tropism, and divided in low-, and high-risk viruses according to correlation with cancers [90]. The high-risk HPV types may be classified as follows: highest risk types (HPV 16, 18, 31, 45), other high-risk types (HPV 33, 35, 39, 51, 52, 56, 58, 59), and probably high-risk types (HPV 26, 53, 66, 68, 73, 82). Oncogenic HPV types 16, 18, 31, 33, and 35 are related to HPV(+) HNC, while HPV-16 is most frequently found in oropharyngeal cancer [91, 92]. Majority of the cases of HPV(+) HNC arise from the oropharyngeal region due to epithelial injury predisposition of its location and lack of protective keratin layer that leads to easy virus exposure of the basal cells [93].

HPVs are circular, non-enveloped, epitheliotrophic, double-stranded DNA viruses belonging to family *Papovaviridae* with an approximately 8000 base pair-sized viral genome carrying early open-reading frame (ORF), late ORF, and noncoding control region between these two regions with histones within a 52–55-nm virion [94]. HPV genome encodes two structural capsid proteins (L1 and L2), two regulatory proteins (E1, E2), three oncoproteins (E5, E6, E7) [94]. The early region encodes the regulatory proteins, E1-E2, E4-E7, which are responsible for gene regulation, replication, and pathogenesis, while the late region encodes the two structural proteins, L1, L2, which form the viral capsid and have no known role in carcinogenesis but are substantial immune response targets to HPV infection. The E4 protein is thought to ease viral particle release into the surroundings and be responsible for G2 arrest in HPV-infected cells [95, 96].

The best-known relation between high-risk HPVs and cancer is established for the uterine cervix. However, HPV is also correlated with vaginal, vulvar, anal, and penile cancers, and especially since 2007, it has also been demonstrated to be a risk factor for oropharyngeal cancer [15, 95, 96]. HPV-16 and HPV-18 remain the main mediating factors in most HPV-related cancers. For instance, they are associated with 70% of cases with cervical cancer [94]. Approximately 50% of penile cancers include HPV DNA, predominantly HPV-16 [93], while HPV-16 accounts for more than 90% of HPV(+) oropharyngeal cancers [74].

The palatine and lingual tonsils are predominant targets of HPV among all other potential sites of HNC. The basal cells are infected by HPV in the stratified squamous epithelium. The reticulated lymphoepithelium of tonsillar crypts expresses programmed death ligand 1 (PD-L1), which suppresses response of T-cells against HPV, and leads to an "immune-privileged" region for viral infection initiation and adaptation to immune resistance [97]. Virus enters through microinjuries in the epithelium, although the receptor and mechanism of this entry remain unknown. Prior to virus entry to the cell by endocytosis, heparin sulfate is considered to mediate the virus particle attachment to the cell [98]. HPV infection of epithelial cells causes different types of viral protein expression and production of 20 to 100 and thousands of viral DNA per cell in the basal layer and superficial layers, respectively [98]. While majority of other virus infections result in the production of progeny from the same target cell, the HPV-infected cells undergo mitosis and continue differentiation [99]. Thus, basal cells are not the only proliferating cells in the infected epithelium since infected suprabasal cells have active cell cycle and differentiation [100].

The three HPV oncoproteins E5, E6, and E7 promote uncontrolled cellular proliferation to lead viral amplification, initiate, and contribute to progression of cancer through the same mechanism and induce genomic instability [101–103]. As in cervical cancer, E6 and E7 oncoproteins are mainly responsible for the malignant transformation and progression in HNCs [101, 102]. Since silencing the E6 and E7 oncogene expression in HPV16(+) human oropharyngeal squamous cell lines led to p53 and Rb tumor suppressor activation and apoptosis induction, these two oncoproteins are thought to be required for maintaining malignant processes [104].

High-risk HPV E7 oncoproteins play a critical role in initiating DNA synthesis by binding and inactivating the Rb and its related pocket proteins p107 and p130 which are tumor suppressor genes by targeting them for degradation [98]. Rb, the most well-known pocket protein family member functions to prevent excessive cell growth by inhibiting cell cycle progression [105]. The Rb inactivation by E7 causes E2F transcription factor overexpression with the cell cycle gene upregulation, leading to the cell transition from G1 to S phase [106]. The inactivation of pRb increases levels of p16/CDKN2A which is an inhibitor of cdk4/cyclin D and cdk6/cyclin D and promotes aberrant cell proliferation [107]. Thus, increased levels of p16/CDKN2A expression correspond as a diagnostic biomarker for transcriptionally active HPV infection and virus-mediated deregulation of cell cycle [108]. E7 oncoproteins also have ability to affect gene transcription by influencing histone acetylation in regulatory regions via either histone acetyl transferases or histone deacetylases [109].

E7-mediated proliferation results in the activation of p53-dependent growth inhibition and apoptosis. To counteract this, HPV E6 causes p53 degradation which leads to apoptosis inhibition and uncontrolled cellular growth as a consequence [101]. E6 transcript produces a 19-kDa protein that binds with a ubiquitin protein ligase (E6AP) that will result in p53 tumor suppressor protein ubiquitination (posttranslational modification) and proteosomal degradation [101]. The p53 regulates the cell cycle by controlling the transition from G1 to the S phase at checkpoint by inducing cyclin inhibitor (p16, p21, and p27) expression [110]. Hence, E6 oncoprotein deregulates cell cycle checkpoints both at G1/S and G2/M in the case of cellular stress such as DNA damage which results in genomic instability. Moreover, E6 protein has the ability to downregulate p53 function either by direct binding or by interacting with the histone acetyltransferases (ADA3) and histone acetyltransferase binding proteins (p300 and CREB) [111, 112]. In addition, it can associate with *ras* and E7 for *in vitro* cell transformation [113]. Furthermore, E6 oncoprotein can activate cellular telomerase by upregulating human telomerase hTERT which leads to cellular immortalization [114]. E6 targets not only p53, but also Bak and Myc proteins which regulate apoptosis [115].

Additionally, the E5 protein works together with E6 and E7 to induce proliferation in infected cells and is considered to have a more minor role in host cell transformation. It also blocks apoptosis in the late process of HPV-induced carcinogenesis [103].

Several studies report that both E6 and E7 bind multiple complementary cooperators that perform oncogenic impacts other than p53 and pRb degradation. Despite the robust growth inducing functions of these HPV oncoproteins, extra oncogenic events are required for malignant development. Although high-risk E6 and E7 cause genomic instability [116], the mutation rate in HPV(+) tumors seem to be lower than in HPV(−) ones [59, 117]. E6 and E7 oncoproteins may lead to chromosomal segregation errors and aneuploidy development during mitosis [118]. Due to the E7 induction of CDK2 activation, multiple immature centrioles are formed which results in several centrosome synthesis rounds [119]. Eventually, E6 and E7 cause these cells with aberrant mitoses to proliferate by inhibiting G2-M checkpoint control and apoptosis [120].

It has been demonstrated that HPV-mediated carcinogenesis causes significantly fewer genomic changes than HPV-independent ones. Particularly, HPV(+) HNC is associated with less mutated p53, higher EGFR expression, and more chromosomal aberrations (3p, 9p, and 17p) [63, 121–123]. It has been confirmed by whole-exome sequencing of HNC that HPV(+) HNC has a distinct genetic entity from HPV(−) HNC which has more mutations compared with HPV(+) ones, independent of smoking [59, 117]. While HPV(+) tumors have no p53 mutation, p53 mutation rate was 78% in HPV(−) cancers [59]. These data indicate that HPV-mediated oncogenesis is correlated with cellular dysregulation to a lesser degree which may be the underlying explanation of better treatment response. HPV(+) tumor differs from HPV(−) HNC not only biologically, but also clinically. They tend to present at earlier T stage with extensive nodal involvement. Despite the fact that distant metastasis may constitute a major problem in HPV(+) tumors, their prognosis is better, especially in locally advanced diseases [124].

6. Mechanisms of improved response to treatment

The prognostic advantage of HPV positivity may be explained to some extent by the patient population features affected with younger age, higher performance status, fewer comorbid diseases, and less tobacco and alcohol exposure. However, after adjustment to these conditions in multivariate analyses, the improved survival of HPV(+) patients still maintains [16, 46].

Actually, these factors only account for approximately 9% of the survival difference between patients with HPV(+) and HPV(−) tumors, which means that the survival difference seems to be largely resulted by HPV status [16, 125]. It is clear that the higher response rate of HPV(+) tumor to therapy is caused by a basic biological difference between HPV(+) and HPV(−) HNCs. It is accepted that intrinsic factors of each individual tumor (e.g., mutations, HPV status) may modulate the microenvironment of tumors [126]. These alterations have the ability to influence immune response, stromal structure, and tumor vasculature [126]. Not only experimental studies but also several clinical studies have demonstrated that patients with HPV/p16(+) tumors had a much better prognosis compared with HPV/p16(−) ones [16].

It has been suggested that the immune system plays a significant role in rejection process of HPV(+) tumors because of viral protein expressions that reveal T-cell responses performing a long-term immunosurveillance. Accumulating evidence over the years appears to reinforce this hypothesis. Spanos et al. [127] showed superior tumor control in HPV(+) cell lines implanted into immunocompetent mice compared with immunocompromised mice [127]. HPV-specific circulating HPV16 E7-specific CD8+ T cells and IFNγ-producing T cells have been defined in patients with HPV(+) HNC [128]. A greater alteration from naive to effector and memory T cells has been shown in patients with HPV(+) compared with both healthy donors and patients with HPV(−) tumors which indicates higher tumor response in HPV(+) patients [129]. In addition, it has been reported that the programmed death-1 (PD-1) positive T-cell presence was associated with improved survival in HPV(+) HNC patients [130]. Moreover, circulating anti-HPV16 antibodies which are suggested to associate with clinical outcome have been detected in HPV(+) HNC patients [92]. Furthermore, radiation may induce expression loss of CD47 which is an important transmembrane cell surface marker in self-identification in HPV(+) cell lines that explains the interaction between the immune system and radiotherapy [131].

Even though radiosensitivity is mainly based on the cell ability to detect DNA damage and repair it, tumor oxygenation status may also be a factor for radiotherapy response [132]. In this context, in the Danish Head and Neck Cancer Group (DAHANCA)-5 study, the ratio of patients with high plasma osteopontin (a marker of hypoxia) levels was greater in HPV(−) tumors than in HPV(+) ones, indicating more hypoxia in HPV(−) group [133]. On the contrary, neither IHC staining for carbonic anhydrase IX (upregulated in hypoxic conditions) nor pO2 level of tumor was found to associate with HPV status of tumor in another study [134].

In two prospective trials investigating the impact of hypoxic modification (using nimorazole or tirapazamine) in HNC, the use of hypoxic cell radiosensitizer provided a trend toward better locoregional control in HPV(−) tumors but had no significant benefit in HPV(+) tumors [53, 135]. Surprisingly, HPV/p16-positive tumors appeared to be insensible to hypoxic modifier and revealed no benefit from nimorazole after which was suggested that HPV/p16(+) HNCs are less hypoxic than HPV(−) ones, and this might contribute to the better prognosis [135]. However, in studies evaluating the hypoxia with imaging markers including (18)F-fluoroazomycin arabinoside positron emission tomography/computed tomography (FAZA PET/CT)), dynamic contrast enhanced-MRI (DCE-MRI), and proton magnetic resonance spectroscopy ((1)H-MRS), no correlation between HPV positivity and intratumoral hypoxia was detected [136, 137]. Additionally, recent *in vitro* evidence comparing radiation response of HPV/p16(+) and (−) cell lines under hypoxia showed no difference regarding gene regulation patterns, while oxygen enhancement ratio (OER) of HPV/p16(+) cells was found similar to HPV/p16(−) ones [138].

Finally, it has been hypothesized that viral oncoproteins play a substantial role in improved treatment sensitivity. It has been shown that low levels of residual wild-type p53 in HPV(+) cells may be activated by radiation, resulting in increased cell death [139]. Recently, Rieckman et al. [140] demonstrated decreased survival fraction, increased double strand breaks levels, and extensive G2 arrest pointing to compromised DNA repair capacity in HPV/p16(+) cell lines compared with HPV(−) cell lines after irradiation [140].

7. Clinical considerations

7.1. Impact of HPV on prognosis (clinical studies)

The changing epidemiology of HPV-positive oropharyngeal cancer formed a new patient population in the clinic that consists of individuals at younger ages without a heavy alcohol or smoking history and with more advanced neck diseases [141]. The natural history of HPV-positive HNC began to be written with many retrospective studies published in the late 1990s to early 2000s. In a study of 42 patients, HPV(+) tonsil cancer revealed higher survival rates compared with HPV(−) ones [142]. In addition, in a German study including 208 HNC sample patients with HPV(+) samples had better survival despite more adverse pathological results [143]. Furthermore, in a Swedish study with 60 patients, HPV(+) oropharyngeal cancer patients were found to have higher 5-year OS rates (53.5% vs. 31.5%) and reduced recurrence risk irrespective of gender, age, or disease stage [144]. Gillison et al. retrospectively analyzed 252 HNC patients in 2000, and patients with HPV(+) HNC from all sites had a 40% reduction in death risk ($p = 0.07$) and a 59% reduction in disease-related death risk ($p = 0.02$) after adjustment for age, nodal status, and alcohol consumption [63]. Finally, a meta-analysis of 37 studies analyzing HPV and HNC reported that HPV(+) oropharyngeal cancer patients had a 28% reduced death risk and a 49% lower disease-failure risk compared with HPV(−) ones in 2007 [145].

In the Danish DAHANCA-5 phase III clinical trial, samples from 156 patients of whom 74 were oropharyngeal cancer patients were collected prospectively. Of oropharyngeal cancer samples, 24 were p16(+) and had a locoregional control benefit (OR, 5.1) compared with those with p16(−) samples [146]. In a phase II prospective trial of 42 oropharyngeal cancer patients of whom pretreatment biopsy HPV-positivity rate was 67%, HPV titer was correlated with improved induction chemotherapy response ($p = 0.001$), chemoradiation response ($p = 0.005$), overall survival ($p = 0.007$), and disease-specific survival (DSS) ($p = 0.008$) [147]. Similarly, in the Trans-Tasman Radiation Oncology Group (TROG), 20.02 trial which retrospectively reviewed for HPV and p16 status, a higher 2-year overall survival rate (91% vs. 74%; HR, 0.36; $p = 0.004$) and failure-free survival (87% vs. 72%; HR, 0.39; $p = 0.003$) were detected in 57% of 185 oropharyngeal cancer patients with p16 positivity compared with HPV(−) patients [53].

Several studies have demonstrated the favorable effect of HPV positivity in oropharyngeal cancer patients [46, 53, 148]. First, in 2008, the Eastern Cooperative Oncology Group (ECOG) 2399 trial which was a phase II prospective study including stages III and IV, M0, oropharynx and larynx cancer patients treated with paclitaxel/carboplatin induction chemotherapy followed by concurrent paclitaxel and radiotherapy showed that patients with HPV(+) oropharyngeal cancer (HPV detection method was p16 IHC) had a 61% lower death risk (HR, 0.39; $p = 0.06$) and a 62% lower progression risk (HR, 0.38; $p = 0.09$) than patients with HPV(−) ones, after adjustments for age, ECOG performance status, and disease stage [46]. Following this, Ang et al. [16] reported the largest retrospective examination of Radiation Therapy Oncology Group (RTOG) 0129 study about HPV effect on survival in oropharyngeal cancer where HPV positivity was tested by ISH. The 3-year overall survival rates were 82.4% and 57.1% in the HPV(+) and HPV(−) subgroups, respectively, while the 3-year progression-free survival rates were similarly better in HPV(+) subgroup compared with HPV(−) ones (73.7% vs. 43.4%). In addition, HPV(+) patients had a 58% lower death risk (HR, 0.42; $p < 0.001$) and a 51% lower progression risk (HR, 0.49; $p < 0.001$). Furthermore, patients were classified into risk-of-death categories (low, moderate, high) based on a recursive partitioning analysis according to HPV status, tumor burden, and tobacco use. The low-risk group included patients with HPV(+) cancer with the exception of smokers with advanced nodal metastasis, while smoker patients with HPV(+) tumors and advanced nodal metastasis or nonsmoker patients HPV(−) tumors of stage T2 or T3 were considered to be at intermediate risk. On the contrary, nonsmoker patients with HPV(−) T4 tumors or smoker patients with HPV(−) tumors consisted of high-risk group while 3-year survival rates of low-, moderate-, and high-risk patients were 93%, 70.8%, and 46.2%, respectively. Importantly, smoking had a negative factor on prognosis, regardless of HPV status [16]. Similarly, in the retrospective analysis of TAX 324 trial, which investigated triple-agent versus double-agent induction chemotherapy confirmed the better prognosis of HPV(+) patients, 5-year overall survival rates were significantly higher in HPV(+) group compared with HPV(−) (82% vs. 35%, $p < 0.0001$). The HPV status was tested using E6/E7 PCR methods in this study [47].

The retrospective subanalysis of 190 patients with oropharyngeal cancer in the RTOG 9003 study, a 4-arm, phase III trial which compared different RT protocols, p16 positivity was found to correlate with T1 stage, better performance status, absence of anemia, and less tobacco consumption. Independently from assigned treatment, the p16(+) oropharyngeal cancer group had better 5-year overall and progression-free survival, lower 5-year locoregional failure but similar 5-year distant metastasis rates compared with p16(−) ones [149]. Additionally, a recently published retrospective analysis of RTOG 0129 and RTOG 0522 revealed that HPV(+)oropharyngeal cancer patients had better overall survival even after disease progression compared with HPV(−) group. Moreover, salvage surgery was detected to provide significantly improved prognosis [150]. Another recent retrospective subanalysis of the phase III trial, IMCL-9815 Bonner trial [53, 54], which evaluated the impact of the role of cetuximab addition to radiotherapy in patients with locally advanced HNC, based on HPV status determined by p16 IHC, p16 positivity was confirmed as a powerful prognostic determinant for oropharyngeal cancer patients [151].

Likewise, surgical reports further confirmed the favorable effect of p16 positivity in oropharyngeal cancer. Rich et al. [148] reported that in a cohort of 84 stage III or IV oropharyngeal cancers, patients who received transoral laser microsurgery (TLM) ± adjuvant therapy, p16 positivity was significantly associated with higher 5-year overall survival (90% vs. 25%, $p < 0.0001$) and disease-specific survival (DSS) rates (94% vs. 50%, $p = 0.0078$) [148]. Furthermore, two recent meta-analysis of clinical trial data of oropharyngeal cancer patients demonstrated hazard ratios for better overall survival of 0.49 and 0.47 correlated with HPV positivity [125, 152]. Overall, patients with HPV(+) tumors have a 60–80% reduced mortality rates, a finding that was confirmed by multiple trials.

The HPV(+) tumors had some unique features. The TAX324 trial analysis showed that HPV(+) patients had T1 or T2 tumors more commonly (49% vs. 20%) and better ECOG performance status (ECOG 0: 77% vs.49%) [47] which was in parallel with the results TROG 02.02 and ECOG 2399 trials [46, 53]. In addition, it has been shown that cystic lymph node metastases were associated with HPV(+) tonsil cancer in a surgical series of neck dissection [153]. Furthermore, Princess Margaret Hospital data of N2-3 HNC patients ($n = 493$) detected that HPV(+) lymph nodes ($n = 257$) were larger (2.9 vs. 2.5 cm), more commonly in cystic structure (38% vs. 6%), regressed more frequently after treatment (36% vs. 41%), and more likely to be eliminated after 36 weeks (90% vs. 0%) compared with HPV(−) ones [154].

7.2. The role of HPV in recurrent/metastatic HNC

The characteristics of metastatic disease in HPV(+) patients differ from HPV(−) ones in terms of sites and time, since metastases is more likely to develop at sites other than lungs and may occur after 2 years following the initial treatment. Locally advanced diseases (T4 and N3-N2C) are the risk factors for metastasis development in HPV(+) disease [16]. Princess Margaret Hospital reviewed the distant metastasis rates in 457 HPV(+) and 167 HPV(−) oropharyngeal cancer cases and found that metastasis rates were similar at 3 years. HPV(+) tumors were more likely to develop metastases after a long interval, such that metastases occurred within 2 years in 24 of 25 HPV(−) cases, while metastasis development were detected 3 years post treatment in 13% of HPV(+) cases. In addition, dissemination pattern was more common in HPV(+) patients (33% vs. 0%). Nevertheless, post-metastases 2-year survival was significantly better in HPV(+) group compared with HPV(−) group (11% vs. 4%, $p = 0.02$) [155]. These findings were confirmed by additional recent retrospective reports showing similar unique metastatic spread patterns [53, 156–158].

Recently, the impact of HPV in recurrent-metastatic HNC was evaluated in large trials. In the phase III EXTREME randomized trial which assessed the benefit of cetuximab addition to platinum + 5-fluorouracil (5-FU) in patients with recurrent-metastatic HNC as first-line therapy, paired tissue samples were analyzed for p16 expression by IHC using a 70% expression cutoff value and HPV via oligonucleotide hybridization test [159]. The p16 and HPV positivity was correlated with higher survival rates compared with p16 and HPV negativity in both cetuximab and control groups [159]. Since the predictive analyses indicated that cetuximab addition to chemotherapy improved survival rates independently from p16 or HPV status, these biomarkers did not have any significance in treatment efficacy prediction. By contrast, in the phase III SPECTRUM randomized trial which assessed the benefit of panitumumab addition to chemotherapy instead of cetuximab in recurrent-metastatic HNC, a nonsignificant difference between HPV(+) and HPV(−) groups was demonstrated. Furthermore, the benefit of panitumumab was not detected in p16(+) group in contrast to p16(−) group [159].

The pooled analysis of patients with recurrent-metastatic HNC from E1395, a phase III trial comparing platinum + 5-fluorouracil with cisplatin + paclitaxel and E3301, a phase II trial evaluating irinotecan + docetaxel demonstrated that patients with HPV(+)/p16(+) disease had better overall survival than HPV(−)/p16(−) ones [160]. Taken together, these three studies indicate the positive impact of HPV positivity on improved survival. The efficiency of anti-EGFR antibodies on survival of HPV(+) and HPV(−) patients remains to be clarified. Hence, further studies including only oropharyngeal cancer patients are required in recurrent-metastatic setting since the impact of HPV positivity at other sides of HNC is not fully known.

7.3. Prognostic factors

Combined with being a nonsmoker, HPV DNA/RNA presence and p16 overexpression are strong prognostic markers [16]. Smoking, the most important risk factor for HNC overall, affects negative survival and response to treatment [161]. In addition, tobacco exposure has been shown to be a significant independent factor for prognosis in patients with HPV(+) oropharyngeal cancer, as it predicted progression and death risk in a dose-dependent pattern. Independently from HPV status and other factors, each pack-year of smoking increases the progression and death risk and the risk of second primary cancers of by 1% and 1.5%, respectively. Furthermore, the risk of death doubles if patients do not quit smoking during radiotherapy [161]. Based on the data of RTOG 0129 trial, a risk stratification for oropharyngeal cancer patients was developed using HPV status, history of smoking (>10 pack-years), and disease stage [16].

Other factors which are correlated with poor prognosis are local extension, disease stage at presentation, cervical node involvement, and rich vascular and lymphatic network [162]. Tumor thickness greater than 5 mm is significantly correlated with occult lymph node metastasis which is suggested to be a stronger determiner of prognosis than TNM staging by some authors. It has been shown that tumor differentiation, angiogenesis, extracapsular extension, and perineural invasion had significant role in prognosis determination [162]. Regarding treatment associated factors, cervical node dissection and disease free margins are important [162], since local relapse rates are 64–84% in patients with positive surgical margins [163].

Concerning the molecular markers, aberrations in chromosomes 3, 9, 11, 13, and 17 and tumor suppressor genes (p53 and pRb) are significant for prognosis [162]. In addition, cytokeratin 8/18 has been shown to be an independent factor correlated with poor prognosis [162, 163]. Furthermore, the absent/low expression of MHC class I, CD44, or CD98 has strong prognostic value for HPV(+) oropharyngeal cancer patients such that MHC class I staining absence defines 3-year disease-free and overall survival with 95–100% probability [164–166]. Moreover, higher

CD8+ tumor infiltrating lymphocyte (TIL) counts is also a prognostic marker for patients with HPV(+) oropharyngeal cancer [167].

HPV16 E6 and E7 in serum were demonstrated to be the most predictive factor in determining the HNC prognosis among the several biomarkers. E6/E7 seropositivity was associated with improved survival, whereas their seronegativity was correlated with poor prognosis irrespective of the DNA or p16 status [168]. Another suggested prognostic factor for survival is pretreatment tumor HPV copy number; higher tumor HPV copy number was correlated with better induction chemotherapy (p = 0.001) and chemoradiotherapy (p = 0.005) response, disease-specific (p = 0.004) and overall survival and (p = 0.008) after adjustment for other significant factors [147]. Similarly, higher viral load was shown to be correlated with improved recurrence-free (p = 0.0037) and overall (p = 0.028) survival in tonsil cancer patients [169]. Furthermore, the presence of both HPV16 and p16 indicated significantly improved prognosis compared with either p16 or HPV16 alone [170].

7.4. Deintensification of treatment in HPV(+) oropharyngeal cancer

Three principal routes have been drawn in treatment deintensification: (1) EGFR inhibitor use (mostly Cetuximab) instead of cisplatin, concurrently with radiotherapy; (2) radiotherapy dose reduction with concurrent chemotherapy (based on induction chemotherapy response); and (3) minimally invasive transoral surgery use followed by reduced adjuvant treatment according to the histopathological properties of the excised tumor.

Since responses to treatment alter even between HPV(+) oropharyngeal cancer patients, defining appropriate patient subgroup is essential. It must be emphasized that all patients with HPV(+) oropharyngeal cancer are not suitable candidates for deintensification approaches. The clinical trial cohorts' analysis indicates some evidence. Some of them suggest that lifetime tobacco use history of >10 pack-years in HPV(+) patients with advanced regional nodal metastasis (N2b, N3) as well as smoking during radiotherapy decreases survival time (3-year overall survival rate of 70.8%) [16, 161]. The Italian study which reported that intermediate-risk patients are not convenient for deintensification trials confirmed these findings [171]. Furthermore, O'Sullivan et al. [27] demonstrated that the 3-year distant control rates of HPV(+) oropharyngeal cancer with advanced T stage (T4) or nodal (N3) was 72% and 78%, respectively [124]. Hence, late recurrences and relapses as distant metastasis are not rare in HPV(+) oropharyngeal cancer. These data indicate the presence of a limit of the biologic advantage provided by HPV positivity and may be helpful in determining patient subgroup that requires chemotherapy use in order to treat early micrometastasis. Both amount of smoking and locoregionally advanced disease have implications in designing deintensification trials for HPV(+) oropharyngeal cancer patients.

Many clinical trials have been planned to evaluate the efficiency of treatment deintensification in HNC patients and recently they have been reviewed by Masterson et al. [152] in detail. Enrolling patients into these trials to define optimum treatment of HPV(+) oropharyngeal cancer is encouraged. Nevertheless, besides as a clinical trial, there is not sufficient data for the treatment reduction or modification according to HPV positivity until we receive the results from these deintensification studies.

7.5. Prevention-vaccination

There are two prophylactic HPV vaccines available commercially; Gardasil® (Merck & Co., Whitehouse Station, NJ, USA) and Cervarix® (GlaxoSmithKline Biologicals, Rixensart, Belgium). The virus-like proteins (VLPs) are used to create HPV major capsid protein L1 neutralizing antibodies. Gardasil is a quadrivalent L1 VLP recombinant vaccine protecting against HPV6, -11, -16, and -18, while Gardasil 9 provides protection against five additional HPV genotypes 16, 18, 31, 33, 45, 52, and 58. In contrast, Cervarix is a bivalent L1 VLP recombinant vaccine against HPV-16 and -18. Both HPV vaccines are highly effective in anogenital HPV infection prevention and consequent anal and cervical cancer development.

Despite the fact that the prophylactic value of vaccination for oropharyngeal cancer has not been proven in randomized trials yet, both the Cervarix and Gardasil vaccines are expected to prevent oropharyngeal HPV16 and -18 infections and consequent oropharyngeal cancer, since HPV16 is the most common type detected in oropharyngeal cancer [172]. The vaccination efficiency was estimated as 93.3% in 7466 women who were aged 18–25 years and randomized to HPV16/18 (Cervarix) vaccine versus hepatitis A vaccine as control for oral HPV 16/18 prevalence evaluation 4 years after vaccination [173]. In addition, cross-sectional study of US population as part of the National Health and Nutrition Examination Survey (NHANES) oral HPV infection prevalence was reduced significantly in 290 vaccinated women compared with 1985 unvaccinated women (0% vs. 0.5%) [54].

Author details

Makbule Tambas[1*], Musa Altun[2] and Deniz Tural[3]

*Address all correspondence to: makbule_tambas@hotmail.com

1 Department of Radiation Oncology, Okmeydani Training and Research Hospital, Istanbul, Turkey

2 Department of Radiation Oncology, Istanbul Faculty of Medicine, Istanbul University, Istanbul, Turkey

3 Department of Medical Oncology, Bakirkoy Dr. Sadi Konuk Education and Research Hospital, Istanbul, Turkey

References

[1] Torre LA, Bray F, Siegel RL, Ferlay J, Lortet-Tieulent J, Jemal A. Global cancer statistics, 2012. CA: A Cancer Journal for Clinicians. 2015;65(2):87–108. Epub 2015/02/06.10.3322/caac.21262

[2] Jemal A, Bray F, Center MM, Ferlay J, Ward E, Forman D. Global cancer statistics. CA: A Cancer Journal for Clinicians. 2011;61(2):69–90. Epub 2011/02/08.10.3322/caac.20107

[3] Ramshankar V, Krishnamurthy A. Human papilloma virus in head and neck cancers-role and relevance in clinical management. Indian Journal of Surgical Oncology. 2013;4(1):59–66. Epub 2014/01/16.10.1007/s13193-012-0196-5

[4] Mehanna H, Paleri V, West CM, Nutting C. Head and neck cancer – part 1: epidemiology, presentation, and prevention. BMJ. 2010;341:c4684. Epub 2010/09/22.10.1136/bmj.c4684

[5] Hashibe M, Brennan P, Chuang SC, Boccia S, Castellsague X, Chen C, et al. Interaction between tobacco and alcohol use and the risk of head and neck cancer: pooled analysis in the International Head and Neck Cancer Epidemiology Consortium. Cancer Epidemiology, Biomarkers & Prevention. 2009;18(2):541–50. Epub 2009/02/05.10.1158/1055-9965.EPI-08-0347

[6] Guha N, Boffetta P, Wunsch Filho V, Eluf Neto J, Shangina O, Zaridze D, et al. Oral health and risk of squamous cell carcinoma of the head and neck and esophagus: results of two multicentric case-control studies. American Journal of Epidemiology. 2007;166(10):1159–73. Epub 2007/09/01.10.1093/aje/kwm193

[7] Mashberg A, Boffetta P, Winkelman R, Garfinkel L. Tobacco smoking, alcohol drinking, and cancer of the oral cavity and oropharynx among U.S. veterans. Cancer. 1993;72(4):1369–75. Epub 1993/08/15.

[8] Johnson S, McDonald JT, Corsten M, Rourke R. Socio-economic status and head and neck cancer incidence in Canada: a case-control study. Oral Oncology. 2010;46(3):200–3. Epub 2010/02/09.10.1016/j.oraloncology.2009.12.004

[9] Chaturvedi AK, Engels EA, Anderson WF, Gillison ML. Incidence trends for human papillomavirus-related and unrelated oral squamous cell carcinomas in the United States. Journal of Clinical Oncology: Official Journal of the American Society of Clinical Oncology. 2008;26(4):612–9. Epub 2008/02/01.10.1200/JCO.2007.14.1713

[10] de Martel C, Ferlay J, Franceschi S, Vignat J, Bray F, Forman D, et al. Global burden of cancers attributable to infections in 2008: a review and synthetic analysis. The Lancet Oncology. 2012;13(6):607–15. Epub 2012/05/12.10.1016/S1470-2045(12)70137-7

[11] Martin-Hernan F, Sanchez-Hernandez JG, Cano J, Campo J, del Romero J. Oral cancer, HPV infection and evidence of sexual transmission. Medicina Oral, Patologia Oral y Cirugia Bucal. 2013;18(3):e439–44. Epub 2013/03/26.

[12] Hammarstedt L, Lindquist D, Dahlstrand H, Romanitan M, Dahlgren LO, Joneberg J, et al. Human papillomavirus as a risk factor for the increase in incidence of tonsillar cancer. International Journal of Cancer. 2006;119(11):2620–3. Epub 2006/09/23.10.1002/ijc.22177

[13] Sturgis EM, Cinciripini PM. Trends in head and neck cancer incidence in relation to smoking prevalence: an emerging epidemic of human papillomavirus-associated cancers? Cancer. 2007;110(7):1429–35. Epub 2007/08/29.10.1002/cncr.22963

[14] Nasman A, Attner P, Hammarstedt L, Du J, Eriksson M, Giraud G, et al. Incidence of human papillomavirus (HPV) positive tonsillar carcinoma in Stockholm, Sweden: an epidemic of viral-induced carcinoma? International Journal of Cancer. 2009;125(2):362–6. Epub 2009/03/31.10.1002/ijc.24339

[15] Attner P, Du J, Nasman A, Hammarstedt L, Ramqvist T, Lindholm J, et al. The role of human papillomavirus in the increased incidence of base of tongue cancer. International Journal of Cancer. 2010;126(12):2879–84. Epub 2009/10/27.10.1002/ijc.24994

[16] Ang KK, Harris J, Wheeler R, Weber R, Rosenthal DI, Nguyen-Tan PF, et al. Human papillomavirus and survival of patients with oropharyngeal cancer. The New England Journal of Medicine. 2010;363(1):24–35. Epub 2010/06/10.10.1056/NEJMoa0912217

[17] Chaturvedi AK, Engels EA, Pfeiffer RM, Hernandez BY, Xiao W, Kim E, et al. Human papillomavirus and rising oropharyngeal cancer incidence in the United States. Journal of Clinical Oncology: Official Journal of the American Society of Clinical Oncology. 2011;29(32):4294–301. Epub 2011/10/05.10.1200/JCO.2011.36.4596

[18] Conway DI, Stockton DL, Warnakulasuriya KA, Ogden G, Macpherson LM. Incidence of oral and oropharyngeal cancer in United Kingdom (1990–1999) – recent trends and regional variation. Oral Oncology. 2006;42(6):586–92. Epub 2006/02/14.10.1016/j.oraloncology.2005.10.018

[19] Hammarstedt L, Dahlstrand H, Lindquist D, Onelov L, Ryott M, Luo J, et al. The incidence of tonsillar cancer in Sweden is increasing. Acta Oto-Laryngologica. 2007;127(9):988–92. Epub 2007/08/23.10.1080/00016480601110170

[20] Braakhuis BJ, Visser O, Leemans CR. Oral and oropharyngeal cancer in the Netherlands between 1989 and 2006: Increasing incidence, but not in young adults. Oral Oncology. 2009;45(9):e85–9. Epub 2009/05/22.10.1016/j.oraloncology.2009.03.010

[21] Marur S, D'Souza G, Westra WH, Forastiere AA. HPV-associated head and neck cancer: a virus-related cancer epidemic. The Lancet Oncology. 2010;11(8):781–9. Epub 2010/05/11.10.1016/S1470-2045(10)70017-6

[22] Ramqvist T, Dalianis T. Oropharyngeal cancer epidemic and human papillomavirus. Emerging Infectious Diseases. 2010;16(11):1671–7. Epub 2010/10/30.10.3201/eid1611.100452

[23] Ramqvist T, Dalianis T. An epidemic of oropharyngeal squamous cell carcinoma (OSCC) due to human papillomavirus (HPV) infection and aspects of treatment and prevention. Anticancer Research. 2011;31(5):1515–9. Epub 2011/05/28.

[24] Ryerson AB, Peters ES, Coughlin SS, Chen VW, Gillison ML, Reichman ME, et al. Burden of potentially human papillomavirus-associated cancers of the oropharynx and

oral cavity in the US, 1998-2003. Cancer. 2008;113(10 Suppl.):2901–9. Epub 2008/11/05.10.1002/cncr.23745

[25] Carvalho AL, Nishimoto IN, Califano JA, Kowalski LP. Trends in incidence and prognosis for head and neck cancer in the United States: a site-specific analysis of the SEER database. International Journal of Cancer. 2005;114(5):806–16. Epub 2004/12/21.10.1002/ijc.20740

[26] Reddy VM, Cundall-Curry D, Bridger MW. Trends in the incidence rates of tonsil and base of tongue cancer in England, 1985-2006. Annals of the Royal College of Surgeons of England. 2010;92(8):655–9. Epub 2010/07/10.10.1308/003588410X12699663904871

[27] Auluck A, Hislop G, Bajdik C, Poh C, Zhang L, Rosin M. Trends in oropharyngeal and oral cavity cancer incidence of human papillomavirus (HPV)-related and HPV-unrelated sites in a multicultural population: the British Columbia experience. Cancer. 2010;116(11):2635–44. Epub 2010/03/26.10.1002/cncr.25087

[28] Hong AM, Grulich AE, Jones D, Lee CS, Garland SM, Dobbins TA, et al. Squamous cell carcinoma of the oropharynx in Australian males induced by human papillomavirus vaccine targets. Vaccine. 2010;28(19):3269–72. Epub 2010/03/17.10.1016/j.vaccine.2010.02.098

[29] Mork J, Moller B, Dahl T, Bray F. Time trends in pharyngeal cancer incidence in Norway 1981-2005: a subsite analysis based on a reabstraction and recoding of registered cases. Cancer Causes & Control. 2010;21(9):1397–405. Epub 2010/05/01.10.1007/s10552-010-9567-9

[30] Blomberg M, Nielsen A, Munk C, Kjaer SK. Trends in head and neck cancer incidence in Denmark, 1978-2007: focus on human papillomavirus associated sites. International Journal of Cancer. 2011;129(3):733–41. Epub 2010/09/30.10.1002/ijc.25699

[31] Lewis A, Kang R, Levine A, Maghami E. The new face of head and neck cancer: the HPV epidemic. Oncology (Williston Park). 2015;29(9):616–26. Epub 2015/09/20.

[32] Mammas IN, Sourvinos G, Zaravinos A, Spandidos DA. Vaccination against human papilloma virus (HPV): epidemiological evidence of HPV in non-genital cancers. Pathology Oncology Research. 2011;17(1):103–19. Epub 2010/07/20.10.1007/s12253-010-9288-0

[33] El-Mofty SK, Zhang MQ, Davila RM. Histologic identification of human papillomavirus (HPV)-related squamous cell carcinoma in cervical lymph nodes: a reliable predictor of the site of an occult head and neck primary carcinoma. Head and Neck Pathology. 2008;2(3):163–8. Epub 2008/09/01.10.1007/s12105-008-0066-1

[34] Vent J, Haidle B, Wedemeyer I, Huebbers C, Siefer O, Semrau R, et al. p16 expression in carcinoma of unknown primary: diagnostic indicator and prognostic marker. Head & Neck. 2013;35(11):1521–6. Epub 2013/01/25.10.1002/hed.23190

[35] Begum S, Gillison ML, Nicol TL, Westra WH. Detection of human papillomavirus-16 in fine-needle aspirates to determine tumor origin in patients with metastatic squamous

cell carcinoma of the head and neck. Clinical Cancer Research: An Official Journal of the American Association for Cancer Research. 2007;13(4):1186–91. Epub 2007/02/24.10.1158/1078-0432.CCR-06-1690

[36] Abogunrin S, Di Tanna GL, Keeping S, Carroll S, Iheanacho I. Prevalence of human papillomavirus in head and neck cancers in European populations: a meta-analysis. BMC Cancer. 2014;14:968. Epub 2014/12/18.10.1186/1471-2407-14-968

[37] Venuti A, Badaracco G, Rizzo C, Mafera B, Rahimi S, Vigili M. Presence of HPV in head and neck tumours: high prevalence in tonsillar localization. Journal of Experimental & Clinical Cancer Research. 2004;23(4):561–6. Epub 2005/03/04.

[38] Koskinen WJ, Chen RW, Leivo I, Makitie A, Back L, Kontio R, et al. Prevalence and physical status of human papillomavirus in squamous cell carcinomas of the head and neck. International Journal of Cancer. 2003;107(3):401–6. Epub 2003/09/25.10.1002/ijc. 11381

[39] Stephen JK, Divine G, Chen KM, Chitale D, Havard S, Worsham MJ. Significance of p16 in site-specific HPV positive and HPV negative head and neck squamous cell carcinoma. Cancer and Clinical Oncology. 2013;2(1):51–61. Epub 2013/08/13.10.5539/cco.v2n1p51

[40] Bussu F, Sali M, Gallus R, Vellone VG, Zannoni GF, Autorino R, et al. HPV infection in squamous cell carcinomas arising from different mucosal sites of the head and neck region. Is p16 immunohistochemistry a reliable surrogate marker? British Journal of Cancer. 2013;108(5):1157–62. Epub 2013/02/14.10.1038/bjc.2013.55

[41] Almadori G, Cadoni G, Cattani P, Posteraro P, Scarano E, Ottaviani F, et al. Detection of human papillomavirus DNA in laryngeal squamous cell carcinoma by polymerase chain reaction. European Journal of Cancer. 1996;32A(5):783–8. Epub 1996/05/01.

[42] Almadori G, Galli J, Cadoni G, Bussu F, Maurizi M. Human papillomavirus infection and cyclin D1 gene amplification in laryngeal squamous cell carcinoma: biologic function and clinical significance. Head & Neck. 2002;24(6):597–604. Epub 2002/07/12.10.1002/hed.10097

[43] Combes JD, Franceschi S. Role of human papillomavirus in non-oropharyngeal head and neck cancers. Oral Oncology. 2014;50(5):370–9. Epub 2013/12/18.10.1016/j.oraloncology.2013.11.004

[44] Isayeva T, Li Y, Maswahu D, Brandwein-Gensler M. Human papillomavirus in non-oropharyngeal head and neck cancers: a systematic literature review. Head and Neck Pathology. 2012;6(Suppl. 1):S104–20. Epub 2012/07/13.10.1007/s12105-012-0368-1

[45] Lingen MW, Xiao W, Schmitt A, Jiang B, Pickard R, Kreinbrink P, et al. Low etiologic fraction for high-risk human papillomavirus in oral cavity squamous cell carcinomas. Oral Oncology. 2013;49(1):1–8. Epub 2012/07/31.10.1016/j.oraloncology.2012.07.002

[46] Fakhry C, Westra WH, Li S, Cmelak A, Ridge JA, Pinto H, et al. Improved survival of patients with human papillomavirus-positive head and neck squamous cell carcinoma

in a prospective clinical trial. Journal of the National Cancer Institute. 2008;100(4):261–9. Epub 2008/02/14.10.1093/jnci/djn011

[47] Posner MR, Lorch JH, Goloubeva O, Tan M, Schumaker LM, Sarlis NJ, et al. Survival and human papillomavirus in oropharynx cancer in TAX 324: a subset analysis from an international phase III trial. Annals of Oncology: Official Journal of the European Society for Medical Oncology/ESMO. 2011;22(5):1071–7. Epub 2011/02/15.10.1093/annonc/mdr006

[48] Lassen P, Eriksen JG, Krogdahl A, Therkildsen MH, Ulhoi BP, Overgaard M, et al. The influence of HPV-associated p16-expression on accelerated fractionated radiotherapy in head and neck cancer: evaluation of the randomised DAHANCA 6 & 7 trial. Radiotherapy and Oncology: Journal of the European Society for Therapeutic Radiology and Oncology. 2011;100(1):49–55. Epub 2011/03/25.10.1016/j.radonc.2011.02.010

[49] Lajer CB, von Buchwald C. The role of human papillomavirus in head and neck cancer. APMIS: Acta Pathologica, Microbiologica, et Immunologica Scandinavica. 2010;118(6–7):510–9. Epub 2010/06/18.10.1111/j.1600-0463.2010.02624.x

[50] Gillison ML, D'Souza G, Westra W, Sugar E, Xiao W, Begum S, et al. Distinct risk factor profiles for human papillomavirus type 16-positive and human papillomavirus type 16-negative head and neck cancers. Journal of the National Cancer Institute. 2008;100(6):407–20. Epub 2008/03/13.10.1093/jnci/djn025

[51] Schwartz SR, Yueh B, McDougall JK, Daling JR, Schwartz SM. Human papillomavirus infection and survival in oral squamous cell cancer: a population-based study. Otolaryngology – Head and Neck Surgery: Official Journal of American Academy of Otolaryngology – Head and Neck Surgery. 2001;125(1):1–9. Epub 2001/07/18.10.1067/mhn.2001.116979

[52] Shiboski CH, Schmidt BL, Jordan RC. Tongue and tonsil carcinoma: increasing trends in the U.S. population ages 20-44 years. Cancer. 2005;103(9):1843–9. Epub 2005/03/18.10.1002/cncr.20998

[53] Rischin D, Young RJ, Fisher R, Fox SB, Le QT, Peters LJ, et al. Prognostic significance of p16INK4A and human papillomavirus in patients with oropharyngeal cancer treated on TROG 02.02 phase III trial. Journal of Clinical Oncology: Official Journal of the American Society of Clinical Oncology. 2010;28(27):4142–8. Epub 2010/08/11.10.1200/JCO.2010.29.2904

[54] Gillison ML, Broutian T, Pickard RK, Tong ZY, Xiao W, Kahle L, et al. Prevalence of oral HPV infection in the United States, 2009-2010. JAMA. 2012;307(7):693–703. Epub 2012/01/28.10.1001/jama.2012.101

[55] Settle K, Posner MR, Schumaker LM, Tan M, Suntharalingam M, Goloubeva O, et al. Racial survival disparity in head and neck cancer results from low prevalence of human papillomavirus infection in black oropharyngeal cancer patients. Cancer Prevention Research (Phila). 2009;2(9):776–81. Epub 2009/07/31.10.1158/1940-6207.CAPR-09-0149

[56] Weinberger PM, Merkley MA, Khichi SS, Lee JR, Psyrri A, Jackson LL, et al. Human papillomavirus-active head and neck cancer and ethnic health disparities. The Laryngoscope. 2010;120(8):1531–7. Epub 2010/06/22.10.1002/lary.20984

[57] Jemal A, Simard EP, Dorell C, Noone AM, Markowitz LE, Kohler B, et al. Annual Report to the Nation on the Status of Cancer, 1975-2009, featuring the burden and trends in human papillomavirus (HPV)-associated cancers and HPV vaccination coverage levels. Journal of the National Cancer Institute. 2013;105(3):175–201. Epub 2013/01/09.10.1093/jnci/djs491

[58] Bouvard V, Baan R, Straif K, Grosse Y, Secretan B, El Ghissassi F, et al. A review of human carcinogens – part B: biological agents. The Lancet Oncology. 2009;10(4):321–2. Epub 2009/04/08.

[59] Stransky N, Egloff AM, Tward AD, Kostic AD, Cibulskis K, Sivachenko A, et al. The mutational landscape of head and neck squamous cell carcinoma. Science. 2011;333(6046):1157–60. Epub 2011/07/30.10.1126/science.1208130

[60] Glombitza F, Guntinas-Lichius O, Petersen I. HPV status in head and neck tumors. Pathology, Research and Practice. 2010;206(4):229–34. Epub 2010/02/09.10.1016/j.prp.2009.11.007

[61] Deng Z, Hasegawa M, Yamashita Y, Matayoshi S, Kiyuna A, Agena S, et al. Prognostic value of human papillomavirus and squamous cell carcinoma antigen in head and neck squamous cell carcinoma. Cancer Science. 2012;103(12):2127–34. Epub 2012/09/04.10.1111/cas.12009

[62] D'Souza G, Gross ND, Pai SI, Haddad R, Anderson KS, Rajan S, et al. Oral human papillomavirus (HPV) infection in HPV-positive patients with oropharyngeal cancer and their partners. Journal of Clinical Oncology: Official Journal of the American Society of Clinical Oncology. 2014;32(23):2408–15. Epub 2014/04/30.10.1200/JCO.2014.55.1341

[63] Gillison ML, Koch WM, Capone RB, Spafford M, Westra WH, Wu L, et al. Evidence for a causal association between human papillomavirus and a subset of head and neck cancers. Journal of the National Cancer Institute. 2000;92(9):709–20. Epub 2000/05/04.

[64] Jay N, Moscicki AB. Human papillomavirus infections in women with HIV disease: prevalence, risk, and management. The AIDS Reader. 2000;10(11):659–68. Epub 2001/02/24.

[65] Cates W, Jr. Estimates of the incidence and prevalence of sexually transmitted diseases in the United States. American Social Health Association Panel. Sexually Transmitted Diseases. 1999;26(4 Suppl.):S2–7. Epub 1999/05/05.

[66] Westra WH. The changing face of head and neck cancer in the 21st century: the impact of HPV on the epidemiology and pathology of oral cancer. Head and Neck Pathology. 2009;3(1):78–81. Epub 2009/03/01.10.1007/s12105-009-0100-y

[67] Herrero R, Castellsague X, Pawlita M, Lissowska J, Kee F, Balaram P, et al. Human papillomavirus and oral cancer: the International Agency for Research on Cancer multicenter study. Journal of the National Cancer Institute. 2003;95(23):1772–83. Epub 2003/12/05.

[68] Anaya-Saavedra G, Ramirez-Amador V, Irigoyen-Camacho ME, Garcia-Cuellar CM, Guido-Jimenez M, Mendez-Martinez R, et al. High association of human papillomavirus infection with oral cancer: a case-control study. Archives of Medical Research. 2008;39(2):189–97. Epub 2008/01/01.10.1016/j.arcmed.2007.08.003

[69] D'Souza G, Agrawal Y, Halpern J, Bodison S, Gillison ML. Oral sexual behaviors associated with prevalent oral human papillomavirus infection. The Journal of Infectious Diseases. 2009;199(9):1263–9. Epub 2009/03/27.10.1086/597755

[70] Syrjanen S, Puranen M. Human papillomavirus infections in children: the potential role of maternal transmission. Critical Reviews in Oral Biology and Medicine: An Official Publication of the American Association of Oral Biologists. 2000;11(2):259–74. Epub 2002/05/11.

[71] D'Souza G, Kreimer AR, Viscidi R, Pawlita M, Fakhry C, Koch WM, et al. Case-control study of human papillomavirus and oropharyngeal cancer. The New England Journal of Medicine. 2007;356(19):1944–56. Epub 2007/05/15.10.1056/NEJMoa065497

[72] Turner CF, Danella RD, Rogers SM. Sexual behavior in the United States 1930-1990: trends and methodological problems. Sexually Transmitted Diseases. 1995;22(3):173–90. Epub 1995/05/01.

[73] Bajos N, Bozon M, Beltzer N, Laborde C, Andro A, Ferrand M, et al. Changes in sexual behaviours: from secular trends to public health policies. AIDS. 2010;24(8):1185–91. Epub 2010/03/20.10.1097/QAD.0b013e328336ad52

[74] Gillison ML, Koch WM, Shah KV. Human papillomavirus in head and neck squamous cell carcinoma: are some head and neck cancers a sexually transmitted disease? Current Opinion in Oncology. 1999;11(3):191–9. Epub 1999/05/18.

[75] Garden AS, Kies MS, Morrison WH, Weber RS, Frank SJ, Glisson BS, et al. Outcomes and patterns of care of patients with locally advanced oropharyngeal carcinoma treated in the early 21st century. Radiation Oncology. 2013;8:21. Epub 2013/01/31.10.1186/1748-717X-8-21

[76] Atula TS, Varpula MJ, Kurki TJ, Klemi PJ, Grenman R. Assessment of cervical lymph node status in head and neck cancer patients: palpation, computed tomography and low field magnetic resonance imaging compared with ultrasound-guided fine-needle aspiration cytology. European Journal of Radiology. 1997;25(2):152–61. Epub 1997/09/01.

[77] Compton AM, Moore-Medlin T, Herman-Ferdinandez L, Clark C, Caldito GC, Wang XI, et al. Human papillomavirus in metastatic lymph nodes from unknown primary head and neck squamous cell carcinoma. Otolaryngology – Head and Neck Surgery:

Official Journal of American Academy of Otolaryngology – Head and Neck Surgery. 2011;145(1):51–7. Epub 2011/04/16.10.1177/0194599811400385

[78] Nishat R, Behura SS, Ramachandra S, Kumar H, Bandyopadhyay A. Human papilloma virus (HPV) induced head & neck squamous cell carcinoma: a comprehensive retrospect. Journal of Clinical and Diagnostic Research. 2015;9(6):ZE01–4. Epub 2015/08/13.10.7860/JCDR/2015/13948.6056

[79] Fischer CA, Kampmann M, Zlobec I, Green E, Tornillo L, Lugli A, et al. p16 expression in oropharyngeal cancer: its impact on staging and prognosis compared with the conventional clinical staging parameters. Annals of Oncology: Official Journal of the European Society for Medical Oncology/ESMO. 2010;21(10):1961–6. Epub 2010/04/29.10.1093/annonc/mdq210

[80] Lewis JS, Jr. p16 Immunohistochemistry as a standalone test for risk stratification in oropharyngeal squamous cell carcinoma. Head and Neck Pathology. 2012;6(Suppl. 1):S75–82. Epub 2012/07/13.10.1007/s12105-012-0369-0

[81] Westra WH. Detection of human papillomavirus (HPV) in clinical samples: evolving methods and strategies for the accurate determination of HPV status of head and neck carcinomas. Oral Oncology. 2014;50(9):771–9. Epub 2014/06/17.10.1016/j.oraloncology.2014.05.004

[82] Shi W, Kato H, Perez-Ordonez B, Pintilie M, Huang S, Hui A, et al. Comparative prognostic value of HPV16 E6 mRNA compared with *in situ* hybridization for human oropharyngeal squamous carcinoma. Journal of Clinical Oncology: Official Journal of the American Society of Clinical Oncology. 2009;27(36):6213–21. Epub 2009/11/04.10.1200/JCO.2009.23.1670

[83] Perrone F, Gloghini A, Cortelazzi B, Bossi P, Licitra L, Pilotti S. Isolating p16-positive/HPV-negative oropharyngeal cancer: an effort worth making. The American Journal of Surgical Pathology. 2011;35(5):774–7; author reply 7–8. Epub 2011/03/26.10.1097/PAS.0b013e3182116a45

[84] Pannone G, Rodolico V, Santoro A, Lo Muzio L, Franco R, Botti G, et al. Evaluation of a combined triple method to detect causative HPV in oral and oropharyngeal squamous cell carcinomas: p16 immunohistochemistry, consensus PCR HPV-DNA, and *in situ* hybridization. Infectious Agents and Cancer. 2012;7:4. Epub 2012/03/02.10.1186/1750-9378-7-4

[85] Cameron JE, Snowhite IV, Chaturvedi AK, Hagensee ME. Human papillomavirus-specific antibody status in oral fluids modestly reflects serum status in human immunodeficiency virus-positive individuals. Clinical and Diagnostic Laboratory Immunology. 2003;10(3):431–8. Epub 2003/05/10.

[86] Clavel C, Masure M, Bory JP, Putaud I, Mangeonjean C, Lorenzato M, et al. Hybrid capture II-based human papillomavirus detection, a sensitive test to detect in routine

high-grade cervical lesions: a preliminary study on 1518 women. British Journal of Cancer. 1999;80(9):1306–11. Epub 1999/07/29.10.1038/sj.bjc.6690523

[87] Gravitt PE, Peyton CL, Apple RJ, Wheeler CM. Genotyping of 27 human papillomavirus types by using L1 consensus PCR products by a single-hybridization, reverse line blot detection method. Journal of Clinical Microbiology. 1998;36(10):3020–7. Epub 1998/09/17.

[88] Schmitt M, Bravo IG, Snijders PJ, Gissmann L, Pawlita M, Waterboer T. Bead-based multiplex genotyping of human papillomaviruses. Journal of Clinical Microbiology. 2006;44(2):504–12. Epub 2006/02/04.10.1128/JCM.44.2.504-512.2006

[89] Lindquist D, Romanitan M, Hammarstedt L, Nasman A, Dahlstrand H, Lindholm J, et al. Human papillomavirus is a favourable prognostic factor in tonsillar cancer and its oncogenic role is supported by the expression of E6 and E7. Molecular Oncology. 2007;1(3):350–5. Epub 2007/12/01.10.1016/j.molonc.2007.08.005

[90] Doorbar J, Quint W, Banks L, Bravo IG, Stoler M, Broker TR, et al. The biology and life-cycle of human papillomaviruses. Vaccine. 2012;30(Suppl. 5):F55–70. Epub 2012/12/05.10.1016/j.vaccine.2012.06.083

[91] Munoz N, Bosch FX, de Sanjose S, Herrero R, Castellsague X, Shah KV, et al. Epidemiologic classification of human papillomavirus types associated with cervical cancer. The New England Journal of Medicine. 2003;348(6):518–27. Epub 2003/02/07.10.1056/NEJMoa021641

[92] Kreimer AR, Clifford GM, Boyle P, Franceschi S. Human papillomavirus types in head and neck squamous cell carcinomas worldwide: a systematic review. Cancer Epidemiology, Biomarkers & Prevention. 2005;14(2):467–75. Epub 2005/03/01.10.1158/1055-9965.EPI-04-0551

[93] Ringstrom E, Peters E, Hasegawa M, Posner M, Liu M, Kelsey KT. Human papillomavirus type 16 and squamous cell carcinoma of the head and neck. Clinical Cancer Research: An Official Journal of the American Association for Cancer Research. 2002;8(10):3187–92. Epub 2002/10/11.

[94] McLaughlin-Drubin ME, Munger K. Oncogenic activities of human papillomaviruses. Virus Research. 2009;143(2):195–208. Epub 2009/06/23.10.1016/j.virusres.2009.06.008

[95] Tertipis N, Villabona L, Nordfors C, Nasman A, Ramqvist T, Vlastos A, et al. HLA-A*02 in relation to outcome in human papillomavirus positive tonsillar and base of tongue cancer. Anticancer Research. 2014;34(5):2369–75. Epub 2014/04/30.

[96] Nordfors C, Grun N, Tertipis N, Ahrlund-Richter A, Haeggblom L, Sivars L, et al. CD8+ and CD4+ tumour infiltrating lymphocytes in relation to human papillomavirus status and clinical outcome in tonsillar and base of tongue squamous cell carcinoma. European Journal of Cancer. 2013;49(11):2522–30. Epub 2013/04/11.10.1016/j.ejca.2013.03.019

[97] Lyford-Pike S, Peng S, Young GD, Taube JM, Westra WH, Akpeng B, et al. Evidence for a role of the PD-1:PD-L1 pathway in immune resistance of HPV-associated head

and neck squamous cell carcinoma. Cancer Research. 2013;73(6):1733–41. Epub 2013/01/05.10.1158/0008-5472.CAN-12-2384

[98] Doorbar J. The papillomavirus life cycle. Journal of Clinical Virology: The Official Publication of the Pan American Society for Clinical Virology. 2005;32(Suppl. 1):S7–15. Epub 2005/03/09.10.1016/j.jcv.2004.12.006

[99] Chow LT, Broker TR, Steinberg BM. The natural history of human papillomavirus infections of the mucosal epithelia. Acta Pathologica, Microbiologica, et Immunologica Scandinavica. 2010;118(6–7):422–49. Epub 2010/06/18.10.1111/j.1600-0463.2010.02625.x

[100] Cheng S, Schmidt-Grimminger DC, Murant T, Broker TR, Chow LT. Differentiation-dependent up-regulation of the human papillomavirus E7 gene reactivates cellular DNA replication in suprabasal differentiated keratinocytes. Genes & Development. 1995;9(19):2335–49. Epub 1995/10/01.

[101] Scheffner M, Werness BA, Huibregtse JM, Levine AJ, Howley PM. The E6 oncoprotein encoded by human papillomavirus types 16 and 18 promotes the degradation of p53. Cell. 1990;63(6):1129–36. Epub 1990/12/21.

[102] Munger K, Werness BA, Dyson N, Phelps WC, Harlow E, Howley PM. Complex formation of human papillomavirus E7 proteins with the retinoblastoma tumor suppressor gene product. The EMBO Journal. 1989;8(13):4099–105. Epub 1989/12/20.

[103] DiMaio D, Mattoon D. Mechanisms of cell transformation by papillomavirus E5 proteins. Oncogene. 2001;20(54):7866–73. Epub 2001/12/26.10.1038/sj.onc.1204915

[104] Rampias T, Sasaki C, Weinberger P, Psyrri A. E6 and e7 gene silencing and transformed phenotype of human papillomavirus 16-positive oropharyngeal cancer cells. Journal of the National Cancer Institute. 2009;101(6):412–23. Epub 2009/03/12.10.1093/jnci/djp017

[105] Indovina P, Marcelli E, Casini N, Rizzo V, Giordano A. Emerging roles of RB family: new defense mechanisms against tumor progression. Journal of Cellular Physiology. 2013;228(3):525–35. Epub 2012/08/14.10.1002/jcp.24170

[106] Strati K, Lambert PF. Role of Rb-dependent and Rb-independent functions of papillomavirus E7 oncogene in head and neck cancer. Cancer Research. 2007;67(24):11585–93. Epub 2007/12/20.10.1158/0008-5472.CAN-07-3007

[107] Khleif SN, DeGregori J, Yee CL, Otterson GA, Kaye FJ, Nevins JR, et al. Inhibition of cyclin D-CDK4/CDK6 activity is associated with an E2F-mediated induction of cyclin kinase inhibitor activity. Proceedings of the National Academy of Sciences of the United States of America. 1996;93(9):4350–4. Epub 1996/04/30.

[108] Klaes R, Friedrich T, Spitkovsky D, Ridder R, Rudy W, Petry U, et al. Overexpression of p16(INK4A) as a specific marker for dysplastic and neoplastic epithelial cells of the cervix uteri. International Journal of Cancer. 2001;92(2):276–84. Epub 2001/04/06.

[109] Brehm A, Nielsen SJ, Miska EA, McCance DJ, Reid JL, Bannister AJ, et al. The E7 oncoprotein associates with Mi2 and histone deacetylase activity to promote cell growth. The EMBO Journal. 1999;18(9):2449–58. Epub 1999/05/06.10.1093/emboj/18.9.2449

[110] Kessis TD, Slebos RJ, Nelson WG, Kastan MB, Plunkett BS, Han SM, et al. Human papillomavirus 16 E6 expression disrupts the p53-mediated cellular response to DNA damage. Proceedings of the National Academy of Sciences of the United States of America. 1993;90(9):3988–92. Epub 1993/05/01.

[111] Patel D, Huang SM, Baglia LA, McCance DJ. The E6 protein of human papillomavirus type 16 binds to and inhibits co-activation by CBP and p300. The EMBO Journal. 1999;18(18):5061–72. Epub 1999/09/16.10.1093/emboj/18.18.5061

[112] Kumar A, Zhao Y, Meng G, Zeng M, Srinivasan S, Delmolino LM, et al. Human papillomavirus oncoprotein E6 inactivates the transcriptional coactivator human ADA3. Molecular and Cellular Biology. 2002;22(16):5801–12. Epub 2002/07/26.

[113] Yamada T, Yamashita T, Nishikawa T, Fujimoto S, Fujinaga K. Biologic activity of human papillomavirus type 16 E6/E7 cDNA clones isolated from SiHa cervical carcinoma cell line. Virus Genes. 1995;10(1):15–25. Epub 1995/01/01.

[114] James MA, Lee JH, Klingelhutz AJ. HPV16-E6 associated hTERT promoter acetylation is E6AP dependent, increased in later passage cells and enhanced by loss of p300. International Journal of Cancer. 2006;119(8):1878–85. Epub 2006/05/19.10.1002/ijc.22064

[115] Pillai MR, Nair MK. Development of a condemned mucosa syndrome and pathogenesis of human papillomavirus-associated upper aerodigestive tract and uterine cervical tumors. Experimental and Molecular Pathology. 2000;69(3):233–41. Epub 2000/12/15.10.1006/exmp.2000.2335

[116] Fan X, Liu Y, Heilman SA, Chen JJ. Human papillomavirus E7 induces rereplication in response to DNA damage. Journal of Virology. 2013;87(2):1200–10. Epub 2012/11/16.10.1128/JVI.02038-12

[117] Agrawal N, Frederick MJ, Pickering CR, Bettegowda C, Chang K, Li RJ, et al. Exome sequencing of head and neck squamous cell carcinoma reveals inactivating mutations in NOTCH1. Science. 2011;333(6046):1154–7. Epub 2011/07/30.10.1126/science.1206923

[118] Duensing S, Lee LY, Duensing A, Basile J, Piboonniyom S, Gonzalez S, et al. The human papillomavirus type 16 E6 and E7 oncoproteins cooperate to induce mitotic defects and genomic instability by uncoupling centrosome duplication from the cell division cycle. Proceedings of the National Academy of Sciences of the United States of America. 2000;97(18):10002–7. Epub 2000/08/16.10.1073/pnas.170093297

[119] Duensing A, Liu Y, Tseng M, Malumbres M, Barbacid M, Duensing S. Cyclin-dependent kinase 2 is dispensable for normal centrosome duplication but required for

oncogene-induced centrosome overduplication. Oncogene. 2006;25(20):2943–9. Epub 2005/12/07.10.1038/sj.onc.1209310

[120] Finzer P, Aguilar-Lemarroy A, Rosl F. The role of human papillomavirus oncoproteins E6 and E7 in apoptosis. Cancer Letters. 2002;188(1–2):15–24. Epub 2002/10/31.

[121] Kumar B, Cordell KG, Lee JS, Worden FP, Prince ME, Tran HH, et al. EGFR, p16, HPV Titer, Bcl-xL and p53, sex, and smoking as indicators of response to therapy and survival in oropharyngeal cancer. Journal of Clinical Oncology: Official Journal of the American Society of Clinical Oncology. 2008;26(19):3128–37. Epub 2008/05/14.10.1200/JCO.2007.12.7662

[122] Licitra L, Perrone F, Bossi P, Suardi S, Mariani L, Artusi R, et al. High-risk human papillomavirus affects prognosis in patients with surgically treated oropharyngeal squamous cell carcinoma. Journal of Clinical Oncology: Official Journal of the American Society of Clinical Oncology. 2006;24(36):5630–6. Epub 2006/12/21.10.1200/JCO.2005.04.6136

[123] Braakhuis BJ, Snijders PJ, Keune WJ, Meijer CJ, Ruijter-Schippers HJ, Leemans CR, et al. Genetic patterns in head and neck cancers that contain or lack transcriptionally active human papillomavirus. Journal of the National Cancer Institute. 2004;96(13):998–1006. Epub 2004/07/09.

[124] O'Sullivan B, Huang SH, Siu LL, Waldron J, Zhao H, Perez-Ordonez B, et al. Deintensification candidate subgroups in human papillomavirus-related oropharyngeal cancer according to minimal risk of distant metastasis. Journal of Clinical Oncology: Official Journal of the American Society of Clinical Oncology. 2013;31(5):543–50. Epub 2013/01/09.10.1200/JCO.2012.44.0164

[125] O'Rorke MA, Ellison MV, Murray LJ, Moran M, James J, Anderson LA. Human papillomavirus related head and neck cancer survival: a systematic review and meta-analysis. Oral Oncology. 2012;48(12):1191–201. Epub 2012/07/31.10.1016/j.oraloncology.2012.06.019

[126] Hanahan D, Weinberg RA. Hallmarks of cancer: the next generation. Cell. 2011;144(5):646–74. Epub 2011/03/08.10.1016/j.cell.2011.02.013

[127] Spanos WC, Nowicki P, Lee DW, Hoover A, Hostager B, Gupta A, et al. Immune response during therapy with cisplatin or radiation for human papillomavirus-related head and neck cancer. Archives of Otolaryngology – Head & Neck Surgery. 2009;135(11):1137–46. Epub 2009/11/18.10.1001/archoto.2009.159

[128] Heusinkveld M, Goedemans R, Briet RJ, Gelderblom H, Nortier JW, Gorter A, et al. Systemic and local human papillomavirus 16-specific T-cell immunity in patients with head and neck cancer. International Journal of Cancer. 2012;131(2):E74–85. Epub 2011/10/25.10.1002/ijc.26497

[129] Turksma AW, Bontkes HJ, van den Heuvel H, de Gruijl TD, von Blomberg BM, Braakhuis BJ, et al. Effector memory T-cell frequencies in relation to tumour stage,

location and HPV status in HNSCC patients. Oral Diseases. 2013;19(6):577–84. Epub 2012/11/28.10.1111/odi.12037

[130] Badoual C, Hans S, Merillon N, Van Ryswick C, Ravel P, Benhamouda N, et al. PD-1-expressing tumor-infiltrating T cells are a favorable prognostic biomarker in HPV-associated head and neck cancer. Cancer Research. 2013;73(1):128–38. Epub 2012/11/09.10.1158/0008-5472.CAN-12-2606

[131] Vermeer DW, Spanos WC, Vermeer PD, Bruns AM, Lee KM, Lee JH. Radiation-induced loss of cell surface CD47 enhances immune-mediated clearance of human papillomavirus-positive cancer. International Journal of Cancer. 2013;133(1):120–9. Epub 2013/01/08.10.1002/ijc.28015

[132] Yoshimura M, Itasaka S, Harada H, Hiraoka M. Microenvironment and radiation therapy. BioMed Research International. 2013;2013:685308. Epub 2013/03/20.10.1155/2013/685308

[133] Overgaard J, Eriksen JG, Nordsmark M, Alsner J, Horsman MR. Plasma osteopontin, hypoxia, and response to the hypoxia sensitiser nimorazole in radiotherapy of head and neck cancer: results from the DAHANCA 5 randomised double-blind placebo-controlled trial. The Lancet Oncology. 2005;6(10):757–64. Epub 2005/10/04.10.1016/S1470-2045(05)70292-8

[134] Kong CS, Narasimhan B, Cao H, Kwok S, Erickson JP, Koong A, et al. The relationship between human papillomavirus status and other molecular prognostic markers in head and neck squamous cell carcinomas. International Journal of Radiation Oncology, Biology, Physics. 2009;74(2):553–61. Epub 2009/05/12.10.1016/j.ijrobp.2009.02.015

[135] Lassen P, Eriksen JG, Hamilton-Dutoit S, Tramm T, Alsner J, Overgaard J. HPV-associated p16-expression and response to hypoxic modification of radiotherapy in head and neck cancer. Radiotherapy and Oncology: Journal of the European Society for Therapeutic Radiology and Oncology. 2010;94(1):30–5. Epub 2009/11/17.10.1016/j.radonc.2009.10.008

[136] Mortensen LS, Johansen J, Kallehauge J, Primdahl H, Busk M, Lassen P, et al. FAZA PET/CT hypoxia imaging in patients with squamous cell carcinoma of the head and neck treated with radiotherapy: results from the DAHANCA 24 trial. Radiotherapy and Oncology: Journal of the European Society for Therapeutic Radiology and Oncology. 2012;105(1):14–20. Epub 2012/10/23.10.1016/j.radonc.2012.09.015

[137] Jansen JF, Carlson DL, Lu Y, Stambuk HE, Moreira AL, Singh B, et al. Correlation of a priori DCE-MRI and (1)H-MRS data with molecular markers in neck nodal metastases: Initial analysis. Oral Oncology. 2012;48(8):717–22. Epub 2012/03/01.10.1016/j.oraloncology.2012.02.001

[138] Sorensen BS, Busk M, Olthof N, Speel EJ, Horsman MR, Alsner J, et al. Radiosensitivity and effect of hypoxia in HPV positive head and neck cancer cells. Radiotherapy and

Oncology: Journal of the European Society for Therapeutic Radiology and Oncology. 2013;108(3):500–5. Epub 2013/08/21.10.1016/j.radonc.2013.06.011

[139] Kimple RJ, Smith MA, Blitzer GC, Torres AD, Martin JA, Yang RZ, et al. Enhanced radiation sensitivity in HPV-positive head and neck cancer. Cancer Research. 2013;73(15):4791–800. Epub 2013/06/12.10.1158/0008-5472.CAN-13-0587

[140] Rieckmann T, Tribius S, Grob TJ, Meyer F, Busch CJ, Petersen C, et al. HNSCC cell lines positive for HPV and p16 possess higher cellular radiosensitivity due to an impaired DSB repair capacity. Radiotherapy and Oncology: Journal of the European Society for Therapeutic Radiology and Oncology. 2013;107(2):242–6. Epub 2013/04/23.10.1016/j.radonc.2013.03.013

[141] Goon PK, Stanley MA, Ebmeyer J, Steinstrasser L, Upile T, Jerjes W, et al. HPV & head and neck cancer: a descriptive update. Head & Neck Oncology. 2009;1:36. Epub 2009/10/16.10.1186/1758-3284-1-36

[142] Portugal LG, Goldenberg JD, Wenig BL, Ferrer KT, Nodzenski E, Sabnani JB, et al. Human papillomavirus expression and p53 gene mutations in squamous cell carcinoma. Archives of Otolaryngology – Head & Neck Surgery. 1997;123(11):1230–4. Epub 1997/11/21.

[143] Andl T, Kahn T, Pfuhl A, Nicola T, Erber R, Conradt C, et al. Etiological involvement of oncogenic human papillomavirus in tonsillar squamous cell carcinomas lacking retinoblastoma cell cycle control. Cancer Research. 1998;58(1):5–13. Epub 1998/01/13.

[144] Mellin H, Friesland S, Lewensohn R, Dalianis T, Munck-Wikland E. Human papillomavirus (HPV) DNA in tonsillar cancer: clinical correlates, risk of relapse, and survival. International Journal of Cancer. 2000;89(3):300–4. Epub 2000/06/22.

[145] Ragin CC, Taioli E. Survival of squamous cell carcinoma of the head and neck in relation to human papillomavirus infection: review and meta-analysis. International Journal of Cancer. 2007;121(8):1813–20. Epub 2007/06/05.10.1002/ijc.22851

[146] Lassen P, Eriksen JG, Hamilton-Dutoit S, Tramm T, Alsner J, Overgaard J. Effect of HPV-associated p16INK4A expression on response to radiotherapy and survival in squamous cell carcinoma of the head and neck. Journal of Clinical Oncology: Official Journal of the American Society of Clinical Oncology. 2009;27(12):1992–8. Epub 2009/03/18.10.1200/JCO.2008.20.2853

[147] Worden FP, Kumar B, Lee JS, Wolf GT, Cordell KG, Taylor JM, et al. Chemoselection as a strategy for organ preservation in advanced oropharynx cancer: response and survival positively associated with HPV16 copy number. Journal of Clinical Oncology: Official Journal of the American Society of Clinical Oncology. 2008;26(19):3138–46. Epub 2008/05/14.10.1200/JCO.2007.12.7597

[148] Rich JT, Milov S, Lewis JS, Jr., Thorstad WL, Adkins DR, Haughey BH. Transoral laser microsurgery (TLM) +/- adjuvant therapy for advanced stage oropharyngeal cancer:

outcomes and prognostic factors. The Laryngoscope. 2009;119(9):1709–19. Epub 2009/07/03.10.1002/lary.20552

[149] Gillison ML, Zhang Q, Ang K, Fu KK, Hammond ME, Jordan R, Trotti A, Spencer S, Rotman M, Chung CH. Analysis of the effect of p16 and tobacco packyears (p-y) on overall (OS) and progression-free survival (PFS) for patients with oropharynx cancer (OPC) in Radiation Therapy Oncology Group (RTOG) protocol 9003. Journal of Clinical Oncology: Official Journal of the American Society of Clinical Oncology. 2010;28:abstract 5510.

[150] Fakhry C, Zhang Q, Nguyen-Tan PF, Rosenthal D, El-Naggar A, Garden AS, et al. Human papillomavirus and overall survival after progression of oropharyngeal squamous cell carcinoma. Journal of Clinical Oncology: Official Journal of the American Society of Clinical Oncology. 2014;32(30):3365–73. Epub 2014/06/25.10.1200/JCO.2014.55.1937

[151] Rosenthal DI, Harari P, Giralt J, Bell D, Raben D, Liu J, Schulten J, Ang KK, Bonner JA. Impact of p16 status on the results of the phase III cetuximab (cet)/radiotherapy (RT). Journal of Clinical Oncology: Official Journal of the American Society of Clinical Oncology. 2014;32:abstract 6001.

[152] Masterson L, Moualed D, Liu ZW, Howard JE, Dwivedi RC, Tysome JR, et al. De-escalation treatment protocols for human papillomavirus-associated oropharyngeal squamous cell carcinoma: a systematic review and meta-analysis of current clinical trials. European Journal of Cancer. 2014;50(15):2636–48. Epub 2014/08/06.10.1016/j.ejca.2014.07.001

[153] Goldenberg D, Begum S, Westra WH, Khan Z, Sciubba J, Pai SI, et al. Cystic lymph node metastasis in patients with head and neck cancer: an HPV-associated phenomenon. Head & Neck. 2008;30(7):898–903. Epub 2008/04/03.10.1002/hed.20796

[154] Huang SH, O'Sullivan B, Xu W, Zhao H, Chen DD, Ringash J, et al. Temporal nodal regression and regional control after primary radiation therapy for N2-N3 head-and-neck cancer stratified by HPV status. International Journal of Radiation Oncology, Biology, Physics. 2013;87(5):1078–85. Epub 2013/11/12.10.1016/j.ijrobp.2013.08.049

[155] Huang SH, Perez-Ordonez B, Weinreb I, Hope A, Massey C, Waldron JN, et al. Natural course of distant metastases following radiotherapy or chemoradiotherapy in HPV-related oropharyngeal cancer. Oral Oncology. 2013;49(1):79–85. Epub 2012/08/25.10.1016/j.oraloncology.2012.07.015

[156] Huang SH, Perez-Ordonez B, Liu FF, Waldron J, Ringash J, Irish J, et al. Atypical clinical behavior of p16-confirmed HPV-related oropharyngeal squamous cell carcinoma treated with radical radiotherapy. International Journal of Radiation Oncology, Biology, Physics. 2012;82(1):276–83. Epub 2010/10/19.10.1016/j.ijrobp.2010.08.031

[157] O'Sullivan B, Huang SH, Perez-Ordonez B, Massey C, Siu LL, Weinreb I, et al. Outcomes of HPV-related oropharyngeal cancer patients treated by radiotherapy alone

using altered fractionation. Radiotherapy and Oncology: Journal of the European Society for Therapeutic Radiology and Oncology. 2012;103(1):49–56. Epub 2012/03/14.10.1016/j.radonc.2012.02.009

[158] McBride SM, Busse PM, Clark JR, Wirth LJ, Ancukiewicz M, Chan AW. Long-term survival after distant metastasis in patients with oropharyngeal cancer. Oral Oncology. 2014;50(3):208–12. Epub 2014/01/07.10.1016/j.oraloncology.2013.10.020

[159] Vermorken JB, Psyrri A, Mesia R, Peyrade F, Beier F, de Blas B, et al. Impact of tumor HPV status on outcome in patients with recurrent and/or metastatic squamous cell carcinoma of the head and neck receiving chemotherapy with or without cetuximab: retrospective analysis of the phase III EXTREME trial. Annals of Oncology: Official Journal of the European Society for Medical Oncology/ESMO. 2014;25(4):801–7. Epub 2014/03/01.10.1093/annonc/mdt574

[160] Mehra R. Analysis of HPV and ERCC1 in recurrent or metastatic squamous cell carcinoma of the head and neck (R/M SCCHN). Journal of Clinical Oncology: Official Journal of the American Society of Clinical Oncology. 2013;31:abstract 6006.

[161] Gillison ML, Zhang Q, Jordan R, Xiao W, Westra WH, Trotti A, et al. Tobacco smoking and increased risk of death and progression for patients with p16-positive and p16-negative oropharyngeal cancer. Journal of Clinical Oncology: Official Journal of the American Society of Clinical Oncology. 2012;30(17):2102–11. Epub 2012/05/09.10.1200/JCO.2011.38.4099

[162] Massano J, Regateiro FS, Januario G, Ferreira A. Oral squamous cell carcinoma: review of prognostic and predictive factors. Oral Surgery, Oral Medicine, Oral Pathology, Oral Radiology, and Endodontics. 2006;102(1):67–76. Epub 2006/07/13.10.1016/j.tripleo.2005.07.038

[163] Jadhav KB, Gupta N. Clinicopathological prognostic implicators of oral squamous cell carcinoma: need to understand and revise. North American Journal of Medical Sciences. 2013;5(12):671–9. Epub 2014/01/10.10.4103/1947-2714.123239

[164] Nasman A, Andersson E, Nordfors C, Grun N, Johansson H, Munck-Wikland E, et al. MHC class I expression in HPV positive and negative tonsillar squamous cell carcinoma in correlation to clinical outcome. International Journal of Cancer. 2013;132(1):72–81. Epub 2012/05/18.10.1002/ijc.27635

[165] Lindquist D, Ahrlund-Richter A, Tarjan M, Tot T, Dalianis T. Intense CD44 expression is a negative prognostic factor in tonsillar and base of tongue cancer. Anticancer Research. 2012;32(1):153–61. Epub 2012/01/04.

[166] Rietbergen MM, Martens-de Kemp SR, Bloemena E, Witte BI, Brink A, Baatenburg de Jong RJ, et al. Cancer stem cell enrichment marker CD98: a prognostic factor for survival in patients with human papillomavirus-positive oropharyngeal cancer. European Journal of Cancer. 2014;50(4):765–73. Epub 2013/12/10.10.1016/j.ejca.2013.11.010

[167] Nasman A, Romanitan M, Nordfors C, Grun N, Johansson H, Hammarstedt L, et al. Tumor infiltrating CD8+ and Foxp3+ lymphocytes correlate to clinical outcome and human papillomavirus (HPV) status in tonsillar cancer. PLoS One. 2012;7(6):e38711. Epub 2012/06/16.10.1371/journal.pone.0038711

[168] Liang C, Marsit CJ, McClean MD, Nelson HH, Christensen BC, Haddad RI, et al. Biomarkers of HPV in head and neck squamous cell carcinoma. Cancer Research. 2012;72(19):5004–13. Epub 2012/09/20.10.1158/0008-5472.CAN-11-3277

[169] Cohen MA, Basha SR, Reichenbach DK, Robertson E, Sewell DA. Increased viral load correlates with improved survival in HPV-16-associated tonsil carcinoma patients. Acta Oto-Laryngologica. 2008;128(5):583–9. Epub 2008/04/19.10.1080/00016480701558880

[170] Weinberger PM, Yu Z, Haffty BG, Kowalski D, Harigopal M, Brandsma J, et al. Molecular classification identifies a subset of human papillomavirus--associated oropharyngeal cancers with favorable prognosis. Journal of Clinical Oncology: Official Journal of the American Society of Clinical Oncology. 2006;24(5):736–47. Epub 2006/01/13.10.1200/JCO.2004.00.3335

[171] Bossi P, Orlandi E, Miceli R, Perrone F, Guzzo M, Mariani L, et al. Treatment-related outcome of oropharyngeal cancer patients differentiated by HPV dictated risk profile: a tertiary cancer centre series analysis. Annals of Oncology: Official Journal of the European Society for Medical Oncology/ESMO. 2014;25(3):694–9. Epub 2014/02/11.10.1093/annonc/mdu004

[172] Dempsey AF, Patel DA. HPV vaccine acceptance, utilization and expected impacts in the U.S.: Where are we now? Human Vaccines. 2010;6(9):715–720. Epub 2010/09/22.10.4161/hv.6.9.12730

[173] Herrero R, Quint W, Hildesheim A, Gonzalez P, Struijk L, Katki HA, et al. Reduced prevalence of oral human papillomavirus (HPV) 4 years after bivalent HPV vaccination in a randomized clinical trial in Costa Rica. PLoS One. 2013;8(7):e68329. Epub 2013/07/23.10.1371/journal.pone.0068329

7

Interventional Techniques for Head and Neck Cancer Pain

Victor M. Silva Ortíz, Guillermo E. Aréchiga Ornelas,
José A. Flores Cantisani,
Juan Ignacio Reyes Torres and
Fernando Cantú Flores

Abstract

One of the most feared consequences of cancer is the possibility of severe and uncontrolled pain in patients with advanced cancer. Patients with head and neck cancer (HNC) have the highest prevalence of pain among patients with cancer, and it is often one of the major reasons for seeking care. A subspecialty approach that incorporates anatomical and technical knowledge to alleviate pain through minimally invasive procedures is relatively recent. The purpose of this chapter is to present different interventional techniques which are used for the treatment of pain in HNC patients when drug treatment is unsuccessful.

Keywords: head, neck, cancer pain, neuropathic pain, interventional pain, pain management

1. Introduction

Interventional procedures in the treatment of head and neck cancer (HNC) pain have been proposed in the past 25 years due to the greater knowledge of the mechanisms of action of pain and its physiological and anatomical basis. There has been development of new techniques to treat refractory pain and treatment strategies with an integral view of the problem. In addition to the progress of knowledge and development of techniques and technologies, education and pain medicine certification programs have been developed around the world [1].

Pain and symptoms associated with HNC is a challenge due to the rich innervation and loss of function caused by tumor invasion or by the treatment of cancer [2].

Pain is the first symptom in 20–50% of patients with cancer; however, in patients with HNC, it can become as high as 85%. Of this, 93% are mixed (nociceptive and neuropathic) and 30% are neuropathic pain due to tumor involving tissues or metastatic disease. In up to 85% of patients, pain is the main cause of medical attention [3]. Compared to other types of cancer, the highest incidence of pain in patients with HNC is due to the intense innervation of anatomical structures.

Common neuropathic syndromes associated with cancer are chemotherapy-induced neuropathy, tumor invasion (leptomeningeal metastases), neuralgias (trigeminal neuralgia or postherpetic neuropathy, glossopharyngeal neuralgia), radiculopathies and plexopathies, paraneoplastic sensory neuropathies, Horner's syndrome, postsurgery neuropathies, and postradiotherapy neuropathies [4, 5].

HNC is generally a disfiguring disease. In addition, it impairs the quality of life (QOL) of patients because it interferes with speech, swallowing, and chewing, the key factors in the patient's autonomy [6].

Not all HNC patients who have pain are due to cancer. Sometimes, it occurs due to medical or surgical treatment. Some studies report cancer-related pain in 52% of the hospitalized patients, of which 50% was due to surgery and 29% directly related to the tumor [7].

One of the adverse effects associated with HNC treatment is orofacial pain. Oral mucositis is the most frequent complaint impairing the QOL of the patient. This is mediated by elevated inflammatory factors, which play a central role in the activation of cytokines, such as TNF-α, that is known to be involved in mediation of neuropathic pain and hyperalgesia. Combined chemotherapy and radiation therapy results in increased frequency, severity and duration of mucositis. The treatment given to patients with HNC represents an important impact on the development of pain and the magnitude of it [7, 2].

Radiotherapy is another important cause of pain in HNC, because it creates a hypoxic environment, and hypoxic nerves are more vulnerable to neuropathic pain. In long term, chronic hypoxia leads to fibrosis in perineural tissues and causes late onset neuropathic pain, even in cancer-free survivors [7, 2].

Approximately 50% of HNC patients report orofacial pain before radiation therapy, 81% during, and 70% at the completion of treatment. Thirty-six percent of HNC patients report pain after 6 months of treatment, and 30% experience pain beyond 6 months. The severity of pain varies among different disease sites and over the treatment course [8]. Pain intensity usually stays the highest during disease treatment (surgery, chemotherapy, radiotherapy) and may take 6 months or more to reach initial levels (pre-treatment).

2. Factors associated with head and neck cancer pain

2.1. Age and gender

Age is an important factor in pain perception, according to studies comparing age groups. The group of patients who reported pain was younger than 65 years. A higher pain scale among females were reported compared to males, however, significantly higher levels of pain among males compared to female was reported also. There are some other factors associated with pain such as improper oral hygiene, depression, and anxiety. The presence of metallic taste was seen as a predictor of spontaneous pain.

2.2. Cancer-related factors

Patients with tumors in the oral cavity have a lower QOL, as well as worse pain, compared to other sites. Patients with end-stage tumors report greater pain compared to stages I and II, as well as an increase in spontaneous pain in patients with nodal disease [8].

3. Interventional management for HNC patients

Trigeminal (CNV) and facial (CNVII) nerves are by far the most frequently affected cranial nerves, alone or in combination. The predilection for these two specific nerves is explained by their wide anatomic distribution in the craniofacial territory and their rich anastomotic connections.

The supply of opioid drugs is insufficient in some countries, or not all the population has access to it; for this reason, it is necessary to have an interventional tool to manage cancer pain. There is a good evidence for the "early integration" of interventional pain treatments for carefully selected head and neck cancer patients, at the same time or even before starting strong opioids.

4. Sphenopalatine ganglion (SPG) block

SPG is located within a triangular structure with a superior base called pterygopalatine fossa, which has a close relationship with the maxillary nerve and very close to the sphenopalatine foramen [9]. It is a complex neural center with multiple connections to trigeminal, facial, and sympathetic systems and consists of somatosensory, sympathetic, and parasympathetic fibers.

The ganglion is located just below the maxillary nerve and receives three nerve roots: The sensory root of the sphenopalatine branches from the maxillary nerve, the motor root from the intermediate nerve (part of the facial nerve) through the major petrosal nerve, and the sympathetic root from the internal carotid plexus.

In 1908, Sluder proposed an inflammatory reaction in the territory of pterygopalatine fossa that may be involved in certain cases of unilateral facial pain associated with rhinorrhea, lacrimation and mucosal congestion. Ruskin later described the blocking technique with local anesthetic to treat a variety of conditions associated with headache [10].

4.1. Indications for SPG block

Some of the indications for the SPG block are trigeminal neuralgia, persistent idiopathic facial pain (previously referred to as atypical facial pain), acute migraine, acute and chronic cluster headache, SP neuralgia, herpes zoster involving the head, and a variety of other facial neuralgias, including tumor invasion.

Sphenopalatine ganglion neuralgia consists mainly of neuropathic symptoms, but is accompanied by sensory, motor, and gustatory manifestations. It is common for the symptoms to be episodes of vasomotor hyperactivity such as lacrimation, discharge and inflammation of the nasal mucosa, and alteration of gustatory sensation of the palate and oropharynx.

The procedure consists of accessing the pterygopalatine fossa by placing local anesthetic with or without steroids, radiofrequency ablation, or pulsed radiofrequency. It may be used for diagnosis or treatment of the conditions described above. It is mandatory that these procedures are performed under radiographic imaging. It is essential that the pterygopalatine fossa is clearly visualized and confirmed before starting the procedure [11]. (See **Figure 1**).

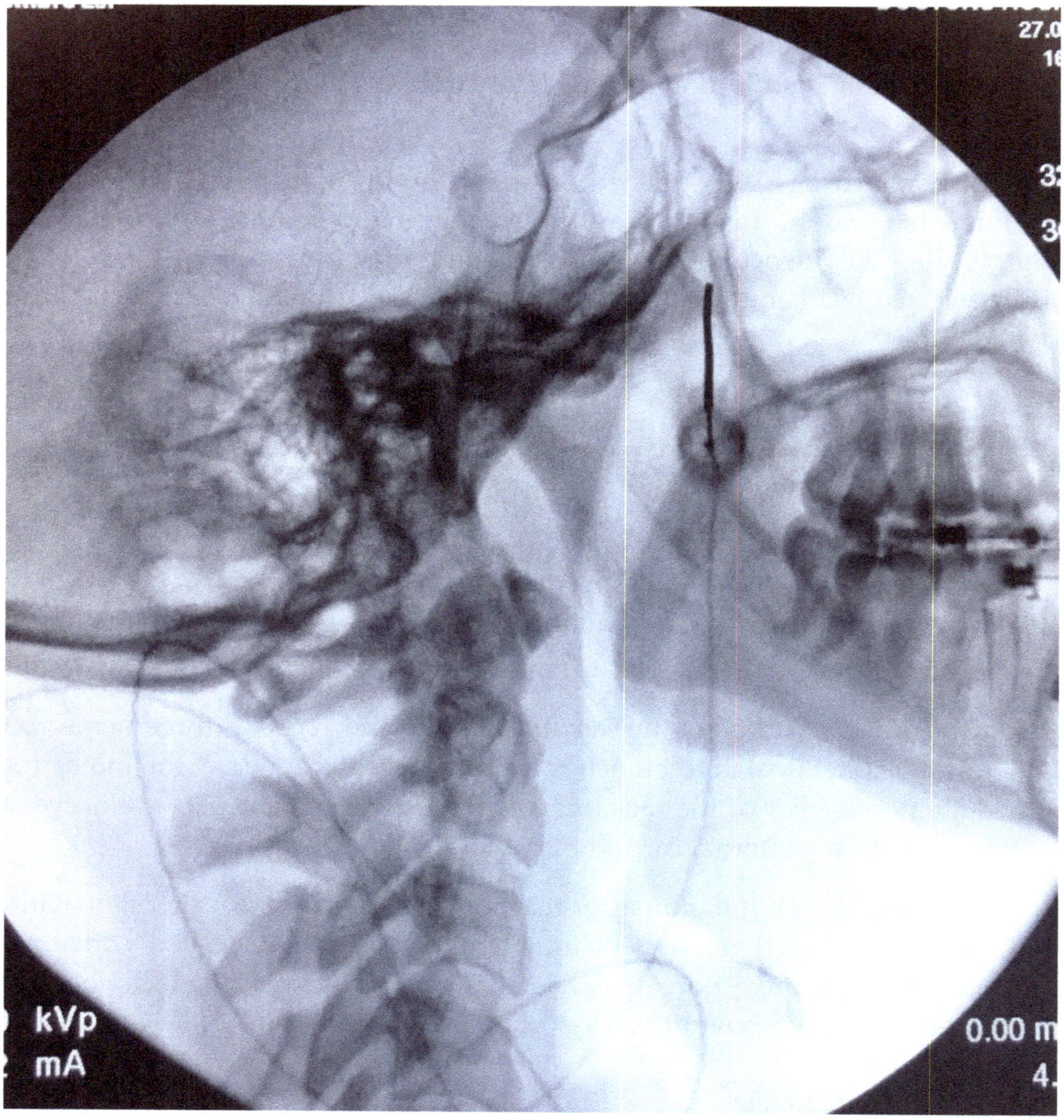

Figure 1. Sphenopalatine ganglion block.

5. Trigeminal ganglion block (Gasserian ganglion)

The trigeminal nerve is the most developed and extensive cranial nerve with a large territory of distribution. This nerve consists of sensitive fibers (touch, pain, temperature) and motor of the face (chewing). It originates in the posterior fossa and lies in the Meckel's cavity (medial cranial fossa), from which originate their three terminal branches: ophthalmic nerve (V1), maxillary (V2), and mandibular nerve (V3).

There are several causes of secondary trigeminal neuralgia, which are tumors compressing the trigeminal nerve, vascular compressions in close relation with the nerve, or tumors in cerebellopontine angle.

The typical clinical presentation of trigeminal neuralgia is sudden, unilateral electrical shock-like pain dispersed among pain-free intervals along the side of the face. Paroxysmal attacks are frequently triggered by chewing, brushing teeth, laughing, talking, and even smiling. It is often referred to as the most excruciating pain syndrome known today affecting quality of life. In contrast, clinical criteria of atypical facial pain consist of persistent facial pain that does not have the characteristics of cranial neuralgias and cannot be attributed to a different disorder [12].

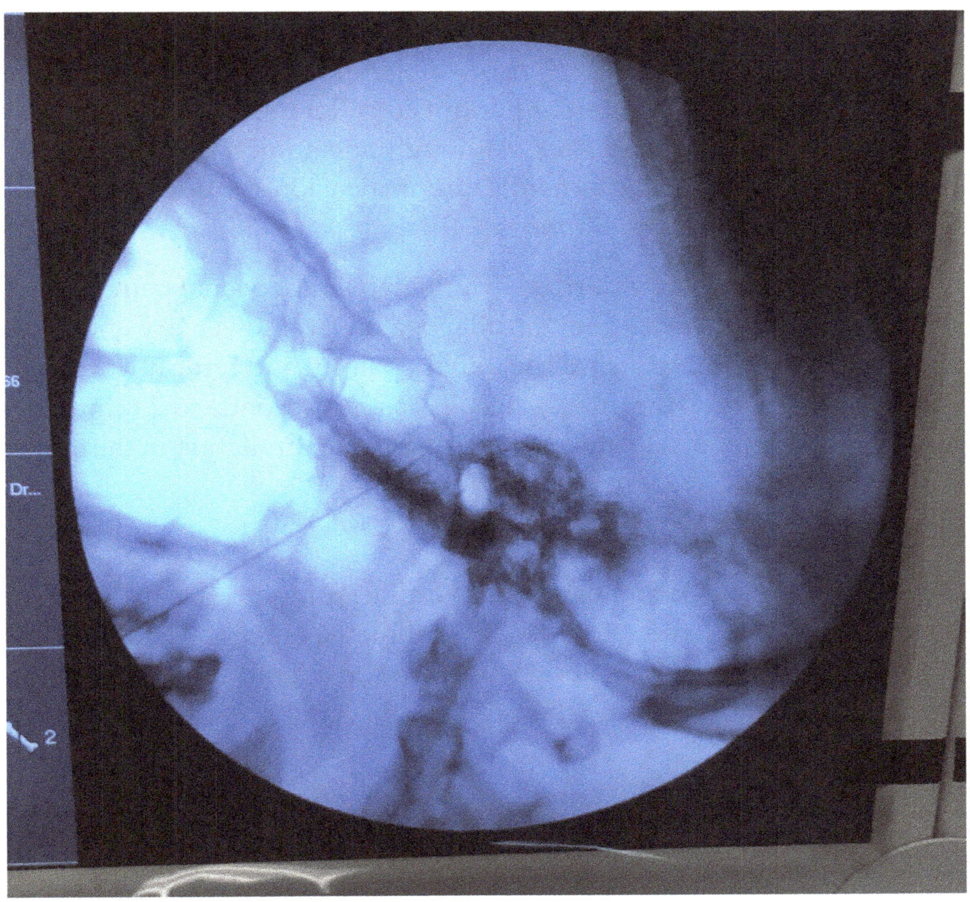

Figure 2. Gasserian ganglion block.

An approach is with fluoroscopy in oblique submental view. In this technique, foramen ovale is visualized; usually medially to the mandibular process, and then the needle is advanced toward the foramen, first in submental view and then in the lateral view to control depth.

One technique used to selectively injure the branches of the trigeminal nerve is continuous radiofrequency. This method allows identifying the affected branch by sensory and motor stimulation with conscious sedation. It is a percutaneous technique using the approach described by Hartel through the foramen ovale. An electrode is introduced through the needle (with an active tip of 2–5 mm) to make the lesion (ranges from 60–90°C). The deliberately damaged nerve is then no longer able to transmit nociceptive signals.

The potential risks of trigeminal rhizotomy include, but are not limited to, facial numbness spreading beyond the required area [causing corneal anesthesia (6%) with its risk of ulceration], weakness of chewing (4%), and a rare chance of neuropathic pain (1%, anesthesia dolorosa) [13].

There is extensive evidence of the use of continuous radiofrequency for the treatment of trigeminal neuralgia, indicated acute pain relief in 97.6% of patients and continued complete pain relief at 5-year follow-up in 57.7% of patients. The effectiveness of pulsed radiofrequency (PRF) for trigeminal neuralgia is still under debate [13]. (See **Figure 2**)

6. Glossopharyngeal nerve block

The glossopharyngeal nerve (GPN) is an important consideration as a pain generator or modulator in cases of pain of the face and neck. Although uncommon as an etiology of head and neck pain (0.57–1.3% of cases of facial pain), tumor invasion can lead to glossopharyngeal neuralgia, like cerebellopontine angle tumors [14].

Glossopharyngeal neuralgia is characterized by unilateral paroxysmal pain in the oropharynx, nasopharynx, larynx, base of the tongue, tonsillar region, and lower jaw and can also radiate to the ipsilateral ear. These attacks are excruciatingly painful and typically described as sharp, stabbing, "shocks of electricity" the attacks usually last for seconds to 2 minutes. It is characteristic that there are triggers such as chewing, yawning, or stimulation in the oral mucosa [15].

6.1. Indications for GPN block

GPN block is beneficial in alleviating pain due to orofacial cancer. It is used for the treatment of glossopharyngeal neuralgia refractory to medical management and for those who are not surgical candidates. Diagnostic GPN block should be considered first to predict the response to radiofrequency or neurolysis in intractable glossopharyngeal neuralgia and cancer-related pain syndromes.

6.1.1. Technique

The patient is placed supine with the head rotated slightly opposite from the affected side. The styloid process is used to identify the course of the GPN, just equidistant to mastoid process and angle of the mandible. Once the styloid apophysis is visualized, the needle is contacted and carefully redirected posteriorly and the contrast medium is injected under continuous "live" fluoroscopy.

Complications are secondary to the close proximity to the internal carotid artery (ICA) and internal jugular vein (IJV) as well as the vagus, accessory, and hypoglossal nerves at the styloid process.

Accidental puncture of the ICA or the IJV can lead to vessel trauma and hematoma formation. Dysphagia can result from blockade of the glossopharyngeal nerve that provides motor innervations to the stylopharyngeus muscle. Blockade of the spinal accessory and hypoglossal nerves can result in temporary weakness of the trapezius muscle and the tongue, respectively. Inadvertent intravascular injection may lead to seizures or cardiovascular collapse. Blockade of the vagus nerve can lead to bradycardia, asystole, reflex tachycardia, and syncope as well as dysphonia secondary to vocal cord paralysis [15].

7. Stellate ganglion block

There are three cervical sympathetic chains: upper cervical ganglion, middle cervical ganglion, and lower cervical ganglion. These ganglions are all connected together. The stellate ganglion is composed of the fusion of the inferior cervical chain and the first thoracic ganglion, this happens in the 80% of the people; in the rest, the first thoracic ganglion is called stellate ganglion [16]. It is located above the muscle longus colli, and this in turn is in the anterolateral aspect of the C6 vertebra.

7.1. Indications for stallate ganglion block

Complex regional pain syndrome (CRPS) I and II, vascular insufficiency—Raynaud's syndrome, vasospasm, vascular disease, postherpetic neuralgia and acute herpes zoster, phantom pain, postmastectomy pain, quinine poisoning, hyperhidrosis of upper extremity, cardiac arrhythmias, angina, vascular headaches, neuropathic pain syndromes, including central pain, cancer pain (neuropathic pain syndromes in cancer pain), atypical facial pain, and trigeminal neuralgia.

7.2. Ultrasound technique

There are many techniques described for stellate ganglion block. We will describe the ultrasound guided block, because this technique allows us to directly visualize the vascular structures, thyroid tissue, vertebral artery, pleura, esophagus, and nerve structures, which are important for the success of the procedure and avoiding catastrophic complications.

Ultrasound-guided C6 stellate ganglion block (C6-SGB) was first described by Kapral et al. [17]. There is a significant variation in the anatomy of stellate ganglion at the level of C_6 and C_7. Ultrasound-guided lateral approach increases the efficacy of SGB by deposition of drug subfascially with real-time imaging.

A high-frequency linear ultrasound transducer is placed over the medial border of the sternocleidomastoid muscle in the transverse position at the level of the cricoid notch (approximately the C6 level). The tip of the needle is placed in the facial plane where the sympathetic chain runs, deep to the prevertebral fascia contributing the posterior fascial layer of the carotid sheath, and superficial to the fascia investing the longus colli muscle. Using ultrasound guidance, the needle can be placed closer to the target in the correct fascial plane, which will minimize the amount of local anesthetic needed and thus improve patient safety [16].

The ultrasound images at this level should reveal the C6 vertebral body with the Chassaignac or the carotid tubercle, the C6 nerve root, the carotid artery, the longus colli muscle, and the short posterior tubercle. If the carotid artery blocks access to the cervical sympathetic chain, the ultrasound transducer can be slowly moved laterally to help delineate a more lateral needle trajectory to avoid the carotid artery.

Complications: Bleeding/hematoma, pneumothorax, hemothorax, vertebral artery injury or inadvertent injection, inadvertent injection into neuraxis, esophageal trauma, tracheal trauma, phrenic nerve injury, brachial plexus injury, recurrent laryngeal nerve injury, and postsympathectomy syndrome.

8. Vertebroplasty for cancer-related cervical vertebral compression fractures

Percutaneous vertebroplasty (PVP) was initially described by Galibert et al. [18] as a treatment for vertebral hemagioma. Later, it was gaining popularity for the treatment of pain of vertebral origin as metastasis or fractures by compression.

The most common targets of spinal metastasis are thoracic vertebrae (60–80%), followed by lumbar (20%) and cervical spine (10%). Although cervical metastases are less prevalent than thoracic and lumbar spine, PVP procedure in cervical vertebrae remains technical challenging, because of the anatomical structures of the neck. The approach can result in serious complications [19].

PVP was recently suggested as an alternative treatment for spinal metastatic patients who were intolerable to surgery and radiotherapy. It is now a well-established procedure comprising a percutaneous injection of a biomaterial, usually polymethyl methacrylate (PMMA), into vertebral body. In most cases, this procedure significantly relieves pain and stabilizes the vertebral body. A significant decrease in visual analogue scale (VAS) and QOL was reported in late-stage cancer patients with multiple cervical spinal metastases, with PVP. The grade of evidence for the treatment of vertebral fractures associated with metastatic disease is 2B + [3].

9. Intrathecal drug delivery systems (IDDS)

The use of intrathecal therapy [IT] to treat patients with cancer pain has increased since its inception in the 1980s. By positioning a catheter in the cerebral spinal fluid, IT therapy may be advantageous over traditional routes because it reduces systemic exposure to the drug and its metabolites as the medication is administered directly to the central nervous system.

To reduce the risk of infection in a long-term intrathecal therapy, it is necessary to implant the device subcutaneously. Occasionally, an intrathecal drug delivery test may be performed by an external catheter. In this way, the infusion of the permanent device is simulated and the dose of the opioid is titrated [20]. This treatment is effective to treat both neuropathic and nociceptive pain of oncological and non-oncological origin.

Related to HNC pain, the ideal opioid for intrathecal infusion should be hydrosoluble, with the intention of having a greater rostral migration.

There are studies that report improvement in pain, mood, function, as well as, an improvement in depression and anxiety in cancer patients at a follow-up of 36 months among patients undergoing intrathecal opioid therapy.

The potential complications of IDDS include opioid-induced hyperalgesia, hypotension, sedation, respiratory depression, inflammatory mass "granuloma at the tip of the catheter,"

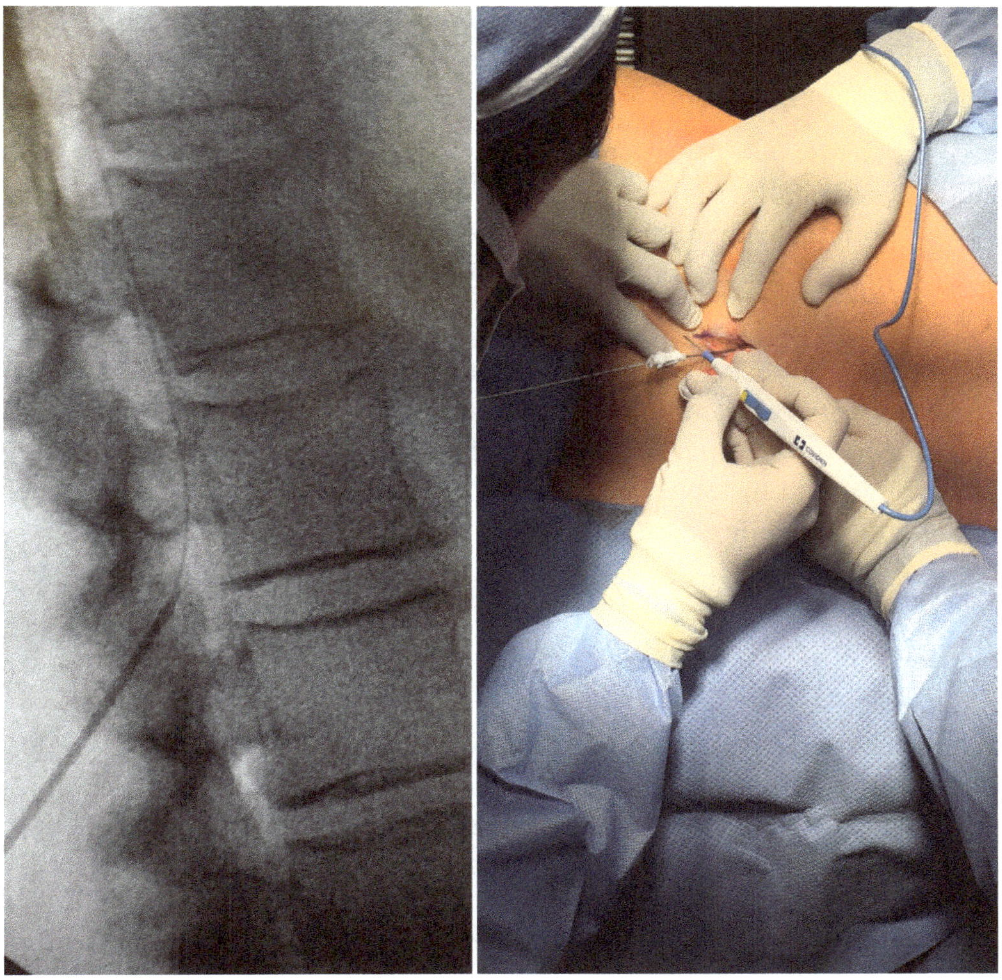

Figure 3. Intrathecal therapy.

hypogonadotropic hypogonadism, and immunologic compromise. The potential for these consequences can be diminished with careful dosing and titration. The patient should be monitored 24 hours after increasing the dose to decrease the risk of respiratory depression and mortality (See **Figure 3**).

10. Peripheral nerve blocks, cervical epidural, and medial branch block

Occipital neuralgia is a debilitating disorder first described in 1821 as recurrent headaches localized in the occipital region. Other symptoms that have been associated with this condition include paroxysmal burning and aching pain in the distribution of the greater, lesser, or third occipital nerves.

10.1. The greater occipital nerve

The HNC-associated headache may be due to entrapment of great occipital nerve (GON), third occipital nerve (TON), or irritation of either of them due to tumor invasion [21, 22]. There are different structures in the cervical region that can cause head and neck pain, due to tumor invasion. The cervicogenic headache is a secondary headache associated with the first cervical segments.

Occipital nerve block is an effective therapeutic tool in treating a variety of headache disorders including occipital neuralgia, migraine, cluster headaches and tumor invasion. The mechanism of action is a result of blockade of nociceptive afferent fibers supplying the posterior head and upper cervical region (C1–C3) which join trigeminal fibers at the trigeminocervical complex [21, 22].

Occipital nerve block and C2–C3 medial branch can be used to treat cervicogenic headache and cancer-related cervical pain, using corticosteroids or radiofrequency. They can be performed percutaneously with an insulated cannula, applying local heat to the sensitive branch with the intention of diminishing the sensitivity. Both nerve blocks are easy to perform and well tolerated with a few side effects.

11. Botulinum neurotoxin (BoNT)

Botulinum neurotoxin derived from *Clostridium botulinum*, not only has been used for cosmetic purposes but also therapeutically for focal dystonia, spasticity, and chronic migraine. There is some evidence that it inhibits the release of peripheral neurotransmitters and inflammatory mediators from sensory nerves; so, its spectrum as a potential treatment for neuropathic pain has grown.

The main mechanism of BoNT is the inhibition of acetylcholine (Ach) release at presynaptic nerve terminals, resulting in a reduction of muscle fiber activity, and the innervated structure becomes paralyzed [23]. It has also been suggested that BoNT acts by inhibiting neurogenic inflammation by interfering with local release of neurotransmitters, such as calcitonin gene-related peptide, substance P and glutamate, as well as expression of transient receptor potencial v member 1 (TRPV1).

BoNT is injected into painful areas of the body. Injection techniques primarily include either intradermal or subcutaneous injections. It is important to mention that there are different reports of BoNT administration in patients with trigeminal neuralgia and other neuralgias in the head and face with significant improvement in VAS and QOL.

12. Conclusions

The increasing need for adequate pain control has led us to enter into interventional pain management. There is good evidence of early integration of interventional treatments in cancer pain [24]. The field of interventional pain management grows very fast throughout the world and is a tool that every physician involved in treatment of cancer must value and offer to patients for a more comprehensive management of the disease.

Author details

Victor M. Silva Ortíz[1]*, Guillermo E. Aréchiga Ornelas[2], José A. Flores Cantisani[3], Juan Ignacio Reyes Torres[4] and Fernando Cantú Flores[1]

*Address all correspondence to: drvictorsilva@gmail.com

1 Pain Management and Palliative Care Department, Hospital Zambrano Hellion, Monterrey, Mexico

2 Pain Management and Palliative Care Department, Hospital General Occidente, Guadalajara, Mexico

3 Pain and Palliative Care, ISSSTELEON, Monterrey, Mexico

4 Pain Management and Palliative Care Department, ISSSTE, Saltillo, Mexico

References

[1] Soto E, Bobr V, Bax JA. Interventional techniques for headaches. Techniques in regional anesthesia and pain management. 2012;**16**:30-40

[2] Epstein JB, Wilkie DJ, Fischer DJ, Kim YO, Villines D. Neuropathic and nociceptive pain in head and neck cancer patients receiving radiation therapy. Head & Neck Oncology. 2009;**1**:26 DOI: 10.1186/1758-3284-1-26

[3] Bhatnagar S, Gupta M. Evidence-based clinical practice guidelines for interventional pain management in cancer pain. Indian Journal of Palliative Care. 2015;**21**:137-147

[4] Kurita GP, Ulrich A, Jensen TS, Werner MU, Sjøgren P. How is neuropathic cancer pain assessed in randomised controlled trials? Pain. 2012;**153**:13-17

[5] Yalcin EES. Neuropathic cancer pain: What we are dealing with? How to manage it? OncoTargets and Therapy. 2014:**7** 599-618

[6] Kolokythas A, Connelly ST, Schmidt BL. Validation of the University of California San Francisco oral cancer pain questionnaire. Journal of Pain.. 2007;**8**(12):950-953

[7] Astrup GL, Rustøen T, Miaskowski C, Paul SM, Bjordal K. Changes in and predictors of pain characteristics in patients with head and neck cancer undergoing radiotherapy Pain. 2015;**156**:967-979

[8] Macfarlane TV, Wirth T, Ranasinghe S, Ah-See KW, Renny N, Hurman D. Head and neck cancer pain: Systematic review of prevalence and associated factors. Journal of Oral & Maxillofacial Research. 2012;**3**(1):e1

[9] Blier Z. Physiology of the sphenopalatine ganglion. American Journal of Physiology. 1930;**93**:398-406

[10] Piagkou M, Demesticha T, Troupis T, Vlasis K, Skandalakis P, Makri A, Mazarakis A, Lappas D, Piagkos G, Johnson EO. The pterygopalatine ganglion and its role in various pain syndromes: From anatomy to clinical practice. Pain Practice. 2012;**12**(5):399-412

[11] Nader A., Kendall MC, De Oliveira GS, Chen JQ, Vanderby B, Rosenow JM, Bernard R, Bendok BK. Ultrasound-guided trigeminal nerve block via the pterygopalatine fossa: An effective treatment for trigeminal neuralgia and atypical facial pain. Pain Physician. 2013;**16**:E537-E545

[12] Zakrzewska JM, Jassim S, Blum JS. A prospective, longitudinal study on patients with trigeminal neuralgia who underwent radiofrequency thermocoagulation of the Gasserian ganglion. Pain. 1999;**79**:51-58

[13] Son B-C, Kim H-S, Kim II-S, Yang S-H, Lee SW. Percutaneous radiofrequency thermocoagulation under fluoroscopic image-guidance for idiopathic trigeminal neuralgia. Journal of Korean Neurosurgical Society. 2011;**50**:446-452

[14] Mehio A-K, Shah SK. Alleviating Head and Neck Pain. Otolaryngologic Clinics of North America. 2009;**42**:143-159 DOI: 10.1016/j.otc.2008.09.013

[15] Ažman J, Pintaric TS, Cvetko E, Vlassakov K. Ultrasound-Guided glossopharyngeal nerve block. A cadaver and a volunteer sonoanatomy study. Regional Anesthesia and Pain Medicine. 2017;**42**:252-258

[16] Narouze S. Ultrasound-Guided stellate ganglion block: Safety and efficacy. Current Pain and Headache Reports. 2014;**18**:424. DOI: 10.1007/s11916-014-0424-5

[17] Kapral S, Krafft P, Gosch M. Ultrasound imaging for stellate ganglion block: Direct visualization of puncture site and local anesthetic spread: A pilot study. Regional Anesthesia and Pain Medicine. 1995;**20**(4):323-328

[18] Galibert P, Deramond H, Rosat P, Le Gars D. Preliminary note on the treatment of vertebral angioma by percutaneous acrylic vertebroplasty. Neurochirurgie. 1987;**33**(2):166-168

[19] Health Quality Ontario. Vertebral Augmentation Involving Vertebroplasty or Kyphoplasty for Cancer- Related Vertebral Compression Fractures: A Systematic Review. Ontario Health Technology Assessment Series. 2016;**16**(11):1-202

[20] Deer TR, Smith HS, Burton AW, Pope JE, Doleys DM, Levy RM, Staats PS, Wallace M, Webster LR, Rauck R, Cousins M. Comprehensive consensus based guidelines on intrathecal drug delivery systems in the treatment of pain caused by cancer pain. Pain Physician. 2011;**14**:E283–E312

[21] Wahezi SE, Silva K, Shaparin N, Lederman A, Emam M, Haramati N, Downie S. Currently recommended TON injectate volumes concomitantly block the GON: Clinical implications for managing cervicogenic headache. Pain Physician. 2016;**19**:E1079-E1086

[22] Nagar VR, Birthi P, Grider JS, Asopa A. Systematic review of radiofrequency ablation and pulsed radiofrequency for management of cervicogenic headache. Pain Physician. 2015;**18**:109-130

[23] Oh H-M, Chung ME. Botulinum toxin for neuropathic pain: A review of the literature. Toxins. 2015;**7**:3127-3154. DOI: 10.3390/toxins7083127

[24] Sommer CL, Wallace MS, Cohen S, Kress M. Pain 2016: Refresher Courses. 16th world congress on pain. IASP Press, Whashington D.C. 2016

8

Thyroid Cancers: Considerations, Classifications, and Managements

Mohammad Hossein Khosravi, Ali Kouhi,
Masoumeh Saeedi, Ali Bagherihagh and
Mohammad Hosein Amirzade-Iranaq

Abstract

Rapidly increasing trend of thyroid cancer incidence has turned this disease into a global concern. An estimated number of 64,300 new cases of thyroid cancer occurred in men and women in 2016, which represents 3.8% of all new cancer cases of USA (https://seer.cancer.gov/statfacts/html/thyro.html). Thus, there is a high possibility for every physician to encounter a case of thyroid cancer during his/her professional lifetime. In this chapter, we clarified epidemiology, different categories, and new approaches toward diagnosis and management of thyroid cancer.

Keywords: thyroid cancer, epidemiology, differentiated thyroid cancer, undifferentiated thyroid cancer, thyroid nodule

1. Detailed epidemiology of thyroid cancer

As the most common endocrine cancer and fifth most common cancer in women, thyroid cancer includes approximately 1–1.5% of all new cases of cancer diagnosed annually in the USA based on previous data [1–3]. Thyroid cancer is more prevalent among women and those with positive family history of thyroid disease. Some prior studies have reported a worldwide increasing trend for thyroid cancer incidence in recent decades [4]. Annual percent change (APC) is a commonly used indicator for the assessment of changes in incidence. Based on US National Cancer Institute's Surveillance, Epidemiology, and End Results (SEER) program, it has been reported 2.4% from 1980 to 1997 and 6.6% from 1997 to 2009 in both genders for thyroid cancer (data available at http://seer.cancer.gov/statfacts/html/thyro.html).

According to 2009–2013 data, the rate of new cases of thyroid cancer was 13.9 per 100,000 men and women per year (**Figure 1**). **Table 1** summarizes number of new cases per 100,000 persons by race/ethnicity and sex. A recently published study on adolescent cancer incidence during 1975–2012 has reported a 2.12% increase for females and 1.59% for males between 15 and 19 years of age [5]. However, there is a study indicating that thyroid cancer incidence trend has slowed following release of American Thyroid Association (ATA) guideline in 2009 [6, 7]. It has been reported that overall thyroid cancer incidence had an increasing trend about 8% per year from 2000 to 2009. But APC showed a deceleration about 3% in men and 2.8% in women, which was confined to tumors less than 2.9 cm of size for women [7].

Also, thyroid cancer-related mortality was estimated to consist 0.3% of all cancer-related deaths in 2016. A 5-year survival rate of 98.1% has been reported for thyroid cancer. Despite increasing trend of incidence, thyroid cancer mortality has a relatively stable rate about 0.5 cases per 100,000 persons both from 1973 to 2002 and 2009 to 2013 [8, 9].

In conclusion, it seems that thyroid cancer has been following an increasing trend in the past decades; although the reason has been remained controversial. Some scientists believe

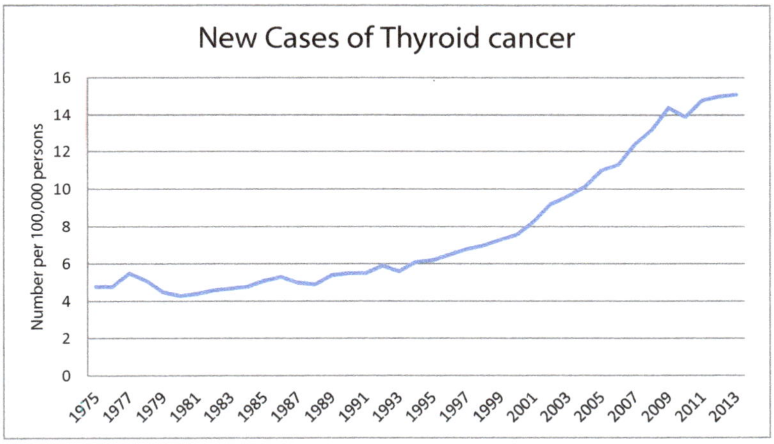

Figure 1. Thyroid cancer incidence in time (http://seer.cancer.gov/statfacts/html/thyro.html).

Races	Male	Female
All races	6.9	20.6
White	7.4	21.9
Black	3.6	12.4
Asian/Pacific Islander	6.5	19.9
American Indian/Alaska Native	3.6	13.6
Hispanic	5.0	18.6
Nonhispanic	7.4	21.3

Table 1. Number of new cases of thyroid cancer per 100,000 persons by race/ethnicity and sex.

that modern diagnostic techniques and strategies or in the other words "overdiagnosis" is in charge for this increasing trend [8, 10]. Others believe that environmental factors such as various irradiations and changes in lifestyle can be considered as the reasons for this true increase [11–14]. Regardless of the nature, this increase has turned thyroid cancer to a world-wide health problem, which involves more attention and efforts toward diagnosis and proper management.

2. Categories of thyroid malignancies

Three are some different classifications for thyroid cancers. Previously and more commonly, thyroid gland malignancies were used to be categorized to three types: differentiated thyroid cancers (such as papillary and follicular thyroid cancers), anaplastic carcinomas, and rare types of thyroid cancer (like medullary thyroid cancer). A newly released classification categorizes thyroid malignancies to two main follicular-derived and neuroendocrine C-cell–derived types [1], which will be discussed in detail in following lines. **Figure 2** illustrates this classification in order for better clarification.

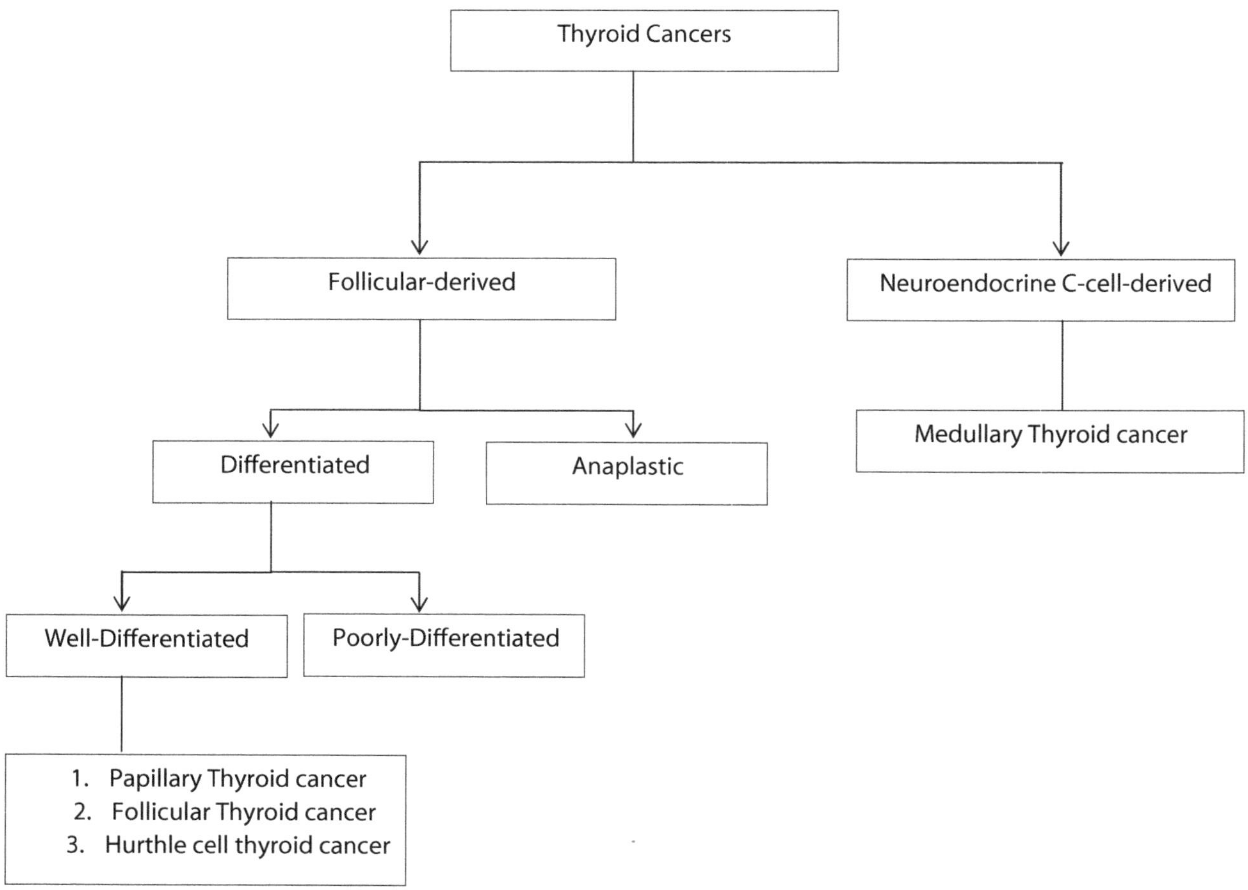

Figure 2. Classification of thyroid malignancies.

2.1. Follicular-derived thyroid cancers

Follicular-derived thyroid cancers have two main subtypes: differentiated and anaplastic cancers.

2.1.1. Differentiated thyroid cancers

Consisting approximately 95% of all thyroid cancers, differentiated thyroid cancer is the most prevalent type of these cancers [15], which is raised from thyroid follicular epithelial cells. There are two main subtypes for differentiated thyroid cancers: well-differentiated and poorly differentiated thyroid cancers. Papillary thyroid cancer, follicular thyroid cancer, and Hurthle cell carcinoma (HCC) are under category of well-differentiated thyroid cancers (WDTC).

2.1.1.1. Papillary thyroid cancer

Accounting for 70–90% of well-differentiated thyroid cancers and 80–85% of follicular cell-derived thyroid cancers [16], papillary thyroid cancers (PTCs) are the most prevalent type of thyroid cancers [17]. Incidence of papillary thyroid cancer has increased along with recent increase in incidence of thyroid cancers. Experts believe that this increase is related to higher detection and diagnosis rates; because PTCs are more easily diagnosed with ultrasound and diagnostic tests such as fine needle aspiration (FNA) cytology in comparison with follicular carcinomas [18].

PTC is mostly diagnosed at the mean age of 45 years old; however the incidence increases with increase in age [19]. Papillary thyroid cancer can also occur in children [19, 20].

There are several known risk and etiologic factors for papillary thyroid carcinoma such as radiation exposure, nitrate, unknown environmental pollutants, and endogenous factors like obesity, high levels of thyroid stimulating hormone (TSH), and presence of Hashimoto's thyroiditis [4]. Based on a meta-analysis, each 5-unit increase in body mass index (BMI), 5 kg increase in weight, 5 cm increase in waist or hip circumference, and 0.1 unit increase in waist-to-hip ratio were associated with 30, 5, 5, and 14% greater risks of thyroid cancer, respectively [21]. Estrogen is also another potential risk factor for papillary thyroid carcinoma, which justifies the sex difference for thyroid nodules and carcinoma [22]. Hepatitis C infection has been mentioned as a potential risk factor for thyroid cancer; however, more studies are needed to confirm this association [23]. It is not exactly clear that which factor(s) are important and mainly contributed to the recent increase in thyroid cancer incidence.

Papillary thyroid cancer has the best overall prognosis [1]; however, there are some static and dynamic prognostic factors, which influence this prognosis [24]. Static prognostic factors help with decision-making on therapeutic strategies and are usually based on patient's background or findings of preoperative imaging studies, intra-operative, and post-operative pathological findings.

Static prognostic factors are subdivided into three classification regarding the time of evaluation; pre-, intra-, and post-operative.

1. Pre- or intra-operative prognostic factors:

- Age: although the age has been considered by approved classification systems like age, metastases, extent and size (AMES); metastasis, age, invasion, completeness, and size (MACIS); and Union for International Cancer Control (UICC) tumor, nodes, metastasis (TNM) classification, its exact role as a prognostic factor has remained controversial [25–27]. Most of the previous studies have indicated that recurrence and mortality are higher in elderly patients [27–33]. On the other hand, it has been reported that younger PTC patients have lower disease-free survival (DFS) than middle-aged patients.

- Gender: prognostic value of male gender has been questioned in recently published studies [24]; however, approved in some previous ones [18]. It has been concluded that male gender has a moderate prognostic value in PTC patients; however, there are studies with contrast findings [34].

- Size of tumor: the fact that larger tumors are associated with higher mortality and poor prognosis has been long determined. AMES has marked tumor size more than 5 cm as high risk and UICC set two cut off at 2 and 4 cm [25, 27]. Most of the recent studies have set the cut off at 3–4 cm according to prognosis of PTC patients [25, 27–30, 35].

- Extrathyroid extension: it is one of the most important prognostic factors for PTC [36]. Grossly significant extrathyroid extension based on intra-operative evidences is one of the most reliable prognostic factors.

- Clinical lymph node metastasis: not only the presence of lymph node metastasis is important, but the number and size of metastasis are also among determining prognostic factors [36].

2. Distant metastasis at diagnosis: it is considered as the strongest predicting factor for carcinoma-related death of PTC patients [18, 24].

Post-operative prognostic factors:

- Ki-67 labeling index: Ki-67 is a molecular marker indicating high level of proliferative activity in carcinoma. Ki-67 labeling index (LI) is generally low in PTC patients; however patients with high Ki-67 labeling index are more likely to show recurrence or persistent disease and to die from carcinoma [24, 37]. High Ki-67 LI is considered as an independent prognostic factor for DFS and cause-specific survival (CSS) [37, 38].

- BRAF V600E mutation: many previous studies have mentioned that PTC with BRAF mutation is more aggressive, associated with more recurrence, and has poorer prognosis [18, 39–42]. It has been shown that PTCs with BRAF V600E mutation and negative for X-linked inhibitor of apoptosis protein (XIAP) have higher chance of recurrence [18]. So, simultaneous evaluation of BRAF V600E mutation and XIAP expression is suggested as a better predictor of cancer recurrence [43].

- Poor differentiation and aggressive variants: patients with poorly differentiated PTC are known for their poor prognosis [24]. Poorly differentiated papillary thyroid carcinoma has been discussed as a separate section.

Dynamic prognostic factors are based on changes in serum thyroglobulin (Tg) and thyroglobulin antibody (TgAb) after total thyroidectomy, which help with estimation of recurrence and cause-specific survival (CSS) of PTC patients.

- Tg-doubling time (Tg-DT): for the first time in 2011, Tg-doubling time was proposed as a dynamic prognostic factor [44]. Tg-DT was recognized as an independent prognostic factor for both DFS and CSS of patients, whereas a short Tg-DT time (less than 1 year) is an indicator of poor prognosis. It was mentioned that Tg-DT is inversely linked to Ki-67 LI and so measurement of Ki-67 may give us information upon post-operative Tg status, Tg-DT, and prognosis of patients [37].

Post-operative Tg status is also related to patients' age; so that a shorter Tg-DT (less than 2 years) is observed in old patients [45]. In conclusion, Tg-DT is a very convenient marker for the prediction of patients' prognosis in real-time and decision-making on use of molecular target agents.

- Pre- and post-operative values of TgAb: Tg-DT is not useful in TgAb positive patients, because serum Tg levels are not reliable in the presence of TgAb. Patients whose TgAb levels decrease less than 50% or increase in post-operative (total thyroidectomy) period are more likely to develop a recurrence of disease [46, 47].

2.1.1.1.1. Staging

American Joint Committee on Cancer (AJCC, https://cancerstaging.org) has divided staging of differentiated thyroid cancers as two groups; in patients under 45 years old and in those 45 years and older. As described previously, younger patients are less likely to die from differentiated thyroid cancers; so all patients younger than 45 years are stage I if they have no distant metastasis and stage II if they have distant metastasis.

Papillary thyroid cancer in patients younger than 45:

- **Stage I (Any T, Any N, M0):** the tumor can be of any size (any T) and may or may not have spread to nearby lymph nodes (any N). It has not spread to distant sites (M0).
- **Stage II (Any T, Any N, M1):** the tumor can be of any size (any T) and may or may not have spread to nearby lymph nodes (any N). It has spread to distant sites (M1).

Papillary thyroid cancer in patients 45 years and older:

Stage I (T1, N0, M0): the tumor is 2 cm or less across and has not grown outside the thyroid (T1). It has not spread to nearby lymph nodes (N0) or distant sites (M0).

Stage II (T2, N0, M0): the tumor is more than 2 cm but not larger than 4 cm across and has not grown outside the thyroid (T2). It has not spread to nearby lymph nodes (N0) or distant sites (M0).

Stage III: one of the following applies:

T3, N0, M0: the tumor is larger than 4 cm across or has grown slightly outside the thyroid (T3), but it has not spread to nearby lymph nodes (N0) or distant sites (M0).

T1–T3, N1a, M0: the tumor is of any size and may have grown slightly outside the thyroid (T1–T3). It has spread to lymph nodes around the thyroid in the neck (N1a) but not to other lymph nodes or to distant sites (M0).

Stage IVA: one of the following applies:

T4a, any N, M0: the tumor is any size and has grown beyond the thyroid gland and into nearby tissues of the neck (T4a). It might or might not have spread to nearby lymph nodes (any N). It has not spread to distant sites (M0).

T1 to T3, N1b, M0: the tumor is any size and might have grown slightly outside the thyroid gland (T1–T3). It has spread to certain lymph nodes in the neck (cervical nodes) or to lymph nodes in the upper chest (superior mediastinal nodes) or behind the throat (retropharyngeal nodes) (N1b), but it has not spread to distant sites (M0).

Stage IVB (T4b, Any N, M0): the tumor is of any size and has grown either back toward the spine or into nearby large blood vessels (T4b). It might or might not have spread to nearby lymph nodes (any N), but it has not spread to distant sites (M0).

Stage IVC (Any T, Any N, M1): the tumor is of any size and might or might not have grown outside the thyroid (any T). It might or might not have spread to nearby lymph nodes (any N). It has spread to distant sites (M1).

2.1.1.1.2. Management

The optimal management of papillary thyroid cancer has remained controversial as the available data on the best approach for management are related to retrospective evaluations, large national registry studies, and meta-analysis but not randomized clinical trials (RCTs) [48–50]. Only RCTs are able to exactly determine the optimal treatment, such as extent of surgery, in PTC patients. It has been estimated that a large number about 3000 to 5000 patients are needed to be randomized for evaluation of cause-specific mortality, which is not actually possible.

Decision-making for primary treatment are depended on preoperative assessments such as clinical, imaging and histological evaluations. Treatment choices are based on location and extent of disease.

Figure 3 illustrates algorithm for primary treatment of patients with differentiated thyroid carcinomas. Recommendations of 2015 American Thyroid Association (ATA) guidelines are excellent reference as they are more conservative than before [51].

According to this guideline, unifocal tumors which are smaller than 4cm with no evidence of extrathyroidal extension or lymph node metastasis are resolvable by lobectomy. Previous studies have shown that bilateral or unilateral resections are associated with similar long-term survival [48, 52–54]. For patients with papillary microcarcinoma (less than 1 cm) without evidence of cervical lymph node metastasis, nonsurgical management is considered as an option [55, 56].

Surgical and pathological findings are applied shortly after surgery for deciscion-making on the possible need for thyroid hormone replacement therapy or radioiodine ablation or both. This assessment is based on well-known TNM staging which determines mortality but

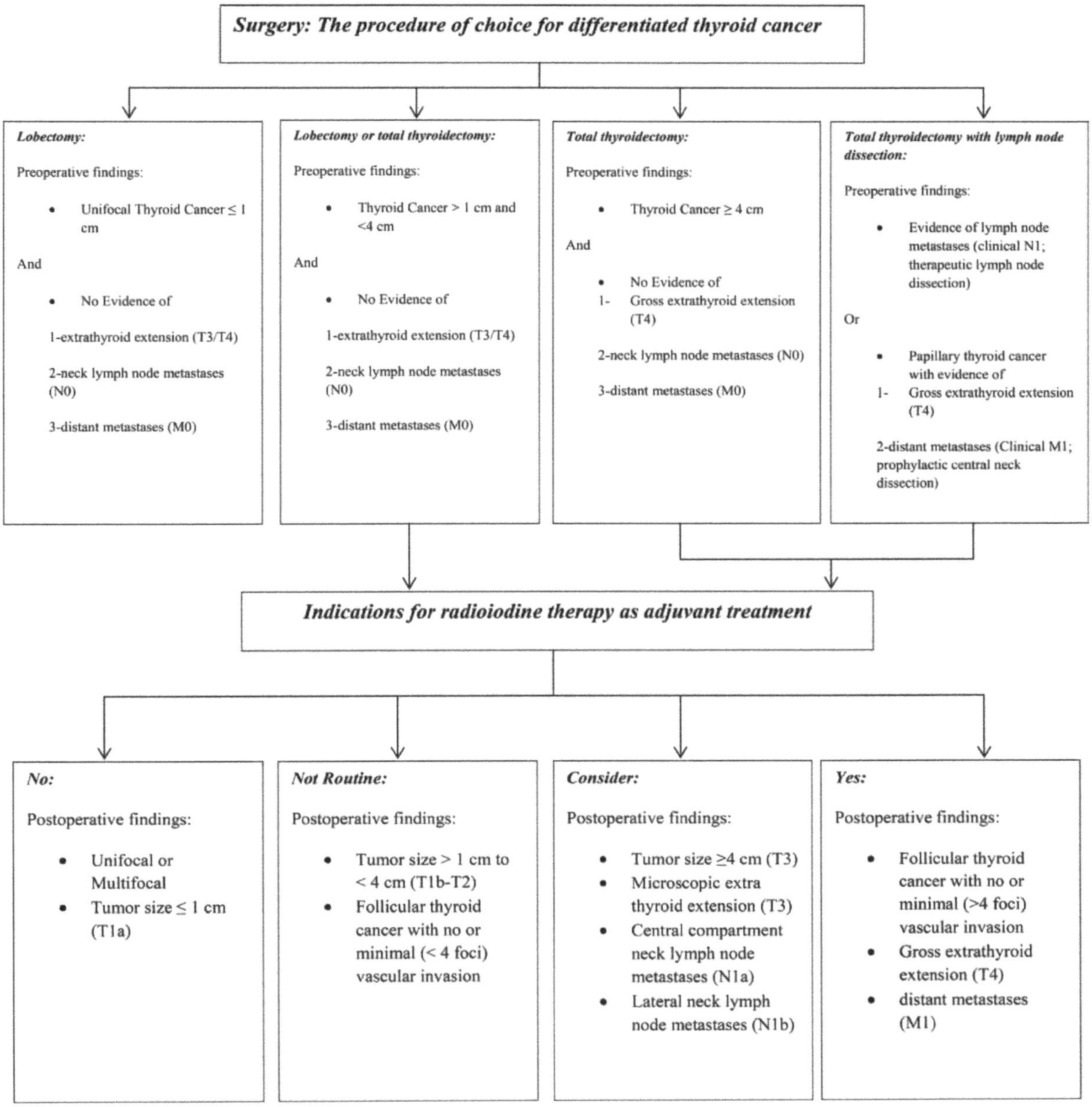

Figure 3. Primary treatment of patients with differentiated thyroid carcinoma.

not the risk of recurrence. Recurrence assessment system proposed by 2015 ATA guideline (**Tables 2** and **3**) is a reliable predictor for the course of differentiated thyroid carcinoma treated with thyroidectomy alone or radioiodine remnant ablation [57–60].

Radioiodine therapy (RAI Tx): Previously application of radioactive iodine was justified by the need for elimination thyroid normal tissue remnants. It is also considered as adjuvant treatment for destroying occult neoplastic cells within the thyroid remnant or throughout the body. This issue has been challenged recently because of short-term morbidity and possible increased risk of second cancers [6, 61]. Recent recommendations believe in individualized use of RAI Tx (**Figure 3**). It can also be used in detection of distant metastasis as well as a treatment. Unfortunately this strategy is not effective in radioiodine refractory patients.

At the time of primary treatment
(1) ATA low risk (≤5% recurrence)
Papillary thyroid cancer
• Intrathyroid tumor
• Clinical N0 or five or fewer lymph node micrometastases (<0.2 cm in largest diameter)
• *V600EBRAF*-mutated microcarcinoma
Follicular thyroid cancer
• Intrathyroid tumor
• Capsular invasion and no or minimal (<4 foci) vascular invasion
(2) ATA intermediate risk (5–20% recurrence)
Papillary thyroid cancer
• Minimal extrathyroid extension
• Aggressive histology
• Vascular invasion
• Clinical N1 or more than five lymph node metastases (<3 cm in largest diameter)
• *V600EBRAF*-mutated, intrathyroid, 1–4 cm, primary tumor
• *V600EBRAF*-mutated microcarcinoma, multifocal with extrathyroid extension
(3) ATA high risk (>20% recurrence)
Papillary thyroid cancer
• Gross extrathyroid extension
• Distant metastases
• Lymph node metastasis at least 3 cm in largest diameter
Follicular thyroid cancer
• >4 foci of vascular invasion

Table 2. Recurrence risk stratification at the time of primary treatment as a function of the response to treatment.

TSH suppression: TSH stimulates proliferation of normal thyrocytes and some malignant cells; so TSH suppression has been used as a treatment after surgery [62]. This approach significantly decreases mortality and recurrence in DTC [63]. The exact amount of needed suppression is not clear but studies show that reducing TSH level to less than 0.1mU/L improves clinical outcome; however moderate reductions are beneficial [64, 65]. This treatment may have some complications like osteoporosis in postmenopausal women or angina and atrial fibrillation in elderly patients; so the risk of complications should be weighed against the risk of proliferation of malignant cells [66].

2.1.1.2. Follicular thyroid cancer

Including approximately 10–15% of well-differentiated thyroid carcinomas, follicular thyroid cancer (FTC) is defined as 'A malignant epithelial tumor showing follicular cell differentiation and lacking the diagnostic nuclear features of papillary thyroid carcinoma' (PTC) [67].

During follow-up
(1) Excellent response (1–4% recurrence)
• Imaging negative for disease recurrence
• Serum thyroglobulin concentration lower than 0.2 ng/mL basal or higher than 1 ng/mL TSH stimulated
(2) Indeterminate response (15–20% recurrence)
• Nonspecific findings on imaging studies
• Serum thyroglobulin 0.2–1 ng/mL basal or 1–10 ng/mL TSH stimulated, or thyroglobulin antibodies stable or decreasing
(3) Biochemical incomplete response (20% recurrence)
• Imaging negative for disease recurrence
• Serum thyroglobulin concentration higher than 1 ng/mL basal or higher than 10 ng/mL TSH stimulated, or increasing thyroglobulin antibody concentrations
(4) Structural incomplete response (50–85% recurrence)
• Structural (neck ultrasound, CT, or MRI) or functional (whole-body scan or ^{18}F-fluorodeoxyglucose PET) evidence of disease in imaging studies

Table 3. Recurrence risk stratification over time as a function of the response to treatment.

Patients' age, size and staging of the tumor, responsiveness to radioiodine therapy and completeness of surgery are among prognostic factors of FTC. Minimally invasive carcinomas have better prognosis than widely invasive carcinomas [68, 69].

2.1.1.2.1. Staging

As a differentiated thyroid cancer, staging of follicular thyroid cancer is the same with papillary thyroid carcinoma based on American Joint Committee on Cancer (AJCC).

2.1.1.2.2. Management

As a differentiated thyroid cancer, management of follicular thyroid carcinoma is compatible with those of papillary thyroid carcinoma.

2.1.1.3. Hurthle cell carcinoma

Oncocytic follicular cells of thyroid, known as Hurthle cells, which were first described by Karl Hürthle are the origin of Hurthle cell carcinoma (HCC) [70, 71]. They can be found in both benign and malignant conditions of thyroid. Histologic differentiation between Hurthle cell adenoma and carcinoma can be definitely made only after the evaluation of resection specimen by the presence or absence of vascular or capsular invasion, which is the hallmark of HCC [72]. HCC represents 3% of all thyroid cancers [73].

There are two types of Hurthle cell carcinoma; minimally invasive carcinomas are fully encapsulated tumors with microscopically identifiable foci of capsular or vascular invasion

(<4 foci) and widely invasive tumors, which have extensive vascular invasion (>4 foci) and extrathyroidal invasion. Patients with minimally invasive carcinomas usually experience a better prognosis [73]. Overall, older patients and those with larger tumor size, extrathyroidal extension, and not undergoing surgery have reduced survival [74]. A previous study indicated that in patients with widely invasive HCC, stages III–IV are independent risk factors for recurrence or death. Five-year risk of recurrence or death was reported 0% in women with stages I–II compared to 17% in men. However, it was 91% among men with stages III–IV disease comparing to 74% of women in the same stage of disease [75].

Stratification of risk of recurrence for HCC based on ATA (American Thyroid Association) guideline [51]:

- Low risk: intrathyroidal encapsulated tumors with minor capsular or vascular invasion (<4 foci) or ≤5 metastatic lymph nodes where the foci of metastases are <0.2 cm.
- Intermediate risk: vascular invasion, minimal extrathyroidal extension, or >5 metastatic lymph nodes (0.2–3 cm).
- High risk: macroscopic extrathyroidal extension, incomplete tumor resection, distant metastases, or metastatic lymph nodes >3 cm.

2.1.1.3.1. Staging

As a differentiated thyroid cancer, staging of follicular thyroid cancer is the same with papillary thyroid carcinoma based on American Joint Committee on Cancer (AJCC).

2.1.1.3.2. Management

As other differentiated thyroid cancers, the main treatment for HCC is surgery. Since the preoperative diagnosis of HCC is impossible by cytology, determining the initial extent of surgery and whether further surgical resection (completion thyroidectomy) involves postoperative histological evaluation [70]. So, the first step is a thyroid lobectomy in the primary surgery unless the pathological features guide us to total thyroidectomy. Presence of dominant contralateral nodule, nodule size greater than 4 cm or preexisting diminished thyroid hormone production requiring thyroid hormone therapy are another indication for total thyroidectomy [51].

TSH suppression: Goal of TSH suppression depends on the risk of recurrence. Completely resected minimally invasive HCC is categorized as low risk and then does not require TSH suppression therapy. Patients with incomplete response to therapy should have TSH levels less than 0.1 mU/L unless there is a contraindication. Patients with incomplete biochemical response to therapy or high-risk HCC and an excellent or indeterminate response to therapy should have TSH levels between 0.1 and 0.5 mU/L considering the risk of TSH suppression and trend of thyroglobulin levels over time.

Radioiodine therapy (*RAI Tx*): Benefit of RAI Tx for HCC patients has remained as a question because a small number of studies have evaluated this treatment. Generally, RAI Tx is not routinely recommended for patients at low risk of recurrence.

External beam radiation therapy (EBRT): In patients with clinically evident gross extrathyroidal extension that is incompletely resected, external beam radiation therapy (EBRT) can be considered as a treatment option. However, potential benefit of radiation should be weighed against potential complications, such as dental decay, tracheal stenosis, esophageal stricture, osteonecrosis, fibrosis, and xerostomia [76].

2.1.1.4. Poorly differentiated thyroid cancer

Introduced by Sakamoto et al., this group of thyroid cancers fall between well-differentiated thyroid cancers (WDTC) and anaplastic thyroid cancer (ATC) in terms of both morphologic appearance and biologic behavior [77, 78]. They account for up to 10% of all thyroid cancers and have a higher incidence in Europe than in the United States with a male-to-female ratio of 1:2 [77, 79, 80]. Poorly differentiated thyroid carcinoma (PDTC) may represent intermediate entities of the progression of WDTC to ATC [78, 81–83]. PDTCs have a high recurrence rate despite appropriate treatment. These types of cancers have more aggressive pattern than typical papillary thyroid cancer.

The most challenging issue in diagnosis of PDTC is lack of a precise definition. So, in 2006 a group of experts set diagnostic criteria for PDTC in Turin, Italy [84]. As the most acceptable criteria, the 2006 Turin criteria are as following:

(1) A solid/trabecular/insular pattern of growth

(2) Absence of conventional nuclear features of papillary carcinoma

(3) Presence of at least one of the following features: convoluted nuclei, mitotic activity (≥3×10 HPF), necrosis

PDTCs are usually at an advanced stage, usually extrathyroidal extension and extensive local invasion, at the time of diagnosis [85]. They can be metastasized to regional lymph nodes (50–85%), and distantly (36–85%), most commonly to the lung (14–54%), and bones (18–33%) [86, 87]. Survival rates are remarkably lower than in patients with WDTC [85, 87, 88]. Patients more than 45 years of age and those with cervical lymph node invasion, tumor necrosis, local recurrence, mitotic index greater than 3 per 10 high-power fields, tumor size greater than 4 cm, and distant metastasis at the time of diagnosis have poorer prognosis [89–92][13, 31–34].

2.1.1.4.1. Management

Since PDTC is rare, the best treatment option for treatment remains inconclusive. Most previous studies are agreed with total thyroidectomy with lymph node dissection because of aggressive nature of these tumors. More than 50% of PDTCs have regional nodal metastasis; so central compartment with modified radical neck dissection is considered [93]. Application of radioiodine therapy (RAI), external beam radiation therapy (EBRT), or chemotherapy has remained controversial [77].

2.1.2. Anaplastic thyroid cancer (undifferentiated thyroid cancer)

Anaplastic thyroid cancer (ATC) is a rare and lethal form of thyroid cancer, which is responsible for 1.7–2% of all thyroid cancers. It usually involves patients in their sixth or seventh decade of life and has a median survival of 5 months and less than 20% of patients are alive 1 year after diagnosis. Geographical prevalence of ATC has a wide range from 1.3 to 9.8% [94–96].

ATC is considered to be originally derived from follicular cells resulted from dedifferentiation. About 80% of ATC presents in patients with long-standing goiter, which is possibly in the setting of an undiagnosed well-differentiated thyroid cancer [95]. In most of the cases, ATC usually presents with a rapidly enlarging neck mass and local symptoms such as neck pain, dysphagia, dyspnea, and hoarseness [97]. Symptoms can be related to invasion of tumor to neighboring structures such as recurrent laryngeal nerve (RLN), parasympathetic chain (causing Horner's syndrome), or even carotid arteries (causing stroke). About 40% of patients usually present with lymphadenopathy and up to 43% have distant metastasis, most commonly to the lung followed by bone and brain at the time of diagnosis [98].

A variety of previous studies have evaluated prognostic factors of ATC [99–102]. These prognostic factors include patients' age, tumor size, and clinical stage. Ages more than 70, acute onset of symptoms, white blood cell count (WBC) more than 10000, tumor size more than 5 cm, T4b and distant metastasis are associated with increased mortality and poor prognosis [102].

A majority of patients will finally die from ATC and should be aware of the prognosis by a thorough discussion in order to have information on the impact of disease on their quality of life and also the potential benefit of participating in clinical trials [97]. The physician should also hold discussions around "do not resuscitate" (DNR) or "allow natural death" (AND) with patients to decrease ambiguity in emergency situations, which require life-supporting procedures such as intubation.

2.1.2.1. Staging

American Joint Committee on Cancer (AJCC) considers all anaplastic thyroid cancers as T4 and Stage IV at the time of diagnosis reflecting the poor prognosis of this cancer.

Stage IVA (T4a, Any N, M0): the tumor is still within the thyroid (T4a). It might or might not have spread to nearby lymph nodes (any N), but it has not spread to distant sites (M0).

Stage IVB (T4b, Any N, M0): the tumor has grown outside the thyroid (T4b). It might or might not have spread to nearby lymph nodes (any N), but it has not spread to distant sites (M0).

Stage IVC (Any T, Any N, M1): the tumor might or might not have grown outside of the thyroid (any T). It might or might not have spread to nearby lymph nodes (any N). It has spread to distant sites (M1).

2.1.2.2. Management

ATC raises both diagnostic and therapeutic challenges. This is because of rarity of the disease and also lack of expression of thyroid and epithelial cell markers in anaplastic cancer cells [103]. In addition, ATC cells present in a variety of histology and morphology abnormalities which causes delay in diagnosis and consequently in treatment. As the diagnosis is established, staging should be done as well as the assessment of airway by fiberoptic laryngoscopy.

Referring the patient to a center with experience with anaplastic thyroid cancer is highly recommended. An expert head and neck surgeon should assess the patient to determine if the primary tumor is resectable. Early after resection, external beam radiation with radiosensitizing drugs, like taxanes with or without platin or anthracycline (chemoradiation). Palliative chemoradiation is suggested for patients with unresectable primary tumors but without distant metastases.

Patients with advanced disease (stage IVC) are the most challenging ones. Treating physician should balance local control of primary tumor and treatment of distant metastases. If the airway is at risk, the chemoradiation should be started. Patients in whom the airway is not at risk or is stabilized by tracheostomy should preferably be enrolled in a clinical trial or undergo systemic chemotherapy by cytotoxic drugs [1].

Recently, targeted treatment has been suggested; for example prescription of *BRAF* inhibitors in patients with $BRAF^{V600E}$-mutated anaplastic thyroid cancer [103]. Dabrafenib, which is a selective BRAF inhibitor, trametinib, lenvatinib, rapamycin, and microtubule inhibitors are among the drugs being evaluated in ATC patients.

Patients and their family members should be informed of poor prognosis of the disease. Some patients should be transferred to a sanatorium if they do not wish to be treated or their performance is poor.

2.2. Neuroendocrine C-cell–derived thyroid cancer

Accounting for 1–2% of all thyroid cancers, medullary thyroid cancer is relatively uncommon [15]. Medullary thyroid cancer (MTC) is originated from parafollicular neuroendocrine cells, in contrast with differentiated thyroid cancer. It occurs either sporadic (in 75% of cases) or in a hereditary form (multiple endocrine neoplasia type 2, MEN2), due to germline mutations in the RET proto-oncogene [104]. As most of the thyroid cancers, MTC usually presents as a solitary thyroid nodule in patients in fourth or sixth decade of life [105]. Since it metastasizes frequently, neck lymphadenopathy is usually the first manifestation. Most (70%) of the patients with palpable MTC have evidence of cervical node involvement at the time of surgery [106]. A classic thyroid nodule associated with flushing and diarrhea is suggestive of widespread metastatic disease. About 25% of MTC cases occur in patients with an inherited multiple endocrine neoplasia syndrome [105].

2.2.1. Staging

Stage I (T1, N0, M0): the tumor is 2 cm or less across and has not grown outside the thyroid (T1). It has not spread to nearby lymph nodes (N0) or distant sites (M0).

Stage II: one of the following applies:

T2, N0, M0: the tumor is more than 2 cm but is not larger than 4 cm across and has not grown outside the thyroid (T2). It has not spread to nearby lymph nodes (N0) or distant sites (M0).

T3, N0, M0: the tumor is larger than 4 cm or has grown slightly outside the thyroid (T3), but it has not spread to nearby lymph nodes (N0) or distant sites (M0).

Stage III (T1–T3, N1a, M0): the tumor is of any size and might have grown slightly outside the thyroid (T1–T3). It has spread to lymph nodes around the thyroid in the neck (N1a) but not to other lymph nodes or to distant sites (M0).

Stage IVA: one of the following applies:

T4a, any N, M0: the tumor is any size and has grown beyond the thyroid gland and into nearby tissues of the neck (T4a). It might or might not have spread to nearby lymph nodes (any N). It has not spread to distant sites (M0).

T1–T3, N1b, M0: the tumor is of any size and might have grown slightly outside the thyroid gland (T1–T3). It has spread to certain lymph nodes in the neck (cervical nodes) or to lymph nodes in the upper chest (superior mediastinal nodes) or behind the throat (retropharyngeal nodes) (N1b), but it has not spread to distant sites (M0).

Stage IVB (T4b, Any N, M0): the tumor is of any size and has grown either back toward the spine or into nearby large blood vessels (T4b). It might or might not have spread to nearby lymph nodes (any N), but it has not spread to distant sites (M0).

Stage IVC (Any T, Any N, M1): the tumor is of any size and might or might not have grown outside the thyroid (any T). It might or might not have spread to nearby lymph nodes (any N). It has spread to distant sites (M1).

2.2.2. Management

As other thyroid cancers, surgery is the mainstay for MTC management; however, imaging and diagnosis before surgery are necessary for determining the best surgical intervention [1]. As the diagnosis of MTC is made, the patient should undergo neck ultrasonography and tumor markers (calcitonin and carcinoembryonic antigen) evaluation.

In addition, it should be determined if the disease is sporadic or associated with MEN 2 syndrome, because patients with MEN 2 may have pheochromocytoma or primary hyperparathyroidism or both. So, biochemical testing should be considered for ruling out pheochromocytoma or primary hyperparathyroidism in MTC patients with unknown status of germline RET mutation. If the patient has primary hyperparathyroidism, a total thyroidectomy should be done including parathyroidectomy. For patients with pheochromocytoma, adrenalectomy should be prioritized to thyroidectomy. Patients with hereditary MTC should be referred to a genetic counselor so that only necessary family members undergo testing for lowering related costs [1]. Family members with germline RET mutation benefit from prophylactic thyroidectomy [105].

If preoperative calcitonin levels are higher than 146 pmol/L, work up should be done for distant metastatic disease [105]. This work up includes neck and chest CT and three-phase MRI of liver with contrast. Axial skeleton MRI is suggested for bone metastasis. Total thyroidectomy with bilateral central neck dissection is preferred for patients with no distant metastasis. Lateral neck dissection is recommended only if metastatic disease is suspected by neck ultrasound and confirmed by FNA cytology.

After surgery, patients need thyroid hormone replacement therapy but not TSH suppression as in high risk differentiated thyroid cancers. Calcitonin and carcinoembryonic antigen (CEA) should be checked not earlier than 3 months after surgery for determining if the patient has persistent disease.

External Beam radiation therapy (EBRT) should be limited in MTC patients, because it can limit further surgical interventions due to fibrosis as well as affecting the quality of life of patients.

Patients should be managed with active surveillance by both ultrasonography and serial evaluation of tumor markers to guide further surgical treatment. Patients with normal levels of tumor markers and imaging after surgery should be followed up annually and those with persistent tumor markers should be observed more closely. Patients with calcitonin and CEA doubling time within 6 months have a shorter overall survival time [107].

3. Assessment and treatment of thyroid nodules

Thyroid nodules are usually the first presenting feature of a thyroid cancer. So evaluation of thyroid nodules is of a great importance.

Size plays a notable role in determining the need of fine needle aspiration (FNA) for a thyroid nodule; however, ultrasound features can provide valuable clues regarding malignancy of nodules [108]. These are hypoechogenicity, a solid internal structure, irregular margins, microcalcifications, taller-than-wide shape, and evidence of extrathyroidal extension or cervical lymphadenopathy for papillary thyroid cancers. Nodules which do not have these characteristics can be followed up without FNA until the nodule remains small [1].

Follicular thyroid cancer and follicular variant of papillary thyroid cancers are more often round and isoechoic with regular margins. A larger size and increased intranodular vascularity on color or power Doppler imaging are also predictive of malignancy [109–112].

The 2015 ATA guideline has bolded the role of ultrasound in diagnosis and approach to thyroid nodules (**Figure 4**) [51]. Concurrent risk factors of thyroid cancer including cough, neck pain, change in voice, presence of a firm mass, history of childhood neck radiation, or familial thyroid cancer should be considered and in these cases FNA is recommended regardless of ultrasound characteristics. ATA recommends biopsy for nodules larger than 1 cm.

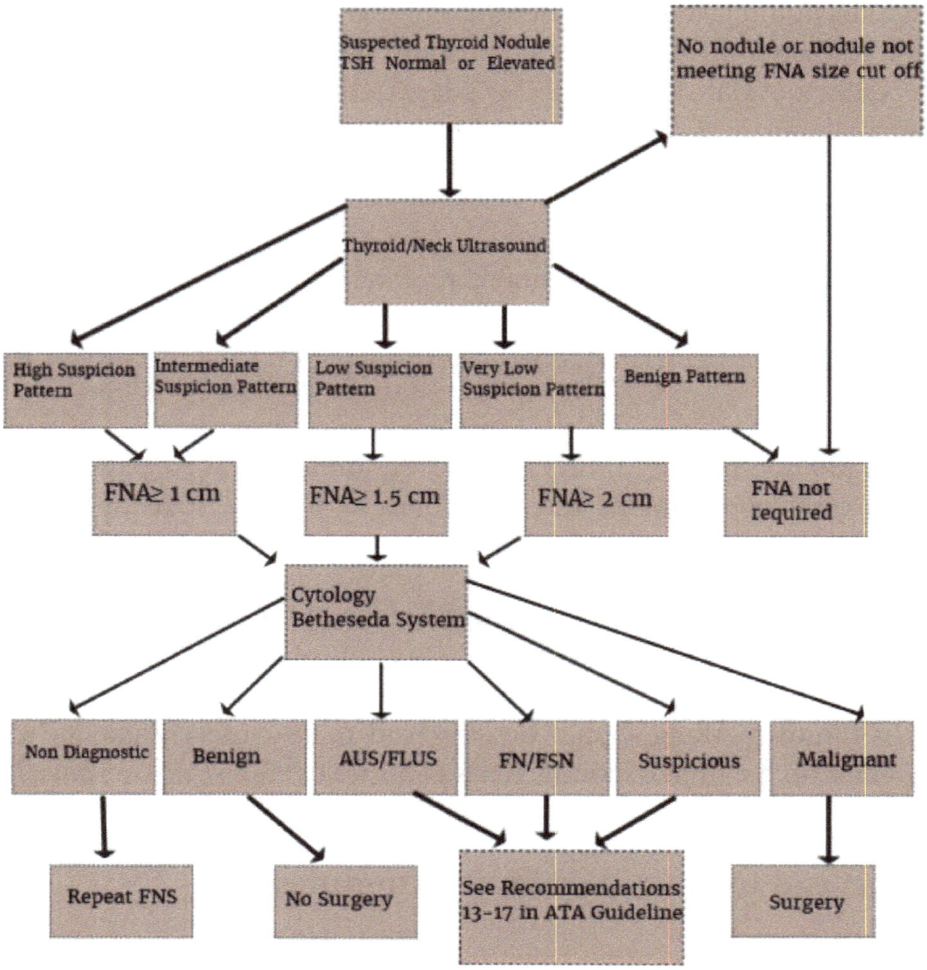

Figure 4. Approach to thyroid nodule based on ATA guideline [51].

Author details

Mohammad Hossein Khosravi[1,2], Ali Kouhi[2,3], Masoumeh Saeedi[2,4], Ali Bagherihagh[2,4]* and Mohammad Hosein Amirzade-Iranaq[5,2]

*Address all correspondence to: ali.bagherihagh@gmail.com

1 Student Research Committee (SRC), Baqiyatallah University of Medical Sciences, Tehran, Iran

2 International Otorhinolaryngology Research Association (IORA), Universal Scientific Education and Research Network (USERN), Tehran, Iran

3 Department of Otolaryngology Head and Neck Surgery, Otorhinolaryngology Research Center, Tehran University of Medical Sciences, Tehran, Iran

4 Department of Otorhinolaryngology-Head and Neck Surgery, Faculty of Medicine, Baqiyatallah University of Medical Sciences, Tehran, Iran

5 Student Research Committee, Shahid Sadoughi University of Medical Sciences, Yazd, Iran

References

[1] Cabanillas ME, McFadden DG, Durante C. Thyroid cancer. The Lancet.388(10061): 2016;2783-95

[2] Curado M-P, Edwards B, Shin HR, Storm H, Ferlay J, Heanue M, et al. Cancer Incidence in Five Continents, Volume IX. IARC Press, International Agency for Research on Cancer; 2007

[3] Jemal A, Siegel R, Xu J, Ward E. Cancer statistics, 2010. CA: A Cancer Journal for Clinicians. 2010;60(5):277-300

[4] Pellegriti G, Frasca F, Regalbuto C, Squatrito S, Vigneri R. Worldwide increasing incidence of thyroid cancer: Update on epidemiology and risk factors. Journal of Cancer Epidemiology. 2013;1-10

[5] Burkhamer J, Kriebel D, Clapp R. The increasing toll of adolescent cancer incidence in the US. PLoS One. 2017;12(2):e0172986

[6] Cooper DS, Doherty GM, Haugen BR, Kloos RT, Lee SL, Mandel SJ, et al. Revised American Thyroid Association management guidelines for patients with thyroid nodules and differentiated thyroid cancer: The American Thyroid Association (ATA) guidelines taskforce on thyroid nodules and differentiated thyroid cancer. Thyroid. 2009;19(11):1167-1214

[7] Shi LL, DeSantis C, Jemal A, Chen AY. Changes in thyroid cancer incidence, post-2009 American Thyroid Association guidelines. The Laryngoscope. 2017. DOI: 10.1002/lary.26473

[8] Davies L, Welch HG. Increasing incidence of thyroid cancer in the United States, 1973-2002. JAMA. 2006;295(18):2164-2167

[9] Davies L, Welch HG. Current thyroid cancer trends in the United States. JAMA Otolaryngology–Head & Neck Surgery. 2014;140(4):317-322

[10] Grodski S, Brown T, Sidhu S, Gill A, Robinson B, Learoyd D, et al. Increasing incidence of thyroid cancer is due to increased pathologic detection. Surgery. 2008;144(6):1038-1043

[11] Aschebrook-Kilfoy B, Ward MH, Sabra MM, Devesa SS. Thyroid cancer incidence patterns in the United States by histologic type, 1992-2006. Thyroid. 2011;21(2):125-134

[12] Chen AY, Jemal A, Ward EM. Increasing incidence of differentiated thyroid cancer in the United States, 1988-2005. Cancer. 2009;115(16):3801-3807

[13] Rego-Iraeta A, Pérez-Méndez LF, Mantinan B, Garcia-Mayor RV. Time trends for thyroid cancer in northwestern Spain: True rise in the incidence of micro and larger forms of papillary thyroid carcinoma. Thyroid. 2009;19(4):333-340

[14] Simard EP, Ward EM, Siegel R, Jemal A. Cancers with increasing incidence trends in the United States: 1999 through 2008. CA: A Cancer Journal For Clinicians. 2012;62(2):118-128

[15] Howlader N NA, Krapcho M, Miller D, Bishop K, Altekruse SF, Kosary CL, Yu M, Ruhl J, Tatalovich Z, Mariotto A, Lewis DR, Chen HS, Feuer EJ, Cronin KA, editors. SEER Cancer Statistics Review, 1975-2013. Bethesda, MD: National Cancer Institute; April 2016. http://seer.cancer.gov/csr/1975_2013/, based on November 2015 SEER data submission, posted to the SEER website

[16] Dralle H, Machens A, Basa J, Fatourechi V, Franceschi S, Hay ID, et al. Follicular cell-derived thyroid cancer. Nature Reviews Disease Primers. 2014;1:15077-

[17] Dideban S, Abdollahi A, Meysamie A, Sedghi S, Shahriari M. Thyroid papillary microcarcinoma: Etiology, clinical manifestations, diagnosis, follow-up, histopathology and prognosis. Iranian Journal of Pathology. 2016;11(1):1

[18] Kim WB. A closer look at papillary thyroid carcinoma. Endocrinology and Metabolism. 2015;30(1):1-6

[19] Longo DL KD, Jameson JL, Fauci AS, Hauser SL, Loscalzo J. Harrison's Principles of Internal Medicine. 16th ed. New York:McGraw-Hill Publishers; 2012

[20] Goldman L AD. Cecil Medicine. 23rd ed. Saunders Elsevier Publishers; 2007

[21] Schmid D, Ricci C, Behrens G, Leitzmann M. Adiposity and risk of thyroid cancer: A systematic review and meta-analysis. Obesity Reviews. 2015;16(12):1042-1054

[22] Derwahl M, Nicula D. Estrogen and its role in thyroid cancer. Endocrine-Related Cancer. 2014;21(5):T273-T283

[23] Wang P, Jing Z, Liu C, Xu M, Wang P, Wang X, et al. Hepatitis C virus infection and risk of thyroid cancer: A systematic review and meta-analysis. Arab Journal of Gastroenterology. 2017;18(1):1-5

[24] Ito Y, Miyauchi A, Kobayashi K, Kihara M, Miya A. Static and dynamic prognostic factors of papillary thyroid carcinoma [Review]. Endocrine Journal. 2014;61(12):1145-1151

[25] Cady B, Rossi R. An expanded view of risk-group definition in differentiated thyroid carcinoma. Surgery. 1988;104(6):947-953

[26] Hay ID, Bergstralh EJ, Goellner JR, Ebersold JR, Grant CS. Predicting outcome in papillary thyroid carcinoma: Development of a reliable prognostic scoring system in a cohort of 1779 patients surgically treated at one institution during 1940 through 1989. Surgery-SAINT LOUIS. 1993;114:1050-

[27] Sobin LHWCe. UICC: TNM Classification of Malignant Tumors. 7th ed. New York: Wiley-Liss; 2009

[28] Ito Y, Ichihara K, Masuoka H, Fukushima M, Inoue H, Kihara M, et al. Establishment of an intraoperative staging system (iStage) by improving UICC TNM classification system for papillary thyroid carcinoma. World Journal of Surgery. 2010;34(11):2570-2580

[29] Ito Y, Kudo T, Kobayashi K, Miya A, Ichihara K, Miyauchi A. Prognostic factors for recurrence of papillary thyroid carcinoma in the lymph nodes, lung, and bone: Analysis of 5,768 patients with average 10-year follow-up. World Journal of Surgery. 2012;36(6):1274-1278

[30] Matsuzu K, Sugino K, Masudo K, Nagahama M, Kitagawa W, Shibuya H, et al. Thyroid lobectomy for papillary thyroid cancer: Long-term follow-up study of 1,088 cases. World Journal of Surgery. 2014;38(1):68-79

[31] Mazurat A, Torroni A, Hendrickson-Rebizant J, Benning H, Nason RW, Pathak KA. The age factor in survival of a population cohort of well-differentiated thyroid cancer. Endocrine Connections. 2013;2(3):154-160

[32] Siironen P, Louhimo J, Nordling S, Ristimäki A, Mäenpää H, Haapiainen R, et al. Prognostic factors in papillary thyroid cancer: An evaluation of 601 consecutive patients. Tumor Biology. 2005;26(2):57-64

[33] Sugitani I, Kasai N, Fujimoto Y, Yanagisawa A. A novel classification system for patients with PTC: Addition of the new variables of large (3 cm or greater) nodal metastases and reclassification during the follow-up period. Surgery. 2004;135(2):139-148

[34] Toniato A, Boschin I, Casara D, Mazzarotto R, Rubello D, Pelizzo M. Papillary thyroid carcinoma: Factors influencing recurrence and survival. Annals of Surgical Oncology. 2008;15(5):1518-1522

[35] Herrera MF, López-Graniel CM, Saldaña J, Gamboa-Domínguez A, Richaud-Patín Y, Vargas-Vorackova F, et al. Papillary thyroid carcinoma in Mexican patients: Clinical aspects and prognostic factors. World Journal of Surgery. 1996;20(1):94-100

[36] Ito Y, Miyauchi A, Kihara M, Kobayashi K, Miya A. Prognostic values of clinical lymph node metastasis and macroscopic extrathyroid extension in papillary thyroid carcinoma [Review]. Endocrine Journal. 2014;61(8):745-750

[37] Miyauchi A, Kudo T, Hirokawa M, Ito Y, Kihara M, Higashiyama T, et al. Ki-67 labeling index is a predictor of postoperative persistent disease and cancer growth and a prognostic indicator in papillary thyroid carcinoma. European Thyroid Journal. 2013;2(1):57-64

[38] Ito Y, Miyauchi A, Kakudo K, Hirokawa M, Kobayashi K, Miya A. Prognostic significance of ki-67 labeling index in papillary thyroid carcinoma. World Journal of Surgery. 2010;34(12):3015-3021

[39] Elisei R, Viola D, Torregrossa L, Giannini R, Romei C, Ugolini C, et al. The BRAF V600E mutation is an independent, poor prognostic factor for the outcome of patients with low-risk intrathyroid papillary thyroid carcinoma: Single-institution results from a large cohort study. The Journal of Clinical Endocrinology & Metabolism. 2012;97(12):4390-4398

[40] Guerra A, Fugazzola L, Marotta V, Cirillo M, Rossi S, Cirello V, et al. A high percentage of BRAFV600E alleles in papillary thyroid carcinoma predicts a poorer outcome. The Journal of Clinical Endocrinology & Metabolism. 2012;97(7):2333-2340

[41] Kwak JY, Kim E-K, Chung WY, Moon HJ, Kim MJ, Choi JR. Association of BRAFV600E mutation with poor clinical prognostic factors and US features in Korean patients with papillary thyroid microcarcinoma 1. Radiology. 2009;253(3):854-860

[42] O'Neill CJ, Bullock M, Chou A, Sidhu SB, Delbridge LW, Robinson BG, et al. BRAF V600E mutation is associated with an increased risk of nodal recurrence requiring reoperative surgery in patients with papillary thyroid cancer. Surgery. 2010;148(6):1139-1146

[43] Yim JH, Kim WG, Jeon MJ, Han JM, Kim TY, Yoon JH, et al. Association between expression of x-linked inhibitor of apoptosis protein and the clinical outcome in a BRAFV600E-prevalent papillary thyroid cancer population. Thyroid. 2014;24(4):689-694

[44] Miyauchi A, Kudo T, Miya A, Kobayashi K, Ito Y, Takamura Y, et al. Prognostic impact of serum thyroglobulin doubling-time under thyrotropin suppression in patients with papillary thyroid carcinoma who underwent total thyroidectomy. Thyroid. 2011;21(7):707-716

[45] Miyauchi A, Kudo T, Kihara M, Higashiyama T, Ito Y, Kobayashi K, et al. Relationship of biochemically persistent disease and thyroglobulin-doubling time to age at surgery in patients with papillary thyroid carcinoma. Endocrine Journal. 2013;60(4):415-421

[46] Kim WG, Yoon JH, Kim WB, Kim TY, Kim EY, Kim JM, et al. Change of serum antithyroglobulin antibody levels is useful for prediction of clinical recurrence in thyroglobulin-negative patients with differentiated thyroid carcinoma. The Journal of Clinical Endocrinology & Metabolism. 2008;93(12):4683-4689

[47] Tsushima Y, Miyauchi A, Ito Y, Kudo T, Masuoka H, Yabuta T, et al. Prognostic significance of changes in serum thyroglobulin antibody levels of pre-and post-total thyroidectomy in thyroglobulin antibody-positive papillary thyroid carcinoma patients. Endocrine Journal. 2013;60(7):871-876

[48] Adam MA, Pura J, Gu L, Dinan MA, Tyler DS, Reed SD, et al. Extent of surgery for papillary thyroid cancer is not associated with survival: An analysis of 61,775 patients. Annals of Surgery. 2014;260(4):601

[49] Bilimoria KY, Bentrem DJ, Ko CY, Stewart AK, Winchester DP, Talamonti MS, et al. Extent of surgery affects survival for papillary thyroid cancer. Annals of Surgery. 2007;246(3):375-384

[50] Lang BH-H, Ng S-H, Lau LL, Cowling BJ, Wong KP, Wan KY. A systematic review and meta-analysis of prophylactic central neck dissection on short-term locoregional recurrence in papillary thyroid carcinoma after total thyroidectomy. Thyroid. 2013;23(9):1087-1098

[51] Haugen BR, Alexander EK, Bible KC, Doherty GM, Mandel SJ, Nikiforov YE, et al. 2015 American Thyroid Association management guidelines for adult patients with thyroid nodules and differentiated thyroid cancer: The American Thyroid Association guidelines task force on thyroid nodules and differentiated thyroid cancer. Thyroid. 2016;26(1):1-133

[52] Barney BM, Hitchcock YJ, Sharma P, Shrieve DC, Tward JD. Overall and cause-specific survival for patients undergoing lobectomy, near-total, or total thyroidectomy for differentiated thyroid cancer. Head & Neck. 2011;33(5):645-649

[53] Haigh PI, Urbach DR, Rotstein LE. Extent of thyroidectomy is not a major determinant of survival in low-or high-risk papillary thyroid cancer. Annals of Surgical Oncology. 2005;12(1):81-89

[54] Mendelsohn AH, Elashoff DA, Abemayor E, St John MA. Surgery for papillary thyroid carcinoma: Is lobectomy enough? Archives of Otolaryngology–Head & Neck Surgery. 2010;136(11):1055-1061

[55] Ito Y, Miyauchi A, Inoue H, Fukushima M, Kihara M, Higashiyama T, et al. An observational trial for papillary thyroid microcarcinoma in Japanese patients. World Journal of Surgery. 2010;34(1):28

[56] Sugitani I, Toda K, Yamada K, Yamamoto N, Ikenaga M, Fujimoto Y. Three distinctly different kinds of papillary thyroid microcarcinoma should be recognized: Our treatment strategies and outcomes. World Journal of Surgery. 2010;34(6):1222-1231

[57] Durante C, Montesano T, Attard M, Torlontano M, Monzani F, Costante G, et al. Long-term surveillance of papillary thyroid cancer patients who do not undergo postoperative radioiodine remnant ablation: Is there a role for serum thyroglobulin measurement? The Journal of Clinical Endocrinology & Metabolism. 2012;97(8):2748-2753

[58] Fabián P, Erika A, Hernán T, Fernanda B, Carolina U. Biochemical persistence in thyroid cancer: Is there anything to worry about? Endocrine. 2014;46(3):532-537

[59] Tuttle RM, Tala H, Shah J, Leboeuf R, Ghossein R, Gonen M, et al. Estimating risk of recurrence in differentiated thyroid cancer after total thyroidectomy and radioactive iodine remnant ablation: Using response to therapy variables to modify the initial risk estimates predicted by the new American Thyroid Association staging system. Thyroid. 2010;20(12):1341-1349

[60] Vaisman F, Shaha A, Fish S, Michael Tuttle R. Initial therapy with either thyroid lobectomy or total thyroidectomy without radioactive iodine remnant ablation is associated with very low rates of structural disease recurrence in properly selected patients with differentiated thyroid cancer. Clinical Endocrinology. 2011;**75**(1):112-119

[61] Sawka AM, Thabane L, Parlea L, Ibrahim-Zada I, Tsang RW, Brierley JD, et al. Second primary malignancy risk after radioactive iodine treatment for thyroid cancer: A systematic review and meta-analysis. Thyroid. 2009;19(5):451-457

[62] Biondi B, Filetti S, Schlumberger M. Thyroid-hormone therapy and thyroid cancer: A reassessment. Nature Reviews Endocrinology. 2005;1(1):32-40

[63] Mazzaferri EL, Kloos RT. Current approaches to primary therapy for papillary and follicular thyroid cancer. The Journal of Clinical Endocrinology & Metabolism. 2001;86(4):1447-1463

[64] Carhill AA, Litofsky DR, Ross DS, Jonklaas J, Cooper DS, Brierley JD, et al. Long-term outcomes following therapy in differentiated thyroid carcinoma: NTCTCS registry analysis 1987-2012. The Journal of Clinical Endocrinology & Metabolism. 2015;100(9):3270-3279

[65] Jonklaas J, Sarlis NJ, Litofsky D, Ain KB, Bigos ST, Brierley JD, et al. Outcomes of patients with differentiated thyroid carcinoma following initial therapy. Thyroid. 2006;16(12):1229-1242

[66] Cooper DS, Biondi B. Subclinical thyroid disease. The Lancet. 2012;379(9821):1142-1154

[67] DeLellis RA. Pathology and genetics of tumours of endocrine organs: Lyon: Oxford: IARC Press; Oxford University Press (distributor), 2004

[68] Livolsi VA. Surgical pathology of the thyroid: Philadelphia:WB Saunders Company; 1990

[69] Rosai J. Tumors of the thyroid gland. Atlas of Tumor Pathology. 1992

[70] Ahmadi S, Stang M. Hürthle cell carcinoma: Current perspectives. OncoTargets and Therapy. 2016;9:6873

[71] Hürthle K. Beiträge zur Kenntniss des Secretionsvorgangs in der Schilddrüse. Archiv für die Gesamte Physiologie des Menschen und der Tiere. 1894;56(1-3):1-44

[72] Montone KT, Baloch ZW, LiVolsi VA. The thyroid Hürthle (oncocytic) cell and its associated pathologic conditions: A surgical pathology and cytopathology review. Archives of Pathology & Laboratory Medicine. 2008;132(8):1241-1250

[73] Hundahl SA, Fleming ID, Fremgen AM, Menck HR. A National Cancer Data Base report on 53,856 cases of thyroid carcinoma treated in the US, 1985-1995. Cancer. 1998;83(12):2638-2648

[74] Goffredo P, Roman SA, Sosa JA. Hurthle cell carcinoma. Cancer. 2013;119(3):504-511

[75] Chindris A-M, Casler JD, Bernet VJ, Rivera M, Thomas C, Kachergus JM, et al. Clinical and molecular features of Hürthle cell carcinoma of the thyroid. The Journal of Clinical Endocrinology & Metabolism. 2014;100(1):55-62

[76] Schlumberger M, Challeton C, De Vathaire F, Travagli J-P. Radioactive iodine treatment and external radiotherapy for lung and bone metastases from thyroid carcinoma. The Journal of Nuclear Medicine. 1996;37(4):598

[77] Patel KN, Shaha AR. Poorly differentiated thyroid cancer. Current Opinion in Otolaryngology & Head and Neck Surgery. 2014;22(2):121-126

[78] Sakamoto A, Kasai N, Sugano H. Poorly differentiated carcinoma of the thyroid. A clinicopathologic entity for a high-risk group of papillary and follicular carcinomas. Cancer. 1983;52(10):1849-1855

[79] Burman KD, Ringel MD, Wartofsky L. Unusual types of thyroid neoplasms. Endocrinology and Metabolism Clinics of North America. 1996;25(1):49-68

[80] Sywak M, Pasieka JL, Ogilvie T. A review of thyroid cancer with intermediate differentiation. Journal of Surgical Oncology. 2004;86(1):44-54

[81] Carcangiu ML, Zamp G, Rosai J. Poorly differentiated ("insular") thyroid carcinoma: A reinterpretation of Langhans' "wuchernde Struma". The American Journal of Surgical Pathology. 1984;8(9):655-668

[82] Nishida T, Katayama S-i, Tsujimoto M, Nakamura J-i, Matsuda H. Clinicopathological significance of poorly differentiated thyroid carcinoma. The American Journal of Surgical Pathology. 1999;23(2):205-211

[83] Sobrinho-Simoes M, Sambade C, Fonseca E, Soares P. Poorly differentiated carcinomas of the thyroid gland: A review of the clinicopathologic features of a series of 28 cases of a heterogeneous, clinically aggressive group of thyroid tumors. International Journal of Surgical Pathology. 2002;**10**(2):123-131

[84] Volante M, Collini P, Nikiforov YE, Sakamoto A, Kakudo K, Katoh R, et al. Poorly differentiated thyroid carcinoma: The Turin proposal for the use of uniform diagnostic criteria and an algorithmic diagnostic approach. The American Journal of Surgical Pathology. 2007;31(8):1256-1264

[85] Bongiovanni M, Sadow PM, Faquin WC. Poorly differentiated thyroid carcinoma: A cytologic-histologic review. Advances in Anatomic Pathology. 2009;16(5):283-289

[86] Chao T-C, Lin J-D, Chen M-F. Insular carcinoma: Infrequent subtype of thyroid cancer with aggressive clinical course. World Journal of Surgery. 2004;28(4):393-396

[87] Sanders Jr EM, LiVolsi VA, Brierley J, Shin J, Randolph GW. An evidence-based review of poorly differentiated thyroid cancer. World Journal of Surgery. 2007;31(5):934-945

[88] Patel KN, Shaha AR. Poorly differentiated and anaplastic thyroid cancer. Cancer Control. 2006;13(2):119

[89] Hannallah J, Rose J, Guerrero MA. Comprehensive literature review: Recent advances in diagnosing and managing patients with poorly differentiated thyroid carcinoma. International Journal of Endocrinology. 2013;1-7

[90] Jung TS, Kim TY, Kim KW, Oh YL, Park DJ, Cho BY, et al. Clinical features and prognostic factors for survival in patients with poorly differentiated thyroid carcinoma and comparison to the patients with the aggressive variants of papillary thyroid carcinoma. Endocrine Journal. 2007;54(2):265-274

[91] Volante M, Cavallo GP, Papotti M. Prognostic factors of clinical interest in poorly differentiated carcinomas of the thyroid. Endocrine Pathology. 2004;15(4):313-317

[92] Walczyk A, Kowalska A, Sygut J. The clinical course of poorly differentiated thyroid carcinoma (insular carcinoma)—Own observations. Endokrynologia Polska. 2010;61(5):467-473

[93] Wreesmann VB, Ghossein RA, Patel SG, Harris CP, Schnaser EA, Shaha AR, et al. Genome-wide appraisal of thyroid cancer progression. The American Journal of Pathology. 2002;161(5):1549-1556

[94] Dijkstra B, Prichard R, Lee A, Kelly L, Smyth P, Crotty T, et al. Changing patterns of thyroid carcinoma. Irish Journal of Medical Science. 2007;176(2):87-90

[95] O'Neill JP, Shaha AR. Anaplastic thyroid cancer. Oral Oncology. 2013;**49**(7):702-706

[96] Smallridge RC, Copland J. Anaplastic thyroid carcinoma: Pathogenesis and emerging therapies. Clinical Oncology. 2010;**22**(6):486-497

[97] Keutgen XM, Sadowski SM, Kebebew E. Management of anaplastic thyroid cancer. Gland Surgery. 2015;**4**(1):44-51

[98] Kebebew E, Greenspan FS, Clark OH, Woeber KA, McMillan A. Anaplastic thyroid carcinoma. Cancer. 2005;**103**(7):1330-1335

[99] Kihara M, Miyauchi A, Yamauchi A, Yokomise H. Prognostic factors of anaplastic thyroid carcinoma. Surgery Today. 2004;**34**(5):394-398

[100] Kim TY, Kim KW, Jung TS, Kim JM, Kim SW, Chung KW, et al. Prognostic factors for Korean patients with anaplastic thyroid carcinoma. Head & Neck. 2007;**29**(8):765-772

[101] Sugitani I, Kasai N, Fujimoto Y, Yanagisawa A. Prognostic factors and therapeutic strategy for anaplastic carcinoma of the thyroid. World Journal of Surgery. 2001;**25**(5):617-622

[102] Sugitani I, Miyauchi A, Sugino K, Okamoto T, Yoshida A, Suzuki S. Prognostic factors and treatment outcomes for anaplastic thyroid carcinoma: ATC Research Consortium of Japan cohort study of 677 patients. World Journal of Surgery. 2012;**36**(6):1247-1254

[103] Hyman DM, Puzanov I, Subbiah V, Faris JE, Chau I, Blay J-Y, et al. Vemurafenib in multiple nonmelanoma cancers with BRAF V600 mutations. New England Journal of Medicine. 2015;**373**(8):726-736

[104] Raue F, Frank-Raue K. Epidemiology and clinical presentation of medullary thyroid carcinoma. Medullary Thyroid Carcinoma. Springer; 2015. pp. 61-90

[105] Wells Jr SA, Asa SL, Dralle H, Elisei R, Evans DB, Gagel RF, et al. Revised American Thyroid Association guidelines for the management of medullary thyroid carcinoma: The American Thyroid Association Guidelines Task Force on medullary thyroid carcinoma. Thyroid. 2015;**25**(6):567-610

[106] Moley JF. Medullary thyroid carcinoma: Management of lymph node metastases. Journal of the National Comprehensive Cancer Network. 2010;**8**(5):549-556

[107] Meijer JA, Le Cessie S, Van Den Hout WB, Kievit J, Schoones JW, Romijn JA, et al. Calcitonin and carcinoembryonic antigen doubling times as prognostic factors in medullary thyroid carcinoma: A structured meta-analysis. Clinical Endocrinology. 2010;**72**(4):534-542

[108] Akhavan A, Jafari SM, Khosravi MH, Khajehpour H, Karimi-Sari H. Reliability of fine-needle aspiration and ultrasound-based characteristics of thyroid nodules for diagnosing malignancy in Iranian patients. Diagnostic Cytopathology. 2016 Apr 1;44(4):269-73

[109] Fukunari N, Nagahama M, Sugino K, Mimura T, Ito K, Ito K. Clinical evaluation of color Doppler imaging for the differential diagnosis of thyroid follicular lesions. World Journal of Surgery. 2004;**28**(12):1261-1265

[110] Lee SH, Baek JS, Lee JY, Lim JA, Cho SY, Lee TH, et al. Predictive factors of malignancy in thyroid nodules with a cytological diagnosis of follicular neoplasm. Endocrine Pathology. 2013;24(4):177-183

[111] Lubitz CC, Faquin WC, Yang J, Mekel M, Gaz RD, Parangi S, et al. Clinical and cytological features predictive of malignancy in thyroid follicular neoplasms. Thyroid. 2010;20(1):25-31

[112] Miyakawa M, Onoda N, Fukuda I, Takano K, Okamoto T, Obara T. Diagnosis of thyroid follicular carcinoma by the vascular pattern and velocimetric parameters using high resolution pulsed and power Doppler ultrasonography. Endocrine Journal. 2005;52(2):207-212

9

Medullary Thyroid Carcinoma: Recent Updates on the Diagnosis and Management

Andrei Cismaru, Iulia Coroian, Gabriel Cismaru and Adrian Udrea

Abstract

Medullary thyroid carcinoma is a hormone-producing malignant tumor that synthesizes calcitonin. MTC can be sporadic or familial. It has a malignant behavior. Our chapter has 3 parts: *1.Updates on the diagnosis of MTC* -in this part we review the clinical findings in MTC: isolated thyroid nodule, palpable cervical lymph nodes and systemic manifestations. Fine needle aspiration, serum calcitonin, computed tomography (CT) and fludeoxyglucose - positron emission tomograpyh (FDG-PET) are summarized. Biomarkers with prognostic value are be described in detail: plasma calcitonin, carcino-embryonic antigen, germ-line RET mutation and matrix metalloproteinase. *2. Updates on the management and treatment of MTC* -we discuss the surgical treatment, radiation therapy, systemic therapy with angiogenesis inhibitors and transcatheter arterial embolization to prevent extension of the tumor. Based on the characteristics of MTC a new approach using gene therapy has been developed to obtain complete remission of the carcinoma. *3. We describe a typical case of MTC* from the oncology department, with cervical lymph nodes and a thyroid nodule. Immunohistochemistry staining showed *calcitonin* in the tumor cells. Thyroid ultrasound with fine needle aspiration biopsy confirmed the MTC. CT images of the cervical lymph nodes and thyroid nodule as well as microscopy images are presented. Chemotherapy with Dacarbazine was initiated with favorable outcome.

Keywords: thyroid, carcinoma, neck, calcitonin, lymph nodes, medullary, chemotherapy

1. Introduction

Medullary thyroid carcinoma (MTC) is a tumor that is derived from the calcitonin-producing cells, which can be either sporadic or hereditary like in MEN2 neoplasia [1]. MTC is suspected after physical examination by measuring plasma calcitonin. For a positive diagnosis, histological confirmation is needed. The tumor extent and presence of metastases are determined using ultrasonography, computed tomography, and magnetic resonance imaging (MRI).

2. Updates on the diagnosis of medullary thyroid carcinoma

2.1. Clinical findings: when should we suspect MTC?

2.1.1. Isolated thyroid nodule

At presentation, most of the time, patients have an isolated thyroid nodule [2], and the diagnosis needs fine needle biopsy with elevated serum calcitonin. An isolated thyroid nodule can be incidentally detected during a carotid ultrasound or a chest CT scan with neck images [3]. Sometimes malignant thyroid nodules might appear in the context of a multinodular goiter.

2.1.2. Palpable cervical lymph nodes

Usually patients with MTC present with a painless thyroid nodule with cervical adenopathies. They are fast growing and fixed to the adjacent structures [4]. Sometimes, the lymph node can be incidentally detected during a carotid ultrasound or a chest or neck computed tomography. Cervical lymph nodes appear early in the course of a MTC and can be found in more than three-fourths of patients. Most of the time, the involvement is ipsilateral and also of the central lymph nodes [5].

2.1.3. Systemic manifestations

A minority of patients present with diarrhea, painful bone metastasis, flushing, or symptoms related to hypercorticism when the adrenocorticotropic hormone (ACTH) production is increased. Typically, MTC metastases occur in the liver, lung bones, lymph nodes, and mediastinum [6].

2.2. Paraclinical examinations: what test should we perform to confirm diagnosis?

2.2.1. Fine needle aspiration (FNA)

It is one of the most important tools for the diagnosis of MTC. The cytological characteristics include isolated cells or cells arranged in isolated groups with two or more round nuclei with eccentric position [7] and presence of fusiform cells and comet-like projections [8]. The sensitivity of FNA is between 46 and 63% with the most frequent negative results given by inadequate function in case of a multinodular goiter or a too small sample for analysis. The washout fluid can be used for calcitonin sampling which increases the sensitivity of the diagnosis. In the doubtful cases, immunohistochemical staining for calcitonin helps the correct diagnosis [9].

2.2.2. Ultrasonography

It is the most commonly used method for lesion assessment and is followed by fine needle biopsy in case of abnormal results. Ultrasonography permits an accurate assessment of the size and characteristics of the nodule, as well as identification of additional abnormal nodules inside the thyroid gland. The most common sonographic features of MTCs are solid composition, hypoechogenicity, and the absence of halo [10]. Calcifications are frequent in MTCs either in the form of macro or microcalcifications. When a lesion with the above characteristics is found, calcitonin should be measured and FNA is performed [11].

2.2.3. Computed tomography (CT) and magnetic resonance imaging (RMI)

These are important for both preoperative and postoperative assessment of MTC. In one of six CTs of the neck, an incidentaloma of the thyroid can be found. But in routine CT and MRI, there is no specific sign to differentiate between malignant and benign thyroid tumor [12]. In patients presenting with cervical lymph nodes, a primary thyroid origin is suggested by the presence of cystic components, calcifications, or hemorrhage appearing as hyperdensity in CT or hyperintensity in MRI. CT and MRI cannot distinguish between different histological types of thyroid cancer and also cannot diagnose multifocal tumors. MRI and CT have a good accuracy for predicting invasion of the trachea [13], larynx, or esophagus [14].

2.2.4. FDG-PET

It is used in the imaging of carcinoids and MTCs. It has a high sensitivity and specificity for MTC and can be used after a successful surgery to detect occult tumor fragments [15]. It has the disadvantage of being positive also in case of infection, inflammation, or other types of thyroid cancers. FDG-PET sensitivity increases with high levels of plasma calcitonin [16] or in case of a short doubling time. It can also be a marker of prognosis of MTC [17].

2.3. Biomarkers with prognostic value

Biomarkers are used in the clinical management of patients with MTC. Some of them are already implemented in the daily management of the disease: plasma calcitonin and CEA are easy to determine but further studies are needed to establish the prognostic of high values. Germline RET mutations are used for the timing of MTC treatment matrix metalloproteinase (MMP)-2 may have a prognostic value.

2.3.1. Plasma calcitonin

Calcitonin is secreted by the thyroid C-cells and is a highly specific marker for MTC. Sometimes, for an unknown reason, MTCs do not secrete calcitonin. The secretion of calcitonin from the C-cells can be increased by pentagastrin or calcium. This test can differentiate between elevated calcitonin from MTC and elevated calcitonin of other causes (smoking, nonC-cell thyroid carcinoma). The doubling time of plasma calcitonin is a good marker for MTC recurrence and survival of patients [18]. A more specific and sensitive method to measure calcitonin is selective venous catheterization of the neck veins and taking a blood sample from near the thyroid nodule. It can exclude other sources of calcitonin rising outside the neck. After surgery, calcitonin is deferred for 6 weeks to allow the postsurgery nadir. A good marker of complete remission is a negative calcitonin after pentagastrin stimulation at 6 weeks after surgery.

2.3.2. Carcinoembryonic antigen (CEA)

It is not specific for MTC but used for prognostic purposes. An elevated CEA levels before surgery are associated with tumor size and recurrences [19]. MTCs that do not secrete calcitonin can be followed by measuring CEA [20].

2.3.3. Germline RET mutation

Germline RET mutation is a well-known MTC biomarker, present in 98% of MEN 2. The presence of RET mutation indicated a familial MTC and the risk of developing MTC is close to 100%. It is used for the follow-up of metastatic and recurrent MTC [21].

2.3.4. Matrix metalloproteinase-2

It participates in angiogenesis and carcinogenesis. In the study of Calvalheiro et al., it was demonstrated a correlation between MMP-2 and the persistence of MTC after a successful treatment [22].

3. Updates on the management and treatment of medullary thyroid carcinoma

3.1. Surgical treatment

MTC has a malignant behavior. There is a general agreement that operation for MTC should obtain complete removal of the neck tumor because adjuvant therapy in MTC has not been proved to be effective. Cervical lymph nodes metastases are often present in initial stages [23]. The appropriate initial treatment is total thyroidectomy with lymph node dissection. Lymphadenectomy comprises central compartment with ipsilateral node dissection, but some centers also perform contralateral lymph node dissection [24]. Where there is a suspicion of mediastinal disease, median sternotomy may be required with mediastinal dissection. Distant metastases can also be treated with surgery such as bone excision and lung resection for metastases.

The parathyroid glands should be preserved during thyroid surgery. In case they are normal, they can be left in place or transplanted in a sternocleidomastoidian muscle [25].

After surgery, plasma calcitonin levels can detect the presence of occult tumor fragments. Elevated calcitonin levels are a sign of persistent MTC after surgery, which can be the case in almost 50% of patients. Furthermore, in a small percentage of patients, several years after thyroidectomy, the plasma calcitonin can increase indicating a recurrent MTC [26]. Measurements should be performed after surgery at 6, 12, 18, 24, 30, 34, and 40 months due to the risk of relapse [27].

3.2. Radiation therapy

In contrast to other forms of thyroid carcinoma, MTC is not sensitive to radioactive iodine or levothyroxine suppressive therapy. External beam radiotherapy is used in an adjuvant therapy in patients with a high risk of local recurrence after surgery. It is also used in palliative therapy in case of bone metastasis [28]. The most important application of radiotherapy is used for painful bone metastases [29].

3.3. Systemic therapy angiogenesis inhibitors

Axitinib, which is a tyrosine kinases inhibitor targeting Vascular endothelial growth factor (VEGF) receptor, was used for MTC treatment. It is associated with a partial response rate of nearly 20% with moderate side effects such as fatigue, proteinuria, and high blood pressure [30]. A second angiogenesis inhibitor AMG-706 was also used in MTC patients, which is an inhibitor of VEGFR [31].

3.4. Transcatheter arterial embolization

Transcatheter arterial embolization can prevent extension of the tumor outside the thyroid gland. However, the method is restricted to visualized primary or metastatic tumors [32]. The small, unvisualized tumors cannot be cured by transcatheter arterial embolization. Another indication of Transcatheter arterial embolization (TAE) is liver metastases with or without adjunction of ethanol injection.

3.5. Percutaneous ethanol injection

It is also able to prevent the extracapsular extension of MTC. The small metastatic tumors that cannot be visualized with recent techniques and have the potential of tissue invasion are not prone to ethanol injection. A combination between transcatheter arterial embolization with ethanol injection and gene therapy could be used in the near future to obtain complete remission [33].

3.6. Gene therapy

Trials of genetic cytokine emerged for treating MTC. Gene therapy using calcitonin gene and adenovirus vector is available; however, the technique is not fully accessible in humans [34]. There are four approaches for gene therapy in MTC: (1) corrective gene therapy to inhibit the RET oncogene; (2) cytoreductive gene therapy using toxin genes to permit ^{131}I uptake; (3) immunomodulatory gene therapy using cytokines; and (4) combined approach [35]. With some improvements for the vector design in terms of efficacy and safety, gene therapy for MTC may soon help to overcome obstacles in the treatment of this type of cancer [36].

3.7. Treatment for MTC metastases

In the case of isolated metastases of the brain, surgical resection should be proposed. If surgery is not possible, radiotherapy should be considered [3].

The liver is the most frequent site of metastases. The liver lesions are multiple and disseminated. Treatment is indicated in the case of large hepatic tumor or rapidly progressive lesions, as well as intense pain or intractable diarrhea [37].

Bone metastasis leads to pain, hypercalcemia, spinal cord compression, and pathological fractures. They associate low survival. Spinal cord compression is treated with emergency surgery and systemic corticoids. Radiotherapy can be used in case of painful metastases or when complete resection cannot be achieved. Intravenous bisphosphonates can be effective to prevent bone fractures, spinal cord compression, and hypercalcemia [38].

Lung metastases that associate hemoptysis or obstruction of the airwaves should be treated with radiotherapy.

4. A case of medullary thyroid carcinoma

We present a case of metastasis to the lung, adrenal glands, and cervical lymphnodes of a medullary thyroid carcinoma. Informed consent was obtained from the patient before the case report submission. A 54-year-old male presented with cervical adenopathies. Computed tomography of the neck and chest showed enlarged laterocervical lymph nodes (**Figure 1**), a left inferior lobe thyroid nodule (**Figure 2**), a tumor of the right pulmonary hilum (**Figure 3**), and bilateral nodules of malignant appearance of adrenal glands (**Figure 4**). Biopsy from the laterocervical lymph nodes was done at first presentation (**Figure 5**).

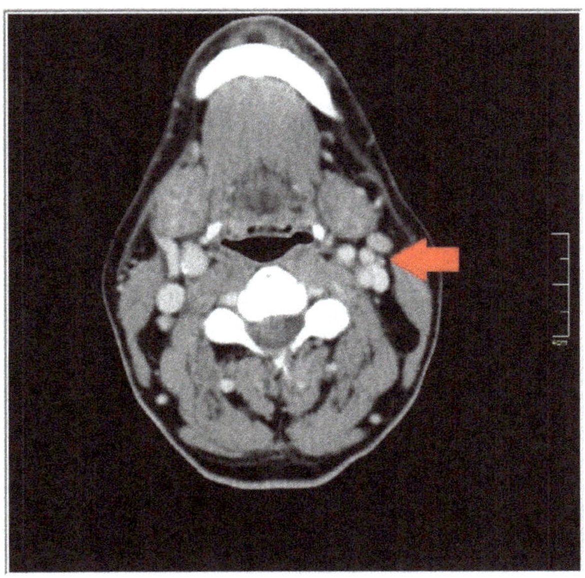

Figure 1. Computer tomography at the level of the neck reveals enlarged laterocervical lymph nodes on the left side.

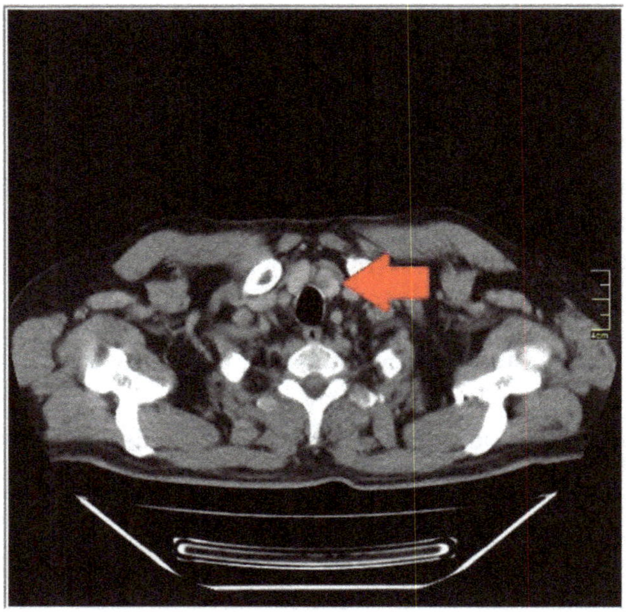

Figure 2. Computer tomography at the level of thyroid gland. On the left side in the inferior lobe, 8, 6/4, 8/7, and 6 mm nodule can be distinguished.

Chemotherapy with taxol + carboplatin-AUC5 (TC) was initiated concomitantly with other diagnostic tools evaluating other sites of the disease. Biopsy of the lung nodule showed neuroendocrine differentiation cancer with negative CK7 staining. Aspiration biopsy of the thyroid nodule showed MTC. All the three biopsies were reassessed and further immunohistochemical staining showed calcitonin in the tumor cells [39], in favor of lung metastases from MTC [40, 41].

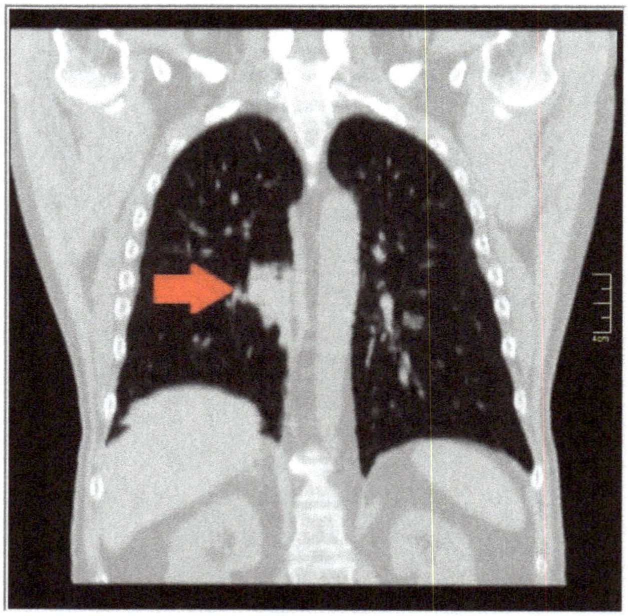

Figure 3. Computer tomography of the chest. On the right lung, a hilar tumor of 4.85 cm can be identified.

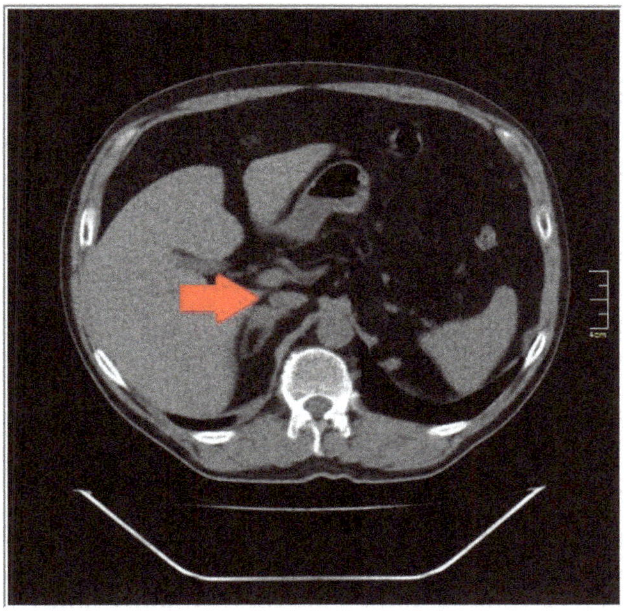

Figure 4. Computer tomography of the abdomen. The scan reveals on the right side an adrenal tumor of 2.8 cm.

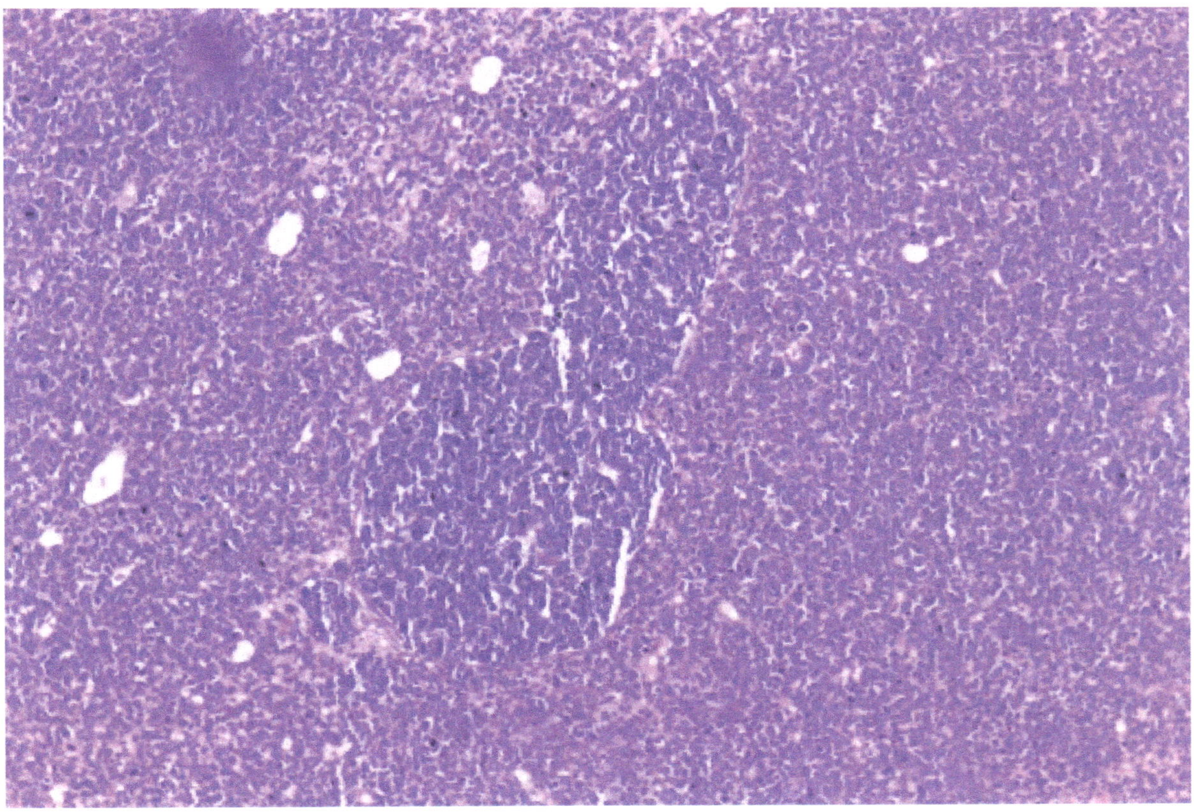

Figure 5. Microscopic examination from adenopathies reveals: lymph nodes occupied by a proliferation of malignant cells, with round/oval nuclei with atypia. The cells are arranged in nests, with fine beads or individual, separated by a fine stroma rich in capillaries. There are areas in which the stroma is rich, loose, myxoid, fibrous, or dense. In some areas, the cells are arranged in palisades with fibrous septa at the interface; the surface looks detached from the basal layer, giving impression of glandular structures.

4.1. Histological examination

The histological examination showed the following:

Lung tumor: *Microscopic examination* reveals fragments of respiratory mucosa with massive infiltration of poorly differentiated tumor cells. *Immunohistochemistry*: Positive; TTF1, CEA, CD56, and calcitonin.

Laterocervical adenopathies: *Microscopic examination reveals* highly malignant tumor cell proliferation, predominantly solid (80% from surface). *Immunohistochemistry*: TTF1 and CEA-positive; S100 and p63 negative; CD30 negative; and Ki-67 present up to 50% in solid areas.

Thyroid nodule: Groups of cells of medium size with immunpositivity for calcitonin in all tumor cells.

4.2. Differential diagnosis

A tongue tumor affecting the salivary glands was excluded through a biopsy from the base of the tongue that found no sign of malignancy. S100, si, and p63 were also negative.

CD30 negative in the laterocervical adenopathy excludes an embryonic carcinoma.

Lung adenocarcinoma with secondary thyroid metastasis is the most important differential diagnosis. Serum calcitonin levels were normal: 3.6/pg/ml (N = 1–11.8/pg/ml), but the thyroid biopsy confirms MTC. Some MTCs may remain within normal ranges of calcitonin. Lung biopsy and immunohistochemistry are in favor of MTC metastases and not adenocarcinoma [42].

4.3. Treatment

Therapy with taxol 175 mg/m^2 + carboplatine-AUC5 (TC) was administered after initial assessment of the biopsies with favorable response (stable disease at thyroid site and partial response at the lung and adrenal glands) after the first three cycles. Three more cycles were delivered, and at relapse, a second-line chemotherapy with dacarbazine 1 g/m^2 was initiated.

Five cycles of paclitaxel and carboplatin (TC) were administrated with a consecutive computer tomography follow-up. The pulmonary tumor showed partial regression and the suprarenal nodule's dimensions decreased.

Chemotherapy had favorable results but showed relapse after sixth cycle of TC.

After dacarbazine three cycles, the dimensions of the thyroid nodule further decreased.

5. Conclusion

The clinical picture of medullary thyroid carcinoma (MTC) is variable and distant metastases are often present at diagnosis. It is essential to know if such is the case as different therapies apply. High calcitonin serum levels provide valuable diagnostic data in MTC with distant metastases but may remain within normal ranges in some cases raising diagnosis difficulties.

Histology with immunohistochemistry can distinguish between primary carcinoma and metastasis.

Author details

Andrei Cismaru[1,2], Iulia Coroian[1,2], Gabriel Cismaru[3]* and Adrian Udrea[2]

*Address all correspondence to: gabi_cismaru@yahoo.com

1 Oncology Department, "Iuliu Hatieganu" University of Medicine and Pharmacy, Cluj-Napoca, Romania

2 Medisprof Oncology Clinic, Cluj-Napoca, Romania

3 5th Department of Internal Medicine, Cardiac Rehabilitation, "Iuliu Hatieganu" University of Medicine and Pharmacy, Cluj-Napoca, Romania

References

[1] Taccaliti A, Silvetti F, Palmonella G, Boscaro M. Genetic alterations in medullary thyroid cancer: Diagnostic and prognostic markers. Current Genomics. 2011;**12**:618-625

[2] Bartolotta TV, Midiri M, Runza G, et al. Incidentally discovered thyroid nodules: Incidence, and greyscale and colour Doppler pattern in an adult population screened by real-time compound spatial sonography. La Radiologia Medica. 2006;**111**:989-998

[3] Moley JF, DeBenedetti MK. Patterns of nodal metastases in palpable medullary thyroid carcinoma: Recommendation for the extent of node dissection. Annals of Surgery. 1999;**229**:880-887

[4] Yoon DY, Chang SK, Choi CS, et al. The prevalence and significance of incidental thyroid nodules identified on computed tomography. Journal of Computer Assisted Tomography. 2008;**32**:810-815

[5] Scollo C, Baudin E, Trvagli JP, et al. Rationale for central and bilateral ymph node dissection in sporadic and hereditary medullary thyroid cancer. The Journal of Clinical Endocrinology and Metabolism. 2003;**88**:2070-2075

[6] Machens A, Hinze R, Thomusch O, Dralle H. Pattern of nodal metastasis for primary and reoperative thyroid cancer. World Journal of Surgery. 2002;**26**:22-28

[7] Papaparaskeva K, Nagel H, Droese M. Cytologic diagnosis of medullary carcinoma of the thyroid gland. Diagnostic Cytopathology. 2000;**22**:351-358

[8] Essig Jr GF, Porter K, Schneider D, Debora A, Lindsey SC, Busonero G, et al. Fine needle aspiration and medullary thyroid carcinoma: The risk of inadequate preoperative evaluation and initial surgery when relying upon FNAB cytology alone. Endocrine Practice. 2013;**19**:920-927

[9] Cooper DS, Doherty GM, Haugen BR, et al. Revised American Thyroid Association management guidelines for patients with thyroid nodules and differentiated thyroid cancer. Thyroid. 2009;**19**:1167-1214

[10] Cai S, Liu H, Li WB, et al. Ultrasonographic features of medullary thyroid carcinoma and their diagnostic values. Chinese Medical Journal. 2010;**123**:3074-3078

[11] Lee S, Shin JH, Han BK, et al. Medullary thyroid carcinoma: Comparison with papillary thyroid carcinoma and application of current sonographic criteria. American Journal of Roentgenology. 2010;**194**:1090-1094

[12] Hoang JK, Vanka J, Ludwig BJ, Glastonbury CM. Evaluation of cervical lymph nodes in head and neck cancer with CT and MRI: Tips, traps, and a systematic approach. American Journal of Roentgenology (AJR). 2013;**200**:W17-25

[13] Wang JC, Takashima S, Takayama F, et al. Tracheal invasion by thyroid carcinoma: Prediction using MR imaging. American Journal of Roentgenology (AJR). 2001;**177**:929-936

[14] Shetty SK, Maher MM, Hahn PF, Halpern EF, Aquino SL. Significance of incidental thyroid lesions detected on CT: Correlation among CT, sonography, and pathology. American Journal of Roentgenology (AJR). 2006;**187**:1349-1356

[15] Eloy JA, Brett EM, Fatterpekar GM, et al. The significance and management of incidental [^{18}F]fluorodeoxyglucose-positron-emission tomography uptake in the thyroid gland in patients with cancer. American Journal of Neuroradiology (AJNR). 2009;**30**:1431-1434

[16] Szakall Jr S, Esik O, Bajzik G, et al. ^{18}F-FDG PET detection of lymph node metastases in medullary thyroid carcinoma. Journal of Nuclear Medicine. 2002;**43**:66-67

[17] Ong SC, Schoder H, Patel SG, et al. Diagnostic accuracy of 18F-FDG PET in restaging patients with medullary thyroid carcinoma and elevated calcitonin levels. Journal of Nuclear Medicine. 2007;**48**:501-507

[18] Miyauchi A, Onishi T, Morimoto S, et al. Relation of doubling time of plasma calcitonin levels to prognosis and recurrence of medullary thyroid carcinoma. Annals of Surgery. 1984;**199**:461-466

[19] Barbet J, Campion L, Kraeber-Bodéré F, Chatal JF; GTE Study Group. Prognostic impact of serum calcitonin and carcinoembryonic antigen doubling-times in patients with medullary thyroid carcinoma. The Journal of Clinical Endocrinology and Metabolism. 2005;**90**:6077-6084

[20] Wells Jr SA, Haagensen Jr DE, Linehan WM, Farrel RE, Dilley WG. The detection of elevated plasma levels of carcinoembryonic antigen in patients with suspected or established medullary thyroid carcinoma. Cancer. 1978;**42**:1498-1503

[21] Wohllk N, Cote GJ, Bugalho MM, et al. Relevance of RET proto-oncogene mutations in sporadic medullary thyroid carcinoma. The Journal of Clinical Endocrinology and Metabolism. 1996;**81**:3740-3745

[22] Cavalhero BG, Junqueira CR, Brandao LG. Expression of matrix metalloproteinase 2 (MMP-2) and tissue inhibitor of metalloproteinase 2 (TIMP-2) in medullary thyroid carcinoma: Prognostic implications. Thyroid. 2008;**18**:865-871

[23] Miyauchi A, Matsuzuka F, Hirai K, Yokozawa T, Kobayashi K, Ito Y, Nakano K, Kuma K, Futami H, Yamaguchi K. Prospective trial of unilateral surgery for nonhereditary medullary thyroid carcinoma in patients without germline RET mutations. World Journal of Surgery. 2002;**26**:1023-1028

[24] Machens A, Holzhausen HJ, Dralle H. Contralateral cervical and mediastinal lymph node metastasis in medullary thyroid cancer: Systemic disease? Surgery. 2006;**139**:28-32

[25] Weber T, Schilling T, Frank-Raue K, Colombo-Benkmann M, Hinz U, Ziegler R, Klar E. Impact of modified radical neck dissection on biochemical cure in medullary thyroid carcinomas. Surgery. 2001;**130**:1044-1049

[26] Kebebew E, Ituarte PH, Siperstein AE, Duh QY, Clark OH. Medullary thyroid carcinoma: Clinical characteristics, treatment, prognostic factors, and a comparison of staging systems. Cancer. 2000;**88**:1139-1148

[27] Brauckhoff M, Machens A, Thanh PN, Lorenz K, Schmeil A, Stratmann M, Sekulla C, Brauckhoff K, Dralle H. Impact of extent of resection for thyroid cancer invading the aerodigestive tract on surgical morbidity, local recurrence, and cancer-specific survival. Surgery. 2010;**148**:1257-1266

[28] Brierley J, Tsang R, Simpson WJ, Gospodarowicz M, Sutcliffe S, Panzarella T. Medullary thyroid cancer: Analyses of survival and prognostic factors and the role of radiation therapy in local control. Thyroid. 1996;**6**:305-310

[29] Brierley JD, Tsang RW. External beam radiation therapy for thyroid cancer. Endocrinology Metabolism Clinics of North America. 2008;**37**:497-509

[30] Brassard M, Neraud B, Trabado S, Salenave S, Brailly-Tabard S, Borget I, Baudin E, Leboulleux S, Chanson P, Schlumberger M, Young J. Endocrine effects of the tyrosine kinase inhibitor vandetanib in patients treated for thyroid cancer. The Journal of Clinical Endocrinology and Metabolism. 2011;**96**:2741-2749

[31] Kim S RL, Cohen EE< Cohen RB. A Phase II study of axitinib (AG-013736), a potent inhibitor of VEGFRs, in patients with advanced thyroid cancer. Journal of Clinical Oncology 2006;**24**(8S):5529-5529

[32] Lorenz K, Brauckhoff M, Behrmann C, Sekulla C, Ukkat J, Brauckhoff K, Gimm O, Dralle H. Selective arterial chemoembolization for hepatic metastases from medullary thyroid carcinoma. Surgery. 2005;**138**:986-993

[33] Isozaki T, Kiba T, Numata K, Saito S, Shimamura T, Kitamura T, Morita K, Tanaka K, Sekihara H. Medullary thyroid carcinoma with multiple hepatic metastases: Treatment with transcatheter arterial embolization and percutaneous ethanol injection. Internal Medicine. 1999;**38**:17-21

[34] Nicklin SA, Baker AH. Tropism-modified adenoviral and adeno-associated viral vectors for gene therapy. Current Gene Therapy. 2002;**2**:273-293

[35] Hinze R, Gimm O, Taubert H, Bauer G, Dralle H, Holzhausen HJ, Rath FW. Regulation of proliferation and apoptosis in sporadic and hereditary medullary thyroid carcinomas and their putative precursor lesions. Virchows Archiv. 2000;**437**:256-263

[36] DeGroot LJ, Zhang R. Clinical review 131. Gene Therapy for thyroid cancer: Where do we stand? The Journal of Clinical Endocrinology and Metabolism. 2001;**86**:2923-2928

[37] Tung WS, Vesely TM, Moley JF. Laparoscopic detection of hepatic metastases in patients with residual or recurrent medullary thyroid cancer. Surgery. 1995;**118**:1024-1029

[38] Even Sapir E. Imaging of malignant bone involvement by morphologic, scintigraphic, and hybrid modalities. Journal of Nuclear Medicine. 2005;**46**:1356-1367

[39] Haraguchi S, Hioki M, Yamashita K, Orii K, Matsumoto K, Shimizu K. Metastasis to the thyroid from lung adenocarcinoma mimicking thyroid carcinoma. The Japanese Journal of Thoracic and Cardiovascular Surgery. 2004;**52**:353-356

[40] Dämmrich J, Ormanns W, Kahaly G, Schrezenmeir J. Multiple peptide hormone producing adenocarcinoma of lung with neurotensin and CRF-like immunoreactivity. Pathology – Research and Practice. 1988;**183**:670-674

[41] Mizukami Y, Saito K, Nonomura A, Michigishi T, Hashimoto T, Nakanuma Y, Matsubara F, Takasakura E. Lung carcinoma metastatic to microfollicular adenoma of the thyroid. A case report. Acta Pathologica Japonica. 1990;**40**:602-608

[42] Alevizaki M, Kyratzoglou E, Bamias A, Tzanela M, Dimopoulos MA, Saltiki K. Metachronous appearance of second malignancies in medullary thyroid carcinoma (MTC) patients: A diagnostic challenge and brief review of the literature. Endocrine. 2013;**44**:610-615

10

Head and Neck Cancer: Epidemiology and Role of MicroRNAs

Muhammad Babar Khawar, Naz Fatima,
Muddasir Hassan Abbasi, Rabia Mehmood,
Saira Kainat Suqaina and Nadeem Sheikh

Abstract

Head and neck cancer (HNC) is referred to the cancers of aerodigestive tract covering number of structures *viz*, oral and nasal cavity, paranasal sinuses, lips, salivary glands, oropharynx, hypopharynx, pharynx, larynx, and local lymph nodes. It is the sixth most common cancer in the world. MicroRNAs (miRNAs) are small single-stranded noncoding RNAs (ncRNAs) of about 19–25 nucleotides. These miRNAs have been reported to influence number of biological activities, i.e., gene regulation, differentiation, organ formation, cell death, cell proliferation, and stress responses. The first ever study involving miRNAs in HNC was published in 2005. Since then, association between dysregulation of miRNAs and head and neck tumorigenesis has been documented by a number of researchers. This chapter has covered a comprehensive state of the art literature review of the recent studies about the role of miRNAs in HNC including oral squamous cell carcinoma (OSCC) and human nasopharyngeal carcinoma. Despite significant improvement in multimodal treatment, the prognosis of advanced HNC is quite poor. Recent studies are promising regarding the potential role of miRNAs as prognostic indicators. Recently, some miRNAs have been discovered as important diagnostic biomarkers. In fact, miRNAs are found circulated stably in different body fluids, i.e., urine, blood, saliva, as well as in breath. Hence, these miRNAs can be assessed easily with noninvasive methods. miRNAs are the key therapeutic targets in addition to their prognostic and diagnostic value. Use of synthetically designed "miRNAs sponges," miR mimics (agomiRs), miR antagonists ("antagomiRs"), and miR inhibitors (antimiRNAs oligonucleotides) is an innovative strategy to modulate oncogenic and tumor-suppressive pathways. Our understanding of miRNAs involvement in HNC is in its infancy. The discovery of miRNAs heralds a complete new paradigm in the understanding of exact molecular pathways involved in HNC development. More detailed studies are required for better understanding and therapeutic targets to treat HNC.

Keywords: biomarker, gene regulation, head and neck cancer, microRNAs, nasopharyngeal carcinoma, noncoding RNAs, oral squamous cell carcinoma (OSCC), therapeutic targets

1. Head and neck cancer epidemiology

Head and neck cancer (HNC) is referred to the cancers of aerodigestive tract covering number of structures *viz*, oral and nasal cavity, paranasal sinuses, lips, salivary glands, oropharynx, hypopharynx, pharynx, larynx, and local lymph nodes [1]. It is the sixth most common cancer in the world with more than 500,000 cases reported annually [2, 3]. HNC has found to be more prevalent among males than females [3]. More than 90% of all the reported cases of HNC are squamous cell carcinomas (HNSCCs) which usually arise from mucosal lining in these sites [1]. Among these cases, 80–90% cases were found to be associated with prolonged usage of alcohol and tobacco [4].

One of the frequently diagnosed malignancies, globally, is head and neck cancer. Frequent relapses and distant metastasis have been observed in patients with advanced disease stages, resulted in an endurance rate of 5 years in almost 60% patients despite of substantial advances in multimodality rehabilitation [5]. Mucosal malignancy of head and neck is a potent melanoma with poor prognosis. The nasal pit, paranasal sinuses, and oral cavity are the most widely recognized areas. Survival rates of 1, 3, and 5 years were 63, 30, and 20%, respectively, around 2000–2007. All interpretations suggested that cigarette smoking is hazardous. Clinical marks and clues are typically nonspecific for it. Surgery is regarded as the backbone of treatment for most mucosal melanomas of the head and neck supplemented with radiotherapy [6]. The relationship amongst alcohol consumption and head and neck disease is quite clear and the outcomes reliably demonstrated an expanded head and neck tumor chance related with alcohol drinking. Bagnardi et al. reported a positive relationship in between alcohol drinking and head and neck cancer risk [7]. In Western nations, around 39% of head and neck malignancy can be ascribed to alcohol utilization (4% for only alcohol drinking and 35% for the joint impact of alcohol and tobacco) [8]. Head and neck squamous cell carcinomas (HNSCCs) cause more than 300,000 deaths globally every year. Locoregional and removed recurrences are more important prognostic indicators and acknowledged surrogate markers of patients' survival. No legitimate biomarker and rescue treatment exist to recognize and treat patients at high-danger of recurrence [9]. Despite of reduction in smoking and alcohol utilization, the rate of oropharyngeal squamous cell carcinoma (OPSCC) is rising. It refers to human papilloma virus (HPV) infection contamination [10]. HPV is an entrenched prognostic marker for OPSCC [11]. Oropharyngeal tumors are firmly connected with HPV-positivity [12]. Oral tumor constitutes the dominant part of head and neck diseases, which is the fifth most basic malignancy around the world, representing 984,430 cases in 2012. During 2000 and 2010, there were 1916 instances of OSCC in New Zealand with a male to female proportion of 1.85:1, and an age-institutionalized rate of 42 for every 1,000,000 people [13]. Liquor utilization, trailed by tobacco, is considered the most common hazard in New Zealand. Given the high pervasiveness of these two hazardous elements and their synergistic impact, it is vital for specialists to boost smoking cessation and limited liquor consumption. More research should be conducted to confirm use of tobacco and water-pipe smoking in New Zealand, particularly because of changing demography and increments in transient populaces. UV radiation is an additionally imperative hazard element [13]. Laryngeal squamous cell carcinoma (LSCC), being a potent threat, is amongst the most regularly analyzed malignant sorts of head and neck SCC around the world. Rates of LSCC have been estimated to escalate recently [14]. Salivary gland pleomorphic adenoma (SGPA) is also one of the most widely recognized types of salivary organ tumor. In China, particularly in the South, nasopharyngeal cancer (NPC) is another widely recognized threatening tumors and hence remained unregistered even by National cancer registries, since little is known about its epidemiology [15]. The occurrence represented around 40% of the world's new cases as indicated by the World Health Organization's GLOBOCAN revealed information of 2012 [16]. Individuals with a family history of NPC have a generously higher danger of NPC [17]. NPC's mortality indicates marked distinction between endemic (highly vulnerable territories), where nonkeratinizing carcinoma (NKC) is pervasive, and nonendemic (safe districts), where the keratinizing squamous cell carcinoma (KSCC) is more frequent. Fluctuations in smoking and alcohol consumption amongst genders and geographic regions may clarify the diverse rates and patterns fully observed for KSCC and partially for NKC. Dietary patterns and improvement in disease management can also be accountable for observed trends [18].

2. MicroRNAs discovery

MicroRNAs (miRNAs) are single-stranded, small RNA molecules whose presence was reported for the first time in 1993 in nematode *Caenorhabditis elegans*. A number of biological activities like gene regulation, differentiation, organ formation, cell death, cell proliferation, and stress responses have been reported to be influenced by these miRNAs [19–22]. These miRNAs were found to regulate translation in larval development through an antisense RNA-RNA interaction [19, 23, 24]. 1600 miRNAs of *Homo sapiens* have been reported and recorded by miRBase database in June 2013 [25]. Since 1970s, studies to determine and understand the function and genetics of gene regulation were performed [26]. *C. elegans* was used as a genetic model and tool to facilitate these kinds of ventures. More than 300 mutants of *C. elegans* with many developmental/birth defects and certain behavioral changes were generated by series of groundbreaking experiments by Brenner and Sulston [26, 27]. One of them was characterized by reverberation of specific cell lineages and showing a flaccid and extremely elongated body [27, 28]. The nature of the gene(s) and the exact mechanism underlying such morphological and behavioral changes were unknown at that time. This mutant was considered as the founding member of the miRNA family and was named as lin-4. Lin-4 was reported to influence specific developmental responses in a variety of cell types of *C. elegans* larva [29, 30]. In 1993, cloning of lin-4 locus took about 2 decades after its early description [23]. Lin-4 locus was found unique having characteristics different from other coding genes. It was found employing site-directed mutagenesis, that lin-4 gene encodes a small RNA molecule instead of a protein. Furthermore, the transcripts of lin-4 were of smaller size compared to other genes as the two transcripts identified were of 22 and 60 nucleotides only. To suffice, lin-4 mRNA transcripts were found to be negatively regulating the lin-14 expression, as it possesses antisense complementarity to a number of sites in 3'untranslated region (UTR) to lin-14 gene [23]. Therefore, these discoveries lead to a novel class of small noncoding RNA molecules, which via antisense-like interaction regulate a number of pathways [31–33]. After 7 years following lin-4 cloning and characterization, a second gene was discovered with similar characters [34]. The study resulted in the isolation of let-7 (21-nt RNA molecule) that was characterized by acting as a heterochronic switch in *C. elegans* development. It was fascinating that the expression of this miRNA was reported in a wide range of animals other than *C. elegans*, including arthropods, mollusks, and mammals [35]. Further studies reported more than 100 different noncoding RNAs (ncRNAs) in a variety of species across the animal phyla [36–38]. A number of important observations were made from these key studies. First, specific small temporal RNAs (stRNAs) express only in few stages of development and are about 22 nt long [38]. Second, cell-type specificity of different stRNAs was determined [38]. For example, miR-1 (a small RNA) exclusively expressed only in cardiac tissues [37]. Presence of homologs of these molecules across a wide range of species is an indication of evolutionary conservation [38]. Abundance and wide existence of these unique molecules represents a novel sequence-specific posttranscriptional gene regulation. So, based on above given account, the small RNAs with similar functions were named as microRNAs (miRNAs) [36–38]. miRNA gene family is increasing day by day since its discovery [39]. Therefore, a number of databases have been generated to cope with the ever-growing list of miRNA genes. The first ever miRNA database is known as "miRBase (http://microrna.sanger.ac.uk/sequences/)" and it has access to clone and register miRNA sequences [40]. The total number of miRNAs is exceeding ten thousands in number up to date.

3. MicroRNAs biology

miRNAs are small ncRNAs of about 19–25 nucleotides and have been discovered recently in all metazoans tested so far [41, 42]. They comprised of a small fraction of expressed genome; however, genes encoding them are present in either introns or exons of coding as well as noncoding genes throughout the genome. miRNAs are involved in regulating number of processes including differentiation, maintenance of homeostasis, migration, programmed cell death, and morphogenesis [42–45]. miRNAs are transcribed with the aid of RNA polymerase II enzyme from the miRNAs genes, which in turn transcribed into primary microRNA transcripts following transformation into pre-miRNAs which are then ultimately results in miRNAs [32, 46–50]. In recent years, a novel class of molecules naming miRNAs has showed a boom. With advancements in genomic technologies and methodologies, miRNAs gene family is rising as new members discovered day by day. In 2005, it was speculated that there are about 1000 miRNAs genes in human genome [51]. However, 2042 mature miRNAs have been reported in miRBase up to date (version 19). miRNAs are characterized by having 21–23 nucleotides in length and are exclusively found in eukaryotes. They show partial complementarity to specific regions in targeted mRNA and hence are involved in gene regulation of 50% of human genome at posttranscriptional level [52]. Each of these noncoding RNAs can have sequence complementary to a large number of transcripts and regulate expression of an enormous number of genes. This can be achieved by multiple mechanisms including an increased mRNA degradation, site-specific cleavage, and translational inhibition [53]. miRNAs dysregulation has been associated with a number of different types of cancer, their initiation, and proliferation, since the first ever study claiming the association between chronic lymphoid leukemia and miR-15a and miR-16-1 in the year 2002 [54–56]. Therefore, they may prove as potent therapeutic targets for cancers including HNSCC as well as biomarkers for timely diagnosis, prognosis, and recurrence of cancers as well. Two different pathways have been reported for the biogenesis of miRNAs. Usually, a canonical pathway is used for their biogenesis as most of the miRNA genes are intergenic (**Figure 1**). These miRNAs when transcribed possess a local hairpin structure and are named as primary transcripts (pri-miRNA) and have characteristics to that of mRNA, as there is a 5′cap and a 3′poly-A tail. Drosha (a protein complex having nuclease activity) and Pasha (an RNA-binding protein) process these pri-miRNAs to pre-miRNAs having 70-nucleotide stem-loop structure. pre-miRNAs are converted into a double-stranded miRNA/miRNA* duplex by an RNase III endonuclease (Dicer) followed by transportation in cytoplasm by Exportin-5. Further, a helicase destabilizes the duplex miRNA/miRNA* to a mature miRNA and miRNA*. Finally, the mature miRNA then integrates into RNA-induced silencing complex (RISC) also called miRNA ribonucleoprotein complex (miRNP).

The resultant miRNP is involved in RNA interference which is initiated by both siRNA and miRNA. In case of intronic stem-loops-derived miRNA, no Drosha activity is involved for the maturation of miRNAs [32, 57] (**Figure 2**).

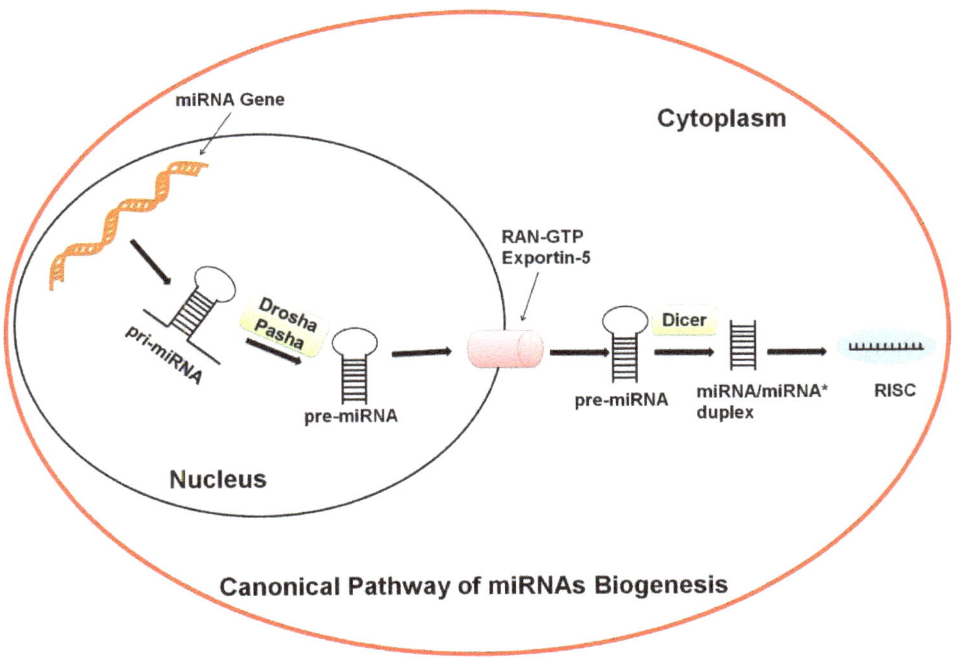

Figure 1. Canonical pathway of miRNAs biogenesis. miRNAs are transcribed into a primary transcript (pri-miRNA) which is processed into pre-miRNAs by Drosha/Pasha complex. After transportation to cytoplasm, these pre-miRNAs are converted into a double-stranded miRNA/miRNA* duplex by Dicer. Further, a helicase destabilizes the duplex miRNA/miRNA* to a mature miRNA and miRNA*. Finally, the mature miRNA then integrates into RISC.

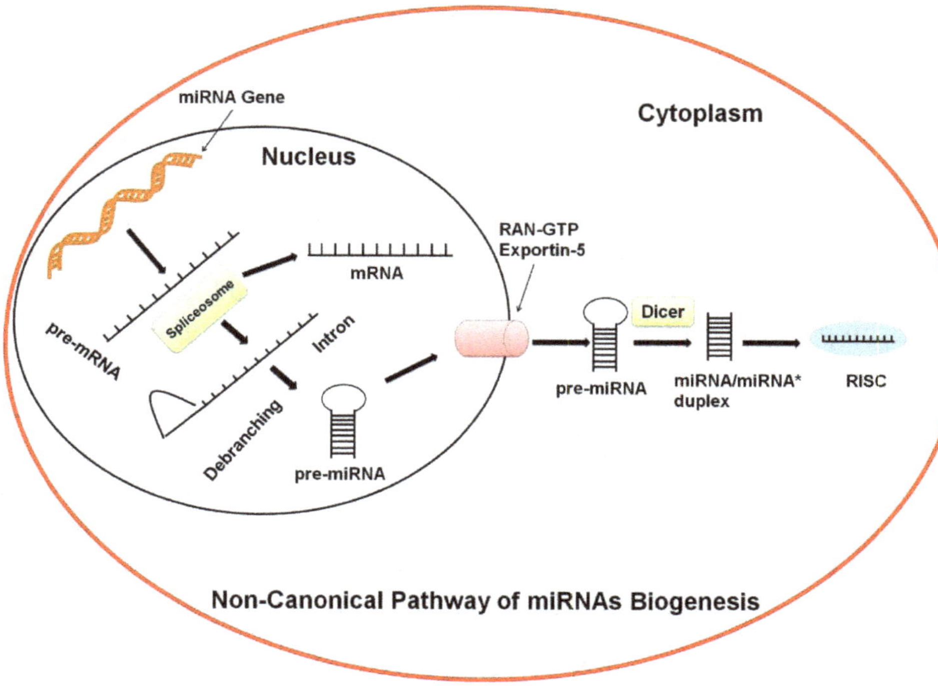

Figure 2. Noncanonical pathway of miRNAs biogenesis. In noncanonical pathway of miRNAs biogenesis, no Drosha activity is involved. Pre-miRNAs are directly produced from the debranching of the introns; and after their transportation, they are processed similar to that produced by canonical pathway.

4. MicroRNAs deregulation in head and neck cancer

The first ever study involving miRNAs in HNC was published in 2005 [58]. miRNAs showed greater cancer-related potential than expected. miRNAs have been associated with all processes of physiological and pathological nature. Expression profiles of miRNAs have reported to be more specific to cancer tissue origin and have greater potential for early diagnosis and provided more information than mRNAs [59, 60]. Association between dysregulation of miRNAs and tumorigenesis in head and neck has been documented previously [61–63]. Many biological and molecular mechanisms cause resistance to the tumors radiotherapy. The principle mechanisms include changes in intracellular pathways that are required in damaging DNA as well as its repair, apoptosis, proliferation, and angiogenesis. The regulation of these perplexing procedures is regularly controlled by microRNAs. miRNAs are short endogenous RNA molecules that posttranscriptionally modulate gene expression. Their impaired expression has been seen in numerous tumors including head and neck cancer. Particular expression patterns of miRNAs have additionally been appeared to anticipate prognosis and therapeutic response in head and neck cancer [64]. Development and progression of different sorts of malignancies in human is attributed to the deregulation of miRNAs. Oncogenic part of miR-214 is proposed in NPC. Bax inhibition initiated by siRNA weakens the advancing impact of miR-214 deregulation on NPC cell apoptosis, recommending that Bax is a downstream effector in miR-214 that is intervened NPC cell proliferation and death. Bax expression level is deregulated in NPC tissues [65]. miR-145 expression in LSCC is downregulated, and its overexpression creates hindrance in multiplication and relocation of Hep-2 cells through cell cycle arrest and apoptotic induction. SOX-2 is overexpressed in tumor samples and exhibit restricted expression in miR-145 overexpressed Hep-2 cells [14]. miRNAs deregulation plays a key role in HNSCC progression [66]. miR-93-5p (HN2092) and miR-425-5p (HN1957) are top candidates of downregulated miRNAs in primary HNSCC cell cultures and blood plasma of patients [67]. miRNAs deregulation plays a noteworthy part in head and neck/oral cancer [68]. miR-10b and miR-196a, not formerly linked with HNSCC, may show a role in oncogenesis through the deregulation of cell proliferation [69]. Deregulation of miRNA genes (such as miR-138) plays a critical part in HNSCC. While downregulation of miR-138 has been observed in HNSCC and other cancer types often; however, the exact role of miR-138 in tumorigenesis is unknown. Current bioinformatics analyses and *in vitro* and *in vivo* researches have recognized a number of functional targets for miR-138. These include genes that take part in necessary biological processes that are exceptionally pertinent to the onset and proliferation of HNSCC, including cell migration, epithelial to mesenchymal transition, cell cycle progression, DNA damage and repair, senescence, and differentiation [70]. Mechanistic target of rapamycin (mTOR) and Insuline like growth factor 1 receptor (IGF1R) signaling pathways depict that the downregulation of miR-99 family adds to HNSCC tumorigenesis [71]. Meta-analysis of various Gene expression omnibus (GEO) datasets revealed that Uracil DNA glycosylation (UNG), Fucosidase alpha-L-2 plasma (FUCA2), Differentially expressed regulation analysis (DERA), Glia maturation factor beta (GMFB), Transferrin (TF) and Sorting nexin 2 (SNX2) were usually downregulated in HNSCC [72]. miRNAs including miR-21 and miR-31 are progressively deregulated in tongue epithelium [73]. Underexpression of miR-375 might play oncogenic roles in HNSCC [74]. miR-29c is considerably deregulated in

Downregulated miRNAs	Sample used	Assay	Type of cancer	Reference
miR-214	Tissue	Luciferase assay qRT-PCR Western blot	NPC	[66]
miR-145	Tissue	qRT-PCR and Western blot analysis	Laryngeal SCC	[14]
miR-425-5p (HN1957)	Blood plasma	qRT-PCR	HNSCC patients	[68]
miR-93-5p (HN2092)	Blood plasma	qRT-PCR	HNSCC patients	[68]
miR-196a	Tissue	Microarray, RT-PCR	HNSCC	[70]
miR-10b	Tissue	Microarray, RT-PCR	HNSCC	[70]
miR-138	Cell lines	RT-PCR	HNSCC	[71]
miR-99 family	Meta analyses	RT-PCR, microarray	HNSCC	[72]
UNG, FUCA2, DERA, GMFB, TF, and SNX2	Cell lines	RT-PCR	Head and neck squamous cell carcinoma	[73]
miR-21 and miR-31	Saliva, Plasma	q-PCR	Tongue epithelium	[74]
miR-375	Tissue	RT-PCR	HNSCC	[75]

Downregulated miRNAs	Sample used	Assay	Type of cancer	Reference
miR-29c	Cell lines, clinical specimens	Microarray, qRT-PCR	NPC	[76]
miR-9	Cell lines, tissues	qRT-PCR	NPC	[76]
miR-378	Cell lines, tissues	qRT-PCR	NPC	[77]
miR-200 family	Cell lines	Microarray	NPC	[78]
miR-451	Tissue	qRT-PCR	NPC	[79]
MiR-99a	Tissue, cell lines	Luciferase assay	Oral cancer	[80]
		qRT-PCR		
		Western blot		
miR-24	Tissue, cell lines	RT-PCR	Oral cancer	[81]
miR-133a, miR-133b, miR-100, miR-138	Tissues	qRT-PCR	TSCC	[82]
miR-16, miR-125b	Tissues	Microarray	OSCC	[83]
miR-133b, miR-138, miR-137, miR-184	Cell lines	qRT-PCR	OSCC	[84]
miR-138, miR-222	Cell lines	Microarray	TSCC	[85, 86]
miR-342, miR-21	Cell line	Microarray	TSCC	[87]
miR-342, miR-346, miR-373	Cell lines	Microarray	HNSCC	[88]
miR-494	Tissue	Microarray	HNSCC	[62]
miR-375	Tissue	Microarray	HNSCC	[89]
miR-125a, miR-125b	Tissue	Microarray	HNSCC	[90]
miR-133a, miR-205	Tissue	Microarray	HNSCC	[91]
miR-125b, miR-375	Tissue	qRT-PCR	HNSCC	[75]

Table 1. Recently identified miRNAs that undergo deregulation in HNC.

NPC. However, there is dearth of knowledge regarding outcome and molecular mechanisms of action of miR-29c downregulation in development and progression of NPC [75]. Some recent studies indicating miRNAs deregulation in HNC are given in **Table 1**.

5. miRNAs as oncogenes in oral squamous cell carcinoma (OSCC)

A number of miRNAs have been reported to act as oncogenes and were found to be upregulated in OSCC. miR-21 was found to be highly expressed and to regulate several biological activities in OSCC [68, 92–94]. Presence of an upregulated level of miR-21 in oral premalignant lesions was an indication that variations in miR-21 level may be prior event in OSCC development [95]. miR-21 plays an oncogenic role in the progression of OSCC by promoting cell proliferation [96], antiapoptotic activity [92], invasion [93, 97], and chemoresistance [98] in both *in vitro* and *in vivo* studies.

Oral squamous cell carcinoma (OSCC) is a typical cause of cancer-related death. A number of efforts have been made in investigating new medications and impressive progress in multimodality treatment; however, remedial tolls have not yet been achieved. The trouble of timely detection and more pervasiveness of metastasis associated with OSCC results in poor prognosis. In recent couple of decades, growing information from tumor biology and clinical trials prompted development of ncRNAs prognostic biomarkers that are believed to be promising biomarkers in this regard. miRNAs are one of the most studied ncRNAs in terms of their biogenesis, function, and significance in carcinogenesis [99]. An association between severity of pathogenesis and increment of miR-31 and miR-21 has been reported through staining in 4NQO-induced injury in tongue epithelium. A dynamic rise in the level of *miR-21*, *miR-31*, and *miR-146a* in saliva and plasma samples was noted. miR-31 was the earliest miRNA to be released in the saliva. A rise in plasma level of miR-146a, miR-372, and miR-184 was found and it was prominent at the most progressive lesion state [73]. miRNA deregulation assists in pathogenesis of various disorders, including human tongue squamous cell carcinoma (TSCC), where they act as powerful oncogenes or tumor suppressors. Widespread miRNA profiling in TSCC samples and further *in vitro* and *in vivo* functional studies unveiled their involvement to hidden molecular mechanisms in initiation, development, progression, metastasis, chemoradioresistance, and relapse of TSCC [100]. An upregulated expression of miR-483-5p in OSCC patient sera might be a novel indicative and prognostic biomarker for this ailment [101]. The upregulation of miR-9 was also detected in primary esophageal squamous cell carcinoma (ESCC) tumor tissue. miR-9 promotes cell migration and tumor metastasis, as these processes effectively retarded when expression of miR-9 was deregulated. Furthermore, it was established that miR-9 interacts with the 3′untranslated region of E-cadherin and downregulates its expression, which leads to β-catenin nuclear translocation and consequently upregulates c-myc and CD-44 expression. Moreover, an ESCC miR-9 results in epithelial-mesenchymal transition (EMT) in ESCC, a key occasion in tumor metastasis [102]. Significantly, low level of miR-29b has been reported. However, overexpression of miR-29b repressed the proliferation, migration, invasion, and progression of TSCC cells, and slowed down the cell death. In addition, miR-29b brings about deregulation of Sp1 by targeting the 3′untranslated part that causes upregulation of phosphatase and tensin homolog (PTEN), and subsequently inhibit phosphorylation of Protein kinase B (AKT). Sp1 knockdown in TSCC cell lines reflected the effects of miR-29b overexpression. miR-29b expression is inversely related to Sp1 expression and positively correlated with PTEN. Thus, miR-29b works as a tumor suppressor, and miR-29b/Sp1/PTEN/AKT alliance may speak of a possible therapeutic target for TSCC prevention [91]. MiR-99a deregulation was confirmed in oral cancer cell lines and clinical specimen as well. Ectopic miR-99a expression resulted in repression of oral cancer cell migration and invasion. Myotubularin-related protein 3 (MTMR3) with one evolutionarily preserved seed locale in the 3′untranslated region was a novel miR-99a target. Draining MTMR3 expression fundamentally diminishes cell proliferation, migration, and invasion. An inverse relation was found among miR-99a and MTMR3 protein in oral cancer lines and clinical patients. miR-99a has been found to suppress oral cancer cell migration and invasion partially through inhibiting MTMR3 expression [103]. Keratinization of tumors and overexpression of miR-21 are major factors responsible for poor prognosis. Interestingly, most of the keratinized tumors were reported to express an elevated miR-21 level [104]. Moreover, an upregulated level of miR-127 and a reduced level of miR-357 have been reported in OSCC [105]. In CD-44 (high) oral CSCs, miR-200s/miR-205s were epigenetically triggered in tumors and their expression was found to be suppressed in the absence of DNA hypermethylation [105]. miRNAs expressions and DNA methylation variations are typical occasion in OSCC, and miR-375, miR-127, miR-137, miR-205, and miR-200 family are promising candidates for future investigations. miR-200/miR-205 downregulation in oral CSCs specify that cell-specific silencing of these miRNAs may enhance tumor expansion and progression [105]. Deregulation of miR-24 was found to be associated with high-grade late stage tumor [92].

6. MicroRNAs in human nasopharyngeal carcinoma (NPC)

Paul Ahlquist's group working at National Cancer Institute (NCI) published the first ever study of global profiling of miRNAs involved in NPC in 2008 [88]. They discovered a number of deregulated miRNAs, using a micro-array-based approach, in laser-capture micro dissected (LCM) 31 NPCs and 10 epithelial samples as control [88]. miRNA downregulation and change in pathways have been involved in NPC which is profoundly invasive and metastatic widespread in Southern China. miR-9 is commonly downregulated in NPC with significant functional consequences. Diminished expression of miR-9 is contrary to clinical stages and denotes the movement from locoregional to metastatic tumors. CpG island hypermethylation adds to inhibition of miR-9 in NPC cell lines and tissues. Ectopic miR-9 expression significantly hinders proliferative, transient, and obtrusive limits of NPC cells, both *in vitro* and *in vivo*. miR-9 strongly reduces expression of CXCR4 in NPC cells. miR-9 works as a tumor-suppressor in NPC, and is interfered by combating CXCR4 expression [106]. NPC is exceptional worldwide, yet profoundly intrusive in later stages. It cannot be identified in normal medical examination at initial stages. Advancement of particular biomarkers ought to spare lives against this sort of ailment. Among them, increased levels of miR-16, miR-21, miR-24, and miR-155 and decreased level of miR-378 have been observed in NPC patients. Plasma miRNA expression and cancer progression are negatively correlated. Blend of miR-16, miR-21, miR-24, miR-378, and miR-155 gives affectability of 87.7% and specificity of 82.0% for marking NPC. Except miR-16, mixture of the rest of four miRNAs gives a similar affectability, however, a somewhat diminished specificity. After treatment, levels of the five miRNAs were reverted to normal levels [88]. Regardless of the fact that enormous miRNAs have been discovered in the previous decade, with the progressions in DNA sequencing, the discovery of some more NPC-related miRNAs is expected. Circulating miRNAs related with NPC are quite compelling, as they present an exploitable instrumentation for early detection, diagnosis, and staging. A few worldwide profiling depicted the altered miRNA expression in a range of head and neck malignancies. In NPC, downregulation of the tumor silencer miRNAs (miR-29c, miR-9, let-7 family, miR-200 family), and overexpression of oncogenic miRNAs, (miR-18a/b, miR-141, miR-155, miR-214) have been observed [107]. miR-9 is the most concerned miRNA in NPC pathogenesis [108], which works in the direction of various crucial cellular processes, facilitating proliferation, apoptosis, incursion, metastasis, angiogenesis, and EMT [109–111]. Restricted expression of miR-9in NPC is related with phenotypes that are more destructive and lesser survival. miR-9 has been appeared to work as a tumor silencer in NPC by focusing on chemokine (CXC theme) receptor 4 (CXCR4) to repress cell multiplication, relocation, and invasion [87]. Similarly, miR-9 directs innate response in NPC through control of various genes that are activated by interferon, and in addition major histocompatibility complex (MHC) class I members [112]. Imperatively, the capacity of miR-9 to work as an individual prognostic biomarker for NPC metastasis has additionally been illustrated, whereas miR-9 expression is related with decreased expansion, movement, and intrusion in NPC cells, and low-levels of miR-9 expression are associated with last stage [106]. Correspondingly, miR-200 family is deregulated in NPC, bringing about expanded cell development, relocation, and intrusion of NPC cells according to suppression of the putative miR-200 targets zinc finger E-box restricting homeobox 2 (ZEB2), beta 1 (CTNNB1), and catenin (cadherin-related protein) bringing about expanded NPC cell development, movement, and invasion. Moreover, diminished miR-200a expression is related with initiating epithelial-mesenchymal transition [89]. Various miRNAs have been reported as tumor silencers/suppressors in NPC, including miR-34c, miR-451, miR-98, miR-216b, miR-375, and miR-26a. miR-375 has been accounted for a potential tumor silencer in NPC, working through restraint of the oncogenic protein metadherin (MTDH). Strangely, NPC cases with MTDH overexpression showed an expanded danger of recurrence of disease [113]. Low miR-451 expression was related with diminished survival in NPC patients, and has been appeared to work by expanding cell development and invasion by focusing on macrophage migration inhibitory factor (MIF) in NPC cells [114]. miR-26a, miR-98, and miR-101 also have been accounted to work as tumor suppressors in NPC [98]. Underexpression of these miRNAs in NPC gives clues about derepression of Enhancer of zeste homolog 2 (EZH2), instigating loss of suppression of targets of EZH2 regulation, comprising cyclins D3, c-Myc, and E2, and cyclin-dependent kinase 6 (CDK6) and CDK4 [115, 116]. Finally, miR-216b has been appeared to increase NPC growth and incursion by pursuing Kirstan rat sarcoma (K-RAS) [117]; on the other hand, miR-34c has been revealed to stifle growth and metastasis by focusing on the proto-oncogene MET [118], both of which are ominously downregulated in primary NPC tissues. In NPC, miR-18a is profoundly overexpressed [119], which results in direct hang-up of the miRNA biogenesis regulatory protein Dicer1, leading to the downregulation of miRNA in NPC [119]. Likewise, miR-18b is overexpressed in NPC, accompanying malady advancement and poor outcome. miR-18b functions to inhibit connective tissue growth factor (CTGF) and thereby augmenting cellular proliferation [120]. Over-articulation of miR-141 in NPC has been connected with more cell growth, relocation, and invasion, and also with loss of cell cycle control and decreased apoptosis. This regulation is thought to happen through downregulation of the supposed target gene phosphatase and tensin homolog (PTEN), bromo-domain 3 (BRD3), and ubiquitin-associated protein 1 (UBAP1) in NPC. Moreover, expression of miR-141 is structured by the oncogenes short palate, lung, nasal epithelium clone 1 (SPLUNC1), and c-Myc [120]. Expression of miR-155 fortifies proliferation, migration, and incursion by regulation of target genes Jumonji Domain 1A (JMJD1A) and BTB and CNC homology 1 (BACH1), and its expression has been strongly related with tumor stage and patient endurance. Interestingly, regulation of miR-155 occurs through the Epstein–Barr virus (EBV)-encoded Latent membrane protein (LMP1) and LMP2A proteins [121]. Furthermore, miR-144 is overexpressed in NPC and inhibits PTEN expression, and brings about expanded cell proliferation, invasion, and metastasis [122]. miR-214 has been firmly connected with augmented metastasis in NPC, both in cell lines and primary human samples, functioning at least in part via inhibition of the tumor suppressor lactotransferrin (LTF) [123]. Besides, miR-214 has been appeared to upgrade proliferation and promote an anti-apoptotic phenotype in NPC cells [124]. In addition to miR-144, miR-155, and miR-214, various other miRNAs that are overexpressed in NPC also contribute considerably to enhance the metastatic phenotype of NPC. miR-30a has been demonstrated both *in vitro* and *in vivo* to build metastasis and intrusion by hindering E-cadherin activity [125]. Moreover, expression of miR-149 was lifted profoundly in metastatic NPC cells, adding increased migration, invasion, and epithelial-mesenchymal phenotypes over E-cadherin inhibition [126]. miR-93 has been accounted to inhibit transforming growth factor-β receptor II (TGFβRII) [127] and disabled homolog-2 (DAB2) [128], in this way directing tumor cell growth incursion and metastasis. Finally, miR-504 is found to be involved as an oncogenic miRNA in NPC, working to specifically target nuclear respiratory factor 1 (NRF1), whereas expanded expression connected with poor reaction to radiation treatment [129].

7. miRNAs as prognostic indicators

Despite significant improvement in multimodal treatment, the prognosis of advanced HNC is quite poor. Recent studies are promising regarding the potential role of miRNAs as prognostic indicators. Downregulation of Let-7 (a family of tumor suppressing miRNAs) has been reported in HNSCCs by many researchers [74, 92, 95, 103, 130–138]. Similarly, underexpression of miR-146a, miR-155, and Let-7 has been correlated with the progression of cancer [138]. Moreover, a decreased level of Let-7 miRNA in nasopharyngeal carcinoma cells was also suggestive of regulating the proliferation of carcinoma cells via c-MYC downregulation [139]. Furthermore, role of Let-7 in the Kirsten rat sarcoma (KRAS) regulation has been demonstrated recently by some studies on nonsmall cell lung cancer [140]. A variant allele in the V-Ki-ras2 Kirsten rat sarcoma viral oncogene homolog (KRAS) 3′untranslated region (KRAS-LCS6) has been demonstrated to be involved in high expression of KRAS and decreased levels of Let-7. Presence of KRAS-LCS6 variant has been reported in Squamous cell head and neck cancer (SCHNC) and was correlated with poor prognosis [130]. TP53, a tumor suppressor gene, encodes a protein product that is involved in cell cycle regulation. It is a major change involved in cancer induction with a remarkable frequency of 53% as reported by Poeta et al. in a hefty cohort of SCHNC. The ratio of TP53 mutations were 75 and 56.7% in patients suffering from hypopharynx and larynx tumor, respectively. Furthermore, a strong association was described between TP53 mutations in SCHNC and high risk of recurrence and poor survival [141]. Ganci et al. has previously reported a strong link among 49 miRNAs and TP53 status. Among them, a more specific correlation of a subset of 12 miRNAs was correlated with a brief recurrence free-survival while four of these were correlated with comparatively lower cancer-specific survival [142]. Expression of some particular miRNAs, such as miR-375 and miR-210, has been correlated with the outcome of SCHNC patients. A low expression of miR-375 results in poor survival and distant metastases while high expression of miR-210 results in locoregional recurrence [143, 144].

8. miRNAs as biomarkers

Diagnosis of HNSCC more frequently occurs in advanced stage when it metastases to regional lymph nodes. Moreover, there is a high risk of recurrence even in patients with a combination of different therapeutic approaches. Therefore, for an early diagnosis, the most important goal would be the detection of biomarkers. Recently, some miRNAs have been discovered to fulfill the goal of diagnosis. In fact, miRNAs are found circulated stably in different body fluids, i.e., urine, blood, saliva, as well as in breath. Hence, these miRNAs can be assessed easily with noninvasive methods.

miRNAs can be utilized as biomarkers or novel therapeutic targets. Further investigation is needed to test its utilization [66]. Circulating miRNAs (miR-425-5p, miR-93-5p) are easily approachable and have turned out to be valuable prognostic markers in cancer patients. The prognostic worth of this exciting perception requires affirmation using an independent patient cohort that includes clinical follow-up data. Changes of miRNAs succeeding radiochemotherapy in the blood plasma are related with the tumor response to therapy, and they might signify novel biomarkers for therapy monitoring [67]. The investigations of microRNA modifications in HNSCC are a fundamental stride to the mechanistic comprehension of tumorigenesis and could prompt the disclosure of clinically pertinent biomarkers [69]. For NPC diagnosis, plasma miRNAs expression proves to be a helpful biomarker [88]. Pathway improvement analysis of these four miRNAs (miR-34c, miR-140, miR-154, and miR-449b) sign posted a role in cell cycle regulation, highlighting a possibly important role for markers of cell cycle enactment as prognostic indicators in NPC [145]. miR-200b expression is mostly connected with distant metastasis, while miR-155 associated with local recurrence. miR-155 and miR-146a were recognized as surrogate markers for tumor-invading lymphocytes in HNSCC [146]. miR-21 expression could be an imperative tool for treatment planning and prognostic predictor for HNSCC patients [147]. Genetic variants of miR-146a and miR-1269b are biomarkers for improvement of oral premalignant lesions (OPLs) and oral squamous cell carcinoma (OPSCC) [148]. hsa-miR-375-3p appears to be a comparatively promising diagnostic marker

miRNA biomarker	Type of cancer	References
miR-34c, miR-140, miR-154, and miR-449b	NPC	[166]
miR-155 and miR-146a	HNSCC	[167]
miR-155		
miR-21	HNSCC	[168]
miR-146a and miR-1269b	Oral premalignant lesions (OPLs) and oral squamous cell carcinoma (OPSCC)	[169]
hsa-miR-375-3p	HNSCC	[170]
miR-182	HNSCC	[171]
miR-30a	NPC	[172]
miR-148a and miR-375	LSCC	[173]

Table 2. A list of miRNAs identified as potent biomarker of HNC.

in HNSCC but is not appropriate for prognosis of patients [149]. Overexpression of TP53 mutation-associated miR-182 may contribute to proliferation and migration of tumour cell in HNSCC, hence suggest a possible biomarker for prognosis of tumour recurrence [150]. miR-30a is a possible biomarker for metastasis in NPC patients [151]. miR-148a and miR-375 are significantly upregulated during LSCC and are conceivable biomarkers for early diagnosis of LSCC [152]. A list of miRNAs is given below which has been identified as potential biomarker by a number of researchers in HNC (**Table 2**).

9. Novel therapeutic targets

miRNAs are key therapeutic agents (depends upon the type of mRNA affected by them) in addition to their prognostic and diagnostic value [21]. miRNAs are efficient molecules to be targeted as they regulate a number of biological activities by interacting with numerous other molecules [53]. Use of synthetically designed "miRNAs sponges" [153], miR mimics (agomiRs) [154], miR antagonists ("antagomiRs") [155, 156], and miR inhibitors (antimiRNAs oligonucleotides) [92] is an innovative strategy to modulate oncogenic and tumor-suppressive pathways. MicroRNAs regulate each step of cell cycle and unraveling their altered expression may prove fruitful in designing new drugs and can open treatment regimes. One piece of evidence is a previous study abduction of miR-122, which has been observed in a novel therapy for HCV patients by Miravirsen (first microRNA targeted drug) in clinical phase2a. This therapy resulted in diminution of HCV RNA levels in a dose-dependent manner [157]. This research has raised a lot of hope for employing miRNAs therapies in number of malignancies despite the disparity of the diseases from cancer. Some other miRNAs therapies are in preclinical and clinical phase 1. These approaches are anxiously awaited to be reported beyond the mere documentations. Few miRNAs, though not verified clinically, are very good applicants for being named for these therapies. Apoptotic pathway is one of the most significant candidates for novel anticancer therapies, as the neoplastic cells usually lose the ability to undergo programmed cell death. Therefore, any powerful proapoptotic agent may directly or indirectly reduce cancer progression by enhancing the apoptosis. *miR-99a* mimics have been shown to decrease cell proliferation by inducing apoptosis in tongue SCC cell line [158]. Moreover, miR-31-3p inhibitor in oral leukoplakia cell lines resulted in decreased cell death [159]. Furthermore, restoration of miR-100 resulted in inhibition of cell migration and proliferation by increasing the apoptosis in HNSCC cell lines [71]. Similarly, cancer cells showed a pronounced cell cycle arrest and enhanced cell death upon transfection with miR-1e [160]. On the other hand, a repression of apoptosis was observed in classical oncogenic *miR-21* [161]. These are only a few well-known examples. A large number of other functionally investigated miRNAs in HNSCCs are directly or indirectly associated with apoptotic pathways promise an era of new and more potent therapeutic factors. miRNAs are utilized in another way in treating the HNSCC patients, as they are capable of highlighting the resistance to either chemotherapy or radiotherapy in patients of HNSCC patients. In addition to it, recently, miRNAs have also been reported to modulate the radiosensitivity and chemoresistance. For instance, let-7 results in inhibition of cancer progression by reduction in cancer-proneness cells and repressing chemoresistance [162]. Similarly, miR-21 in HA/CD44-activated head and neck cancer cells may prove a significant drug target to overcome chemoresistance and apoptosis as it is involved in regulation of Nanog/Stat-3 signaling pathway [111]. Furthermore, transfection of pre-miR-98 in HNSCC cell lines led to an enhanced resistance to doxorubicin and cisplatin by downregulating the *HMGA2* expression [163].

Nevertheless, for an efficient and target specific miRNAs-based drug delivery system, there lies enormous challenges [22, 53]. To access the targeted sites, therapeutic RNA must travel across the plasma membrane to enter in cytoplasm by leaving the circulatory system and avoiding endosomal vesicles to entering in the cell [53]. Moreover, nonconjugated therapeutic RNA molecules are either cleared by the kidney (<50kDa) or by the immune cells (7-20kDa) [53]. Levels of mature miRNAs may be modulated or reduced by delivery of synthetic double-stranded hairpin exogenously by complexing with lipids or proteins. Delivery of miR-34a may prove effective in HNSCC cells as suppression of cellular proliferation and apoptosis was observed in two cancer cell lines (colon) and experimental lung metastasis of murine melanoma upon miR-34a delivery [164, 165]. Use of unmodified dsRNAs in environments, where local administration is possible, is of limited value *in vivo* as they are likely to be degraded by nucleases [166]. A high expression of these miRNAs from well-defined transcription start and termination sites can be achieved using a viral vector with Pol III promoters for stable miR reintroduction; however, they are not cell-specific [53, 165, 167]. In contrast, for a tissue-specific approach or for ectopic expression of miRNAs, RNA Pol II promoters may be used for pri-miRNAs expression [168]. For an effective reintroduction of dysregulated miRNAs, later techniques may be utilized in HNSCC, e.g., miR-375 [132]. However, use of a viral system for reintroduction of miRNAs possesses a number of risks [53]. One of the major risks is that the delivered molecules integrate to an unpredictable site of host DNA and may activate proto-oncogene and results in insertional mutagenesis [53]. These methods also have certain limitations as insertion of retroviral vectors is limited only to actively dividing cells and use of other units, like adenoviral vectors, may activate a severe immune response in host body [53, 169]. AntagomiRs (recently identified chemically engineered oligonucleotides) are commonly utilized today for silencing of host miRNAs [53, 156]. These AntagomiRs reverted the effects of upregulation of miRNAs in HNSCC, i.e., decreased cell viability and enhanced programmed cell death was observed in KB cells overexpressing miRNA-155 upon introduction of antagomir-155 in nude mice [155]. Moreover, to boost the efficient delivery of these antagomiR, they are delivered intravenously by complexing with a recently identified molecule the interfering nanoparticle (iNOP) [170]. Systemic delivery of iNop complexed with antimir-122 in mice did not initiate any immune response and successfully silenced the miRNA-122 with long lasting effects [170]. Chemically modified antimiRNAs oligonucleotides (AMOs) that are highly specific and efficient in binding to targeted RNA are another choice for miRNAs silencing but they do not have any specific delivery system [92, 164]. An enhanced apoptosis, limited survival, and proliferation were observed in tongue SCC cell lines upon inhibition of miRNA-21 with AMO [92]. Moreover, a pronounced apoptosis and decreased cell proliferation was observed in nude mice upon repeated injections of miR-21-AMO which ultimately resulting in tumor suppression [92]. In HNSCC, miRNAs sponges or miRNAs masks can also be used to inhibit oncomiRNAs. miRNAs sponges block specific miRNAs attachment to their targets by expressing an mRNA having a number of tandem-binding sites for entire family of targeted miRNAs, thus blocking their effects [53, 153]. On the other hand, miRNAs-masking antisense oligonucleotides technology shows its effect by destabilizing the association between specific miR-mRNA pairs, as it comprised of complementary antisense oligonucleotides to miRNAs interacting site in the 3′UTR of a targeted mRNA [53, 167]. This methodology has advantage over others as there are few off-target/undesirable effects and may be helpful in cancer therapy as multiple pathways are targeted there simultaneously [53]. Furthermore, miRNAs may enhance sensitivity to radiotherapy [168]. In addition to it, some epigenetic drugs may also revert irregular methylation or acetylation of a tumoral phenotype by restoration of tumor-suppressive miRNAs expression [53]. Most of above-mentioned techniques are in experimental phases. Our future approach should aim to aberrant miRNAs networks, as multiple miRNAs along with multiple miRNAs-transcriptome interactions are involved in cancer pathogenesis. To achieve this aim, miRNAs biogenesis machinery or regulatorypathways must be targeted [53, 169]. However, exploration of the full potential ofthese drugs is highly recommended.

10. Future challenges

For last 3 decades, dysregulation of tumor suppressor genes and protein-coding oncogenes were thought to be involved in cancer. However, discovery of noncoding genes, i.e., miRNAs raised a question on the notion that this mechanism is solely responsible for cancer. To unveil the involvement of miRNAs in cancer, massive efforts have been made but still enormous challenges lie ahead. Detection of the exact pathways and genes regulated by these miRNAs will be of prime importance. A better understanding of the wide-ranging effects of these novel molecules will equip the researchers in the selection of specific pathways for treatment of cancers. Our understanding of miRNAs involvement in HNC is in its infancy. However, studies have been confirmed the dysregulation of a number of miRNAs in both benign and malignant HNC. There are real prospects that miRNAs in near future may be used as prognostic and diagnostics of HNC to improve its treatment strategies. Growing evidences make these miRNAs viable targets for the development of new and better anticancer therapies. However, before translation to be carried out in clinical settings, a more clear insight of efficacy and "off-target" effects of miRNAs is necessarily suggested. It is quite fascinating that recently a number of miRNAs including miR-21, miR-155, and let-7b have been nominated as key players of human carcinogenesis including head and neck tumors. The discovery of miRNAs heralds a complete new paradigm in the understanding of exact molecular pathways involved in HNC development. More detailed studies are required for better understanding and therapeutic targets to treat HNC.

However, a number of efforts have been made but truly comprehensive profiling of miRNAs is still needed in HNSCC. Even, technology utilized for profiling also needs to be improved. Use of Polymerase chain reaction (PCR) and microarrays is a common practice for profiling but for a better picture and more deep insight next-generation sequencing (NGS), cross-platform analysis and new approaches like NanoString nCounter system must be applied. Functional studies are growing, highlighting the potentially targetable miRNAs and some related pathways. Tumor cells survival and their development have been reported to be affected by the forced expression or even the inhibition of a number of miRNAs *in vitro*, representing a new class of novel therapeutic targets [158, 171, 172]. To deliver therapeutic miRNAs, delivery of pre-miR-107 and siRNA nanoparticles proves to be an effective strategy [173, 174]. Therefore, the future of tumor biology seems quite bright.

Author details

Muhammad Babar Khawar[1], Naz Fatima[1], Muddasir Hassan Abbasi[1,3], Rabia Mehmood[1], Saira Kainat Suqaina[1] and Nadeem Sheikh[1,2]*

*Address all correspondence to: s_nadeem77@yahoo.com

1 Cell & Molecular Biology Lab, Department of Zoology, University of the Punjab, Lahore, Pakistan

2 Centre of Applied Molecular Biology, University of the Punjab, Lahore, Pakistan

3 Department of Zoology, Govt. College of Science, Lahore, Pakistan

References

[1] Alibek K, Kakpenova A, Baiken Y. Role of infectious agents in the carcinogenesis of brain and head and neck cancers. Infectious Agents and Cancer. 2013;**8**:1

[2] Warnakulasuriya S. Global epidemiology of oral and oropharyngeal cancer. Oral Oncology. 2009;**45**:309-316

[3] Vokes EE, Weichselbaum RR, Lippman SM, Hong WK. Head and neck cancer. New England Journal of Medicine. 1993;**328**:184-194

[4] Nagadia R, Pandit P, Coman WB, Cooper-White J, Punyadeera C. miRNAs in head and neck cancer revisited. Cellular Oncology. 2013;**36**:1-7

[5] Courthod G, Franco P, Palermo L, Pisconti S, Numico G. The role of microRNA in head and neck cancer: Current knowledge and perspectives. Molecules. 2014;**19**:5704-5716

[6] Ascierto PA, Accorona R, Botti G, Farina D, Fossati P, Gatta G, Gogas H, Lombardi D, Maroldi R, Nicolai P, Ravanelli M, Vanella V. Mucosal melanoma of the head and neck. Critical Reviews in Oncology/Hematology. 2017;**112**:136-152

[7] Bagnardi V, Rota M, Botteri E, Tramacere I, Islami F, Fedirko V, Scotti L, Jenab M, Turati F, Pasquali E, Pelucchi C, Galeone C, Bellocco R, Negri E, Corrao G, Boffetta P, La VC. Alcohol consumption and site-specific cancer risk: A comprehensive dose-response meta-analysis. British Journal of Cancer. 2015;**112**:580-593

[8] Hashibe M, Brennan P, Chuang SC, Boccia S, Castellsague X, Chen C, Curado MP, Dal ML, Daudt AW, Fabianova E, Fernandez L, Wunsch-Filho V, Franceschi S, Hayes RB, Herrero R, Kelsey K, Koifman S, La VC, Lazarus P, Levi F, Lence JJ, Mates D, Matos E, Menezes A, McClean MD, Muscat J, Eluf-Neto J, Olshan AF, Purdue M, Rudnai P, Schwartz SM, Smith E, Sturgis EM, Szeszenia-Dabrowska N, Talamini R, Wei Q, Winn DM, Shangina O, Pilarska A, Zhang ZF, Ferro G, Berthiller J, Boffetta P. Interaction between tobacco and alcohol use and the risk of head and neck cancer: Pooled analysis in the International Head and Neck Cancer Epidemiology Consortium. Cancer Epidemiology, Biomarkers & Prevention. 2009;**18**:541-550

[9] Citron F, Armenia J, Franchin G, Polesel J, Talamini R, D'Andrea S, Sulfaro S, Croce CM, Klement W, Otasek D, Pastrello C, Tokar T, Jurisica I, French D, Bomben R, Vaccher E, Serraino D, Belletti B, Vecchione A, Barzan L, Baldassarre G. An integrated approach identifies mediators of local recurrence in Head & Neck Squamous Carcinoma. Clinical Cancer Research. 2017: clincancers-2814. DOI: 10.1158/1078-0432.CCR-16-2814

[10] Qureishi A, Mawby T, Fraser L, Shah KA, Moller H, Winter S. Current and future techniques for human papilloma virus (HPV) testing in oropharyngeal squamous cell carcinoma. European Archives of Oto-Rhino-Laryngology. 2017; Mar **11**:1-9.

[11] Fakhry C, Westra WH, Wang SJ, van ZA, Zhang Y, Rettig E, Yin LX, Ryan WR, Ha PK, Wentz A, Koch W, Richmon JD, Eisele DW, D'Souza G. The prognostic role of sex, race, and human papillomavirus in oropharyngeal and nonoropharyngeal head and neck squamous cell cancer. Cancer. 2017;**123**(9):1566-1575

[12] Peterson CE, Khosla S, Jefferson GD, Davis FG, Fitzgibbon ML, Freels S, Johnson TP, Hoskins K, Joslin CE. Measures of economic advantage associated with HPV-positive head and neck cancers among non-Hispanic black and white males identified through the National Cancer Database. Journal of Cancer Epidemiology. 2017;**48**:1-7

[13] Yakin M, Gavidi RO, Cox B, Rich A. Oral cancer risk factors in New Zealand. The New Zealand Medical Journal. 2017;**130**:30-38

[14] Karatas OF, Yuceturk B, Suer I, Yilmaz M, Cansiz H, Solak M, Ittmann M, Ozen M. Role of miR-145 in human laryngeal squamous cell carcinoma. Head Neck. 2016; **38**:260-266

[15] Valstar MH, de RM, van den Broek EC, Stuiver MM, van Dijk BA, van Velthuysen ML, Balm AJ, Smeele LE. Salivary gland pleomorphic adenoma in the Netherlands: A nationwide observational study of primary tumor incidence, malignant transformation, recurrence, and risk factors for recurrence. Oral Oncology. 2017;**66**:93-99

[16] Ferlay J, Soerjomataram I, Dikshit R, Eser S, Mathers C, Rebelo M, Parkin DM, Forman D, Bray F. Cancer incidence and mortality worldwide: Sources, methods and major patterns in GLOBOCAN 2012. International Journal of Cancer. 2015;**136**:E359-E386

[17] Liu Z, Chang ET, Liu Q, Cai Y, Zhang Z, Chen G, Huang QH, Xie SH, Cao SM, Shao JY, Jia WH, Zheng Y, Liao J, Chen Y, Lin L, Liang L, Ernberg I, Vaughan TL, Adami HO, Huang G, Zeng Y, Zeng YX, Ye W. Quantification of familial risk of nasopharyngeal carcinoma in a high-incidence area. Cancer. 2017. 10.1002/cncr.30643

[18] Carioli G, Negri E, Kawakita D, Garavello W, La VC, Malvezzi M. Global trends in nasopharyngeal cancer mortality since 1970 and predictions for 2020: Focus on low-risk areas. International Journal of Cancer. 2017;**140**(10):2256-2264

[19] Malumbres M. miRNAs and cancer: An epigenetics view. Molecular Aspects of Medicine. 2013;**34**:863-874

[20] Li B, Hu Y, Ye F, Li Y, Lv W, Xie X. Reduced miR-34a expression in normal cervical tissues and cervical lesions with high-risk human papillomavirus infection. International Journal of Gynecological Cancer. 2010;**20**:597-604

[21] Lajer CB, Garnaes E, Friis-Hansen L, Norrild B, Therkildsen MH, Glud M, Rossing M, Lajer H, Svane D, Skotte L. The role of miRNAs in human papilloma virus (HPV)-associated cancers: Bridging between HPV-related head and neck cancer and cervical cancer. British Journal of Cancer. 2012;**106**:1526-1534

[22] Wu BH, Xiong Xp, Jia J, Zhang WF. MicroRNAs: New actors in the oral cancer scene. Oral Oncology. 2011;**47**:314-319

[23] Lee RC, Feinbaum RL, Ambros V. The *C. elegans* heterochronic gene lin-4 encodes small RNAs with antisense complementarity to lin-14] Cell. 1993;**75**:843-854

[24] Michael J. McCullough, Gareema Prasad, Sarah Zhao and Camile S. Farah (2012). The Changing Aetiology of Oral Cancer and the Role of Novel Biomarkers to Aid in Early Diagnosis, Oral Cancer, Dr. Kalu U. E. Ogbureke (Ed.), InTech, DOI: 10.5772/36526. Available from: https://www.intechopen.com/books/oral-cancer/the-changing-aetiology-of-oral-cancer-and-the-role-of-novel-biomarkers-to-aid-in-early-diagnosis

[25] John K, Wu J, Lee BW, Farah CS. MicroRNAs in head and neck cancer. International Journal of Dentistry. 2013;**2013**

[26] Brenner S. The genetics of Caenorhabditis elegans. Genetics. 1974;**77**:71-94

[27] Sulston JE, Brenner S. The DNA of *Caenorhabditis elegans*. Genetics. 1974;**77**:95-104

[28] Horvitz HR, Sulston JE. Isolation and genetic characterization of cell-lineage mutants of the nematode *Caenorhabditis elegans*. Genetics. 1980;**96**:435-454

[29] Chalfie M, Horvitz HR, Sulston JE. Mutations that lead to reiterations in the cell lineages of *C. elegans*. Cell. 1981;**24**:59-69

[30] Ambros V, Horvitz HR. The lin-14 locus of *Caenorhabditis elegans* controls the time of expression of specific postembryonic developmental events. Genes & Development. 1987;**1**:398-414

[31] Stefani G, Slack FJ. Small non-coding RNAs in animal development. Nature Reviews Molecular Cell Biology. 2008;**9**:219-230

[32] Carthew RW, Sontheimer EJ. Origins and mechanisms of miRNAs and siRNAs. Cell. 2009;**136**:642-655

[33] Ghildiyal M, Zamore PD. Small silencing RNAs: An expanding universe. Nature Reviews Genetics. 2009;**10**:94-108

[34] Reinhart BJ, Slack FJ, Basson M, Pasquinelli AE, Bettinger JC, Rougvie AE, Horvitz HR, Ruvkun G. The 21-nucleotide let-7 RNA regulates developmental timing in *Caenorhabditis elegans*. Nature. 2000;**403**:901-906

[35] Pasquinelli AE, Reinhart BJ, Slack F, Martindale MQ, Kuroda MI, Maller B, Hayward DC, Ball EE, Degnan B, Muller P. Conservation of the sequence and temporal expression of let-7 heterochronic regulatory RNA. Nature. 2000;**408**:86-89

[36] Lau NC, Lim LP, Weinstein EG, Bartel DP, An abundant class of tiny RNAs with probable regulatory roles in *Caenorhabditis elegans*. Science. 2001;**294**:858-862

[37] Lee RC, Ambros V. An extensive class of small RNAs in *Caenorhabditis elegans*. Science. 2001;**294**:862-864

[38] Lagos-Quintana M, Rauhut R, Lendeckel W, Tuschl T. Identification of novel genes coding for small expressed RNAs. Science. 2001;**294**:853-858

[39] Griffiths-Jones S. The microRNA registry. Nucleic Acids Research. 2004;**32**:D109-D111

[40] Griffiths-Jones S, Saini HK, van Dongen S, Enright AJ. miRBase: Tools for microRNA genomics. Nucleic Acids Research. 2008;**36**:D154-D158

[41] Zeng Y, Cullen BR. The biogenesis and function of MicroRNAs. Gene Expression and Regulation. 2006;481-492

[42] Hwang HW, Mendell JT. MicroRNAs in cell proliferation, cell death, and tumorigenesis. British Journal of Cancer. 2006;**94**:776-780

[43] Williams AH, Liu N, Van Rooij E, Olson EN. MicroRNA control of muscle development and disease. Current Opinion in Cell Biology. 2009;**21**:461-469

[44] Carleton M, Cleary MA, Linsley PS. MicroRNAs and cell cycle regulation. Cell Cycle. 2007;**6**:2127-2132

[45] Berezikov E, Guryev V, van de Belt J, Wienholds E, Plasterk RH, Cuppen E. Phylogenetic shadowing and computational identification of human microRNA genes. Cell. 2005;**120**:21-24

[46] Kim VN, Nam JW. Genomics of microRNA. TRENDS in Genetics. 2006;**22**:165-173

[47] Kim VN. MicroRNA biogenesis: Coordinated cropping and dicing. Nature Reviews Molecular Cell Biology. 2005;**6**:376-385

[48] Kim VN, Han J, Siomi MC. Biogenesis of small RNAs in animals. Nature Reviews Molecular Cell Biology. 2009;**10**:126-139

[49] Rodriguez A, Griffiths-Jones S, Ashurst JL, Bradley A. Identification of mammalian microRNA host genes and transcription units. Genome Research. 2004;**14**:1902-1910

[50] Gregory RI, Yan Kp, Amuthan G, Chendrimada T, Doratotaj B, Cooch N, Shiekhattar R. The Microprocessor complex mediates the genesis of microRNAs. Nature. 2004;**432**:235-240

[51] Bentwich I, Avniel A, Karov Y, Aharonov R, Gilad S, Barad O, Barzilai A, Einat P, Einav U, Meiri E. Identification of hundreds of conserved and nonconserved human microRNAs. Nature Genetics. 2005;**37**:766-770

[52] Friedman RC, Farh KK-H, Burge CB, Bartel DP. Most mammalian mRNAs are conserved targets of microRNAs. Genome Research. 2009;**19**:92-105

[53] Iorio MV, Croce CM. MicroRNA dysregulation in cancer: Diagnostics, monitoring and therapeutics. A comprehensive review. EMBO Molecular Medicine. 2012;**4**:143-159

[54] Calin GA, Dumitru CD, Shimizu M, Bichi R, Zupo S, Noch E, Aldler H, Rattan S, Keating M, Rai K. Frequent deletions and down-regulation of micro-RNA genes miR15 and miR16 at 13q14 in chronic lymphocytic leukemia. Proceedings of the National Academy of Sciences. 2002;**99**:15524-15529

[55] Calin GA, Croce CM. MicroRNA signatures in human cancers. Nature Reviews Cancer. 2006;**6**:857-866

[56] Volinia S, Calin GA, Liu CG, Ambs S, Cimmino A, Petrocca F, Visone R, Iorio M, Roldo C, Ferracin M. A microRNA expression signature of human solid tumors defines cancer gene targets. Proceedings of the National academy of Sciences of the United States of America. 2006;**103**:2257-2261

[57] Bartel DP. MicroRNAs: Genomics, biogenesis, mechanism, and function. Cell. 2004;**116**: 281-297

[58] Jiang J, Lee EJ, Gusev Y, Schmittgen TD. Real-time expression profiling of microRNA precursors in human cancer cell lines. Nucleic Acids Research. 2005;**33**:5394-5403

[59] Lujambio A, Lowe SW. The microcosmos of cancer. Nature. 2012;**482**:347-355

[60] MacFarlane LA, Murphy R. MicroRNA: Biogenesis, function and role in cancer. Current Genomics. 2010;**11**:537-561

[61] Chang SS, Jiang WW, Smith I, Poeta LM, Begum S, Glazer C, Shan S, Westra W, Sidransky D, Califano JA. MicroRNA alterations in head and neck squamous cell carcinoma. International Journal of Cancer. 2008;**123**:2791-2797

[62] Chen HC, Chen GH, Chen YH, Liao WL, Liu CY, Chang KP, Chang YS, Chen SJ. MicroRNA deregulation and pathway alterations in nasopharyngeal carcinoma. British Journal of Cancer. 2009;**100**:1002-1011

[63] Jakymiw A, Patel RS, Deming N, Bhattacharyya I, Shah P, Lamont RJ, Stewart CM, Cohen DM, Chan EK. Overexpression of dicer as a result of reduced let-7 MicroRNA levels contributes to increased cell proliferation of oral cancer cells. Genes, Chromosomes and Cancer. 2010;**49**:549-559

[64] Ahmad P, Sana J, Slavik M, Slampa P, Smilek P, Slaby O. MicroRNAs involvement in radioresistance of head and neck cancer. Disease Markers. 2017;**2017**:8245345

[65] He J, Tang Y, Tian Y. MicroRNA214 promotes proliferation and inhibits apoptosis via targeting Bax in nasopharyngeal carcinoma cells. Journal of Molecular Medicine. 2015;**12**:6286-6292

[66] Masood Y, Kqueen CY, Rajadurai P. Role of miRNA in head and neck squamous cell carcinoma. Expert Review of Anticancer Therapy. 2015;**15**:183-197

[67] Summerer I, Niyazi M, Unger K, Pitea A, Zangen V, Hess J, Atkinson MJ, Belka C, Moertl S, Zitzelsberger H. Changes in circulating microRNAs after radiochemotherapy in head and neck cancer patients. Radiation Oncology. 2013;**8**:296

[68] Chen D, Cabay RJ, Jin Y, Wang A, Lu Y, Shah-Khan M, Zhou X. MicroRNA deregulations in head and neck squamous cell carcinomas. Journal of Oral & Maxillofacial Research. 2013;**4**:e2

[69] Severino P, Bruggemann H, Andreghetto FM, Camps C, Klingbeil MF, de Pereira WO, Soares RM, Moyses R, Wunsch-Filho V, Mathor MB, Nunes FD, Ragoussis J, Tajara EH. MicroRNA expression profile in head and neck cancer: HOX-cluster embedded microRNA-196a and microRNA-10b dysregulation implicated in cell proliferation. BMC Cancer. 2013;**13**:533

[70] Jin Y, Chen D, Cabay RJ, Wang A, Crowe DL, Zhou X. Role of microRNA-138 as a potential tumor suppressor in head and neck squamous cell carcinoma. International Review of Cell and Molecular Biology. 2013;**303**:357-385

[71] Chen Z, Jin Y, Yu D, Wang A, Mahjabeen I, Wang C, Liu X, Zhou X. Down-regulation of the microRNA-99 family members in head and neck squamous cell carcinoma. Oral Oncology. 2012;**48**:686-691

[72] Pashaei E, Guzel E, Ozgurses ME, Demirel G, Aydin N, Ozen M. A Meta-Analysis: Identification of common Mir-145 target genes that have similar behavior in different GEO datasets. PLoS One. 2016;**11**:e0161491

[73] Kao YY, Tu HF, Kao SY, Chang KW, Lin SC. The increase of oncogenic miRNA expression in tongue carcinogenesis of a mouse model. Oral Oncology. 2015;**51**:1103-1112

[74] Hui AB, Lenarduzzi M, Krushel T, Waldron L, Pintilie M, Shi W, Perez-Ordonez B, Jurisica I, O'Sullivan B, Waldron J. Comprehensive MicroRNA profiling for head and neck squamous cell carcinomas. Clinical Cancer Research. 2010;**16**:1129-1139

[75] Liu N, Tang LL, Sun Y, Cui RX, Wang HY, Huang BJ, He QM, Jiang W, Ma J. MiR-29c suppresses invasion and metastasis by targeting TIAM1 in nasopharyngeal carcinoma. Cancer Letters. 2013;**329**:181-188

[76] Lu J, Luo H, Liu X, Peng Y, Zhang B, Wang L, Xu X, Peng X, Li G, Tian W, He ML, Kung H, Li XP. miR-9 targets CXCR4 and functions as a potential tumor suppressor in nasopharyngeal carcinoma. Carcinogenesis. 2014;**35**:554-563

[77] Liu X, Luo HN, Tian WD, Lu J, Li G, Wang L, Zhang B, Liang BJ, Peng XH, Lin SX, Peng Y, Li XP. Diagnostic and prognostic value of plasma microRNA deregulation in nasopharyngeal carcinoma. Cancer Biology & Therapy. 2013;**14**:1133-1142

[78] Xia H, Ng SS, Jiang S, Cheung WK, Sze J, Bian XW, Kung HF, Lin MC. miR-200a-mediated downregulation of ZEB2 and CTNNB1 differentially inhibits nasopharyngeal carcinoma cell growth, migration and invasion. Biochemical and Biophysical Research Communications. 2010;**391**:535-541

[79] Alajez NM, Shi W, Hui AB, Bruce J, Lenarduzzi M, Ito E, Yue S, O'Sullivan B, Liu FF. Enhancer of Zeste homolog 2 (EZH2) is overexpressed in recurrent nasopharyngeal carcinoma and is regulated by miR-26a, miR-101, and miR-98. Cell Death and Disease. 2010;**1**:e85

[80] Jia LF, Huang YP, Zheng YF, Lyu MY, Wei SB, Meng Z, Gan YH. miR-29b suppresses proliferation, migration, and invasion of tongue squamous cell carcinoma through PTEN-AKT signaling pathway by targeting Sp1. Oral Oncology. 2014;**50**:1062-1071

[81] Zheng X, Li J, Peng C, Zhao J, Chi J, Meng X, Yun X, Li D, Yu Y, Gao M, Li Y. MicroRNA-24 induces cisplatin resistance by targeting PTEN in human tongue squamous cell carcinoma. Oral Oncology. 2015;**51**:998-1003

[82] Wong TS, Liu XB, Wong BY, Ng RW, Yuen AP, Wei WI. Mature miR-184 as potential oncogenic microRNA of squamous cell carcinoma of tongue. Clinical Cancer Research. 2008;**14**:2588-2592

[83] Yu T, Wang XY, Gong RG, Li A, Yang S, Cao YT, Wen YM, Wang CM, Yi XZ. The expression profile of microRNAs in a model of 7,12-dimethyl-benz[a]anthrance-induced oral carcinogenesis in Syrian hamster. Journal of Experimental & Clinical Cancer Research. 2009;**28**:64

[84] Kozaki K, Imoto I, Mogi S, Omura K, Inazawa J. Exploration of tumor-suppressive microRNAs silenced by DNA hypermethylation in oral cancer. Cancer Research. 2008;**68**:2094-2105

[85] Liu X, Yu J, Jiang L, Wang A, Shi F, Ye H, Zhou X. MicroRNA-222 regulates cell invasion by targeting matrix metalloproteinase 1 (MMP1) and manganese superoxide dismutase 2 (SOD2) in tongue squamous cell carcinoma cell lines. Cancer Genomics Proteomics. 2009;**6**:131-139

[86] Liu X, Jiang L, Wang A, Yu J, Shi F, Zhou X. MicroRNA-138 suppresses invasion and promotes apoptosis in head and neck squamous cell carcinoma cell lines. Cancer Letters. 2009;**286**:217-222

[87] Yu ZW, Zhong LP, Ji T, Zhang P, Chen WT, Zhang CP. MicroRNAs contribute to the chemoresistance of cisplatin in tongue squamous cell carcinoma lines. Oral Oncology. 2010;**46**:317-322

[88] Tran N, McLean T, Zhang X, Zhao CJ, Thomson JM, O'Brien C, Rose B. MicroRNA expression profiles in head and neck cancer cell lines. Biochemical and Biophysical Research Communications. 2007;**358**:12-17

[89] Avissar M, Christensen BC, Kelsey KT, Marsit CJ. MicroRNA expression ratio is predictive of head and neck squamous cell carcinoma. Clinical Cancer Research. 2009;**15**:2850-2855

[90] Ramdas L, Giri U, Ashorn CL, Coombes KR, El-Naggar A, Ang KK, Story MD. miRNA expression profiles in head and neck squamous cell carcinoma and adjacent normal tissue. Head Neck. 2009;**31**:642-654

[91] Childs G, Fazzari M, Kung G, Kawachi N, Brandwein-Gensler M, McLemore M, Chen Q, Burk RD, Smith RV, Prystowsky MB, Belbin TJ, Schlecht NF. Low-level expression of microRNAs let-7d and miR-205 are prognostic markers of head and neck squamous cell carcinoma. American Journal of Pathology. 2009;**174**:736-745

[92] Li J, Huang H, Sun L, Yang M, Pan C, Chen W, Wu D, Lin Z, Zeng C, Yao Y. MiR-21 indicates poor prognosis in tongue squamous cell carcinomas as an apoptosis inhibitor. Clinical Cancer Research. 2009;**15**:3998-4008

[93] Kawakita A, Yanamoto S, Yamada Si, Naruse T, Takahashi H, Kawasaki G, Umeda M. MicroRNA-21 promotes oral cancer invasion via the Wnt/beta-catenin pathway by targeting DKK2. Pathology & Oncology Research. 2014;**20**:253-261

[94] Hedback N, Jensen DH, Specht L, Fiehn AM, Therkildsen MH, Friis-Hansen L, Dabelsteen E, von Buchwald C. MiR-21 expression in the tumor stroma of oral squamous cell carcinoma: An independent biomarker of disease free survival. PloS One. 2014;**9**:e95193

[95] Brito JA, Gomes CC, Guimaraes AL, Campos K, Gomez RS. Relationship between microRNA expression levels and histopathological features of dysplasia in oral leukoplakia. Journal of Oral Pathology & Medicine. 2014;**43**:211-216

[96] Mydlarz W, Uemura M, Ahn S, Hennessey P, Chang S, Demokan S, Sun W, Shao C, Bishop J, Krosting J. Clusterin is a gene-specific target of microRNA-21 in head and neck squamous cell carcinoma. Clinical Cancer Research. 2014;**20**:868-877

[97] Reis PP, Tomenson M, Cervigne NK, Machado J, Jurisica I, Pintilie M, Sukhai MA, Perez-Ordonez B, Grenman R, Gilbert RW. Programmed cell death 4 loss increases tumor cell invasion and is regulated by miR-21 in oral squamous cell carcinoma. Molecular Cancer. 2010;**9**:1

[98] Bourguignon LY, Earle C, Wong G, Spevak CC, Krueger K. Stem cell marker (Nanog) and Stat-3 signaling promote MicroRNA-21 expression and chemoresistance in hyaluronan/CD44-activated head and neck squamous cell carcinoma cells. Oncogene. 2012; **31**:149-160

[99] Yu T, Li C, Wang Z, Liu K, Xu C, Yang Q, Tang Y, Wu Y. Non-coding RNAs deregulation in oral squamous cell carcinoma: Advances and challenges. Clinical and Translational Oncology. 2016;**18**:427-436

[100] Karatas OF, Oner M, Abay A, Diyapoglu A. MicroRNAs in human tongue squamous cell carcinoma. From pathogenesis to therapeutic implications. Oral Oncology. 2017;**67**:124-130

[101] Xu H, Yang Y, Zhao H, Yang X, Luo Y, Ren Y, Liu W, Li N. Serum miR-483-5p: A novel diagnostic and prognostic biomarker for patients with oral squamous cell carcinoma. Tumour Biology. 2016;**37**:447-453

[102] Song Y, Li J, Zhu Y, Dai Y, Zeng T, Liu L, Li J, Wang H, Qin Y, Zeng M, Guan XY, Li Y. MicroRNA-9 promotes tumor metastasis via repressing E-cadherin in esophageal squamous cell carcinoma. Oncotarget. 2014;**5**:11669-11680

[103] Kuo YZ, Tai YH, Lo HI, Chen YL, Cheng HC, Fang WY, Lin SH, Yang CL, Tsai ST, Wu LW. MiR-99a exerts anti-metastasis through inhibiting myotubularin-related protein 3 expression in oral cancer. Oral Disease. 2014;**20**:e65–e75

[104] Jung HM, Phillips BL, Patel RS, Cohen DM, Jakymiw A, Kong WW, Cheng JQ, Chan EK. Keratinization-associated miR-7 and miR-21 regulate tumor suppressor reversion-inducing cysteine-rich protein with kazal motifs (RECK) in oral cancer. Journal of Biological Chemistry. 2012;**287**:29261-29272

[105] Wiklund ED, Gao S, Hulf T, Sibbritt T, Nair S, Costea DE, Villadsen SB, Bakholdt V, Bramsen JB, Sorensen JA, Krogdahl A, Clark SJ, Kjems J. MicroRNA alterations and associated aberrant DNA methylation patterns across multiple sample types in oral squamous cell carcinoma. PLoS One. 2011;**6**:e27840

[106] Lu J, Xu X, Liu X, Peng Y, Zhang B, Wang L, Luo H, Peng X, Li G, Tian W, He M, Li X. Predictive value of miR-9 as a potential biomarker for nasopharyngeal carcinoma metastasis. British Journal of Cancer. 2014;**110**:392-398

[107] Spence T, Bruce J, Yip KW, Liu FF. MicroRNAs in nasopharyngeal carcinoma. Chinese Journal of Clinical Oncology. 2016;**5**:17

[108] Yuva-Aydemir Y, Simkin A, Gascon E, Gao FB. MicroRNA-9: Functional evolution of a conserved small regulatory RNA. RNA Biology. 2011;**8**:557-564

[109] Gwak JM, Kim HJ, Kim EJ, Chung YR, Yun S, Seo AN, Lee HJ, Park SY. MicroRNA-9 is associated with epithelial-mesenchymal transition, breast cancer stem cell phenotype, and tumor progression in breast cancer. Breast Cancer Research and Treatment. 2014;**147**:39-49

[110] Ma L, Young J, Prabhala H, Pan E, Mestdagh P, Muth D, Teruya-Feldstein J, Reinhardt F, Onder TT, Valastyan S, Westermann F, Speleman F, Vandesompele J, Weinberg RA. miR-9, a MYC/MYCN-activated microRNA, regulates E-cadherin and cancer metastasis. Nature Cell Biology. 2010;**12**:247-256

[111] Yu T, Liu K, Wu Y, Fan J, Chen J, Li C, Yang Q, Wang Z. MicroRNA-9 inhibits the proliferation of oral squamous cell carcinoma cells by suppressing expression of CXCR4 via the Wnt/beta-catenin signaling pathway. Oncogene. 2014;**33**:5017-5027

[112] Gao F, Zhao ZL, Zhao WT, Fan QR, Wang SC, Li J, Zhang YQ, Shi JW, Lin XL, Yang S, Xie RY, Liu W, Zhang TT, Sun YL, Xu K, Yao KT, Xiao D. miR-9 modulates the expression of interferon-regulated genes and MHC class I molecules in human nasopharyngeal carcinoma cells. Biochemical and Biophysical Research Communications. 2013;**431**:610-616

[113] Hui AB, Bruce JP, Alajez NM, Shi W, Yue S, Perez-Ordonez B, Xu W, O'Sullivan B, Waldron J, Cummings B, Gullane P, Siu L, Liu FF. Significance of dysregulated metadherin and microRNA-375 in head and neck cancer. Clinical Cancer Research. 2011;**17**:7539-7550

[114] Liu N, Jiang N, Guo R, Jiang W, He QM, Xu YF, Li YQ, Tang LL, Mao YP, Sun Y, Ma J. MiR-451 inhibits cell growth and invasion by targeting MIF and is associated with survival in nasopharyngeal carcinoma. Molecular Cancer. 2013;**12**:123

[115] Lu J, He ML, Wang L, Chen Y, Liu X, Dong Q, Chen YC, Peng Y, Yao KT, Kung HF, Li XP. MiR-26a inhibits cell growth and tumorigenesis of nasopharyngeal carcinoma through repression of EZH2. Cancer Research. 2011;**71**:225-233

[116] Yu L, Lu J, Zhang B, Liu X, Wang L, Li SY, Peng XH, Xu X, Tian WD, Li XP. miR-26a inhibits invasion and metastasis of nasopharyngeal cancer by targeting EZH2. Oncology Letters. 2013;**5**:1223-1228

[117] Deng M, Tang H, Zhou Y, Zhou M, Xiong W, Zheng Y, Ye Q, Zeng X, Liao Q, Guo X, Li X, Ma J, Li G. miR-216b suppresses tumor growth and invasion by targeting KRAS in nasopharyngeal carcinoma. Journal of Cell Science. 2011;**124**:2997-3005

[118] Li YQ, Ren XY, He QM, Xu YF, Tang XR, Sun Y, Zeng MS, Kang TB, Liu N, Ma J. MiR-34c suppresses tumor growth and metastasis in nasopharyngeal carcinoma by targeting MET. Cell Death ad Disease. 2015;**6**:e1618

[119] Luo Z, Dai Y, Zhang L, Jiang C, Li Z, Yang J, McCarthy JB, She X, Zhang W, Ma J, Xiong W, Wu M, Lu J, Li X, Li X, Xiang J, Li G. miR-18a promotes malignant progression by impairing microRNA biogenesis in nasopharyngeal carcinoma. Carcinogenesis. 2013;**34**:415-425

[120] Yu X, Zhen Y, Yang H, Wang H, Zhou Y, Wang E, Marincola FM, Mai C, Chen Y, Wei H, Song Y, Lyu X, Ye Y, Cai L, Wu Q, Zhao M, Hua S, Fu Q, Zhang Y, Yao K, Liu Z, Li X, Fang W. Loss of connective tissue growth factor as an unfavorable prognosis factor activates miR-18b by PI3K/AKT/C-Jun and C-Myc and promotes cell growth in nasopharyngeal carcinoma. Cell Death and Disease. 2013;**4**:e634

[121] Du ZM, Hu LF, Wang HY, Yan LX, Zeng YX, Shao JY, Ernberg I. Upregulation of MiR-155 in nasopharyngeal carcinoma is partly driven by LMP1 and LMP2A and downregulates a negative prognostic marker JMJD1A. PLoS One. 2011;**6**:e19137

[122] Zhang LY, Lee VH-F, Wong AMG, Kwong DL-W, Zhu YH, Dong SS, Kong KL, Chen J, Tsao SW, Guan XY. MicroRNA-144 promotes cell proliferation, migration and invasion in nasopharyngeal carcinoma through repression of PTEN. Carcinogenesis. 2012;bgs346

[123] Deng M, Ye Q, Qin Z, Zheng Y, He W, Tang H, Zhou Y, Xiong W, Zhou M, Li X, Yan Q, Ma J, Li G. miR-214 promotes tumorigenesis by targeting lactotransferrin in nasopharyngeal carcinoma. Tumour Biology. 2013;**34**:1793-1800

[124] Zhang ZC, Li YY, Wang HY, Fu S, Wang XP, Zeng MS, Zeng YX, Shao JY. Knockdown of miR-214 promotes apoptosis and inhibits cell proliferation in nasopharyngeal carcinoma. PLoS One. 2014;**9**:e86149

[125] Wang HY, Li YY, Fu S, Wang XP, Huang MY, Zhang X, Shao Q, Deng L, Zeng MS, Zeng YX, Shao JY. MicroRNA-30a promotes invasiveness and metastasis in vitro and in vivo through epithelial-mesenchymal transition and results in poor survival of nasopharyngeal carcinoma patients. Experimental Biology and Medicine (Maywood). 2014;**239**:891-898

[126] Luo Z, Zhang L, Li Z, Jiang C, Dai Y, Liu X, Zheng Y, Yu H, Xiang J, Li G. miR-149 promotes epithelial-mesenchymal transition and invasion in nasopharyngeal carcinoma cells. Zhong Nan Da Xue Xue Bao Yi Xue Ban. 2011;**36**:604-609

[127] Lyu X, Fang W, Cai L, Zheng H, Ye Y, Zhang L, Li J, Peng H, Cho WC, Wang E, Marincola FM, Yao K, Cai H, Li J, Li X. TGFbetaR2 is a major target of miR-93 in nasopharyngeal carcinoma aggressiveness. Molecular Cancer. 2014;**13**:51

[128] Xu YF, Mao YP, Li YQ, Ren XY, He QM, Tang XR, Sun Y, Liu N, Ma J. MicroRNA-93 promotes cell growth and invasion in nasopharyngeal carcinoma by targeting disabled homolog-2. Cancer Letters. 2015;**363**:146-155

[129] Zhao L, Tang M, Hu Z, Yan B, Pi W, Li Z, Zhang J, Zhang L, Jiang W, Li G, Qiu Y, Hu F, Liu F, Lu J, Chen X, Xiao L, Xu Z, Tao Y, Yang L, Bode AM, Dong Z, Zhou J, Fan J, Sun L, Cao Y. miR-504 mediated down-regulation of nuclear respiratory factor 1 leads to radio-resistance in nasopharyngeal carcinoma. Oncotarget. 2015;**6**:15995-16018

[130] Christensen BC, Moyer BJ, Avissar M, Ouellet LG, Plaza SL, McClean MD, Marsit CJ, Kelsey KT. A let-7 microRNA-binding site polymorphism in the KRAS 30–UTR is associated with reduced survival in oral cancers. Carcinogenesis. 2009;**30**:1003-1007

[131] Fletcher AM, Heaford AC, Trask DK. Detection of metastatic head and neck squamous cell carcinoma using the relative expression of tissue-specific mir-205. Translational Oncology. 2008;**1**:202-208

[132] Lajer CB, Nielsen FC, Friis-Hansen L, Norrild B, Borup R, Garnaes E, Rossing M, Specht L, Therkildsen MH, Nauntofte B. Different miRNA signatures of oral and pharyngeal squamous cell carcinomas: A prospective translational study. British Journal of Cancer. 2011;**104**:830-840

[133] Liu CJ, Tsai MM, Hung PS, Kao SY, Liu TY, Wu KJ, Chiou SH, Lin SC, Chang KW. miR-31 ablates expression of the HIF regulatory factor FIH to activate the HIF pathway in head and neck carcinoma. Cancer Research. 2010;**70**:1635-1644

[134] Kikkawa N, Hanazawa T, Fujimura L, Nohata N, Suzuki H, Chazono H, Sakurai D, Horiguchi S, Okamoto Y, Seki N. miR-489 is a tumour-suppressive miRNA target PTPN11 in hypopharyngeal squamous cell carcinoma (HSCC). British Journal of Cancer. 2010;**103**:877-884

[135] Nohata N, Hanazawa T, Kikkawa N, Sakurai D, Fujimura L, Chiyomaru T, Kawakami K, Yoshino H, Enokida H, Nakagawa M. Tumour suppressive microRNA-874 regulates novel cancer networks in maxillary sinus squamous cell carcinoma. British Journal of Cancer. 2011;**105**:833-841

[136] Ramdas L, Giri U, Ashorn CL, Coombes KR, ElΓÇÉNaggar A, Ang KK, Story MD. miRNA expression profiles in head and neck squamous cell carcinoma and adjacent normal tissue. Head & Neck. 2009;**31**:642-654

[137] Rentoft M, Fahlen J, Coates PJ, Laurell G, Sjostrom B, Ryden P, Nylander K. miRNA analysis of formalin-fixed squamous cell carcinomas of the tongue is affected by age of the samples. International Journal of Oncology. 2011;**38**:61

[138] Scapoli L, Palmieri A, Muzio LL, Pezzetti F, Rubini C, Girardi A, Farinella F, Mazzotta M, Carinci F. MicroRNA expression profiling of oral carcinoma identifies new markers of tumor progression. International Journal of Immunopathology and Pharmacology. 2010;**23**:1229-1234

[139] Wong TS, Man O-Y, Tsang CM, Tsao SW, Tsang RK-Y, Chan JY-W, Ho WK, Wei WI, To VS-H. MicroRNA let-7 suppresses nasopharyngeal carcinoma cells proliferation through downregulating c-Myc expression. Journal of Cancer Research and Clinical Oncology. 2011;**137**:415-422

[140] Chin LJ, Ratner E, Leng S, Zhai R, Nallur S, Babar I, Muller RU, Straka E, Su L, Burki EA. A SNP in a let-7 microRNA complementary site in the KRAS 3 untranslated region increases non-small cell lung cancer risk. Cancer Research. 2008;**68**:8535-8540

[141] Poeta ML, Manola J, Goldwasser MA, Forastiere A, Benoit N, Califano JA, Ridge JA, Goodwin J, Kenady D, Saunders J. TP53 mutations and survival in squamous-cell carcinoma of the head and neck. New England Journal of Medicine. 2007;**357**:2552-2561

[142] Ganci F, Sacconi A, Ben-Moshe NB, Manciocco V, Sperduti I, Strigari L, Covello R, Benevolo M, Pescarmona E, Domany E. Expression of TP53 mutation-associated microRNAs predicts clinical outcome in head and neck squamous cell carcinoma patients. Annals of Oncology. 2013;**24**:3082-3088

[143] Harris T, Jimenez L, Kawachi N, Fan JB, Chen J, Belbin T, Ramnauth A, Loudig O, Keller CE, Smith R. Low-level expression of miR-375 correlates with poor outcome and metastasis while altering the invasive properties of head and neck squamous cell carcinomas. The American Journal of Pathology. 2012;**180**:917-928

[144] Gee HE, Camps C, Buffa FM, Patiar S, Winter SC, Betts G, Homer J, Corbridge R, Cox G, West CM. hsa-miR-210 is a marker of tumor hypoxia and a prognostic factor in head and neck cancer. Cancer. 2010;**116**:2148-2158

[145] Bruce JP, Hui AB, Shi W, Perez-Ordonez B, Weinreb I, Xu W, Haibe-Kains B, Waggott DM, Boutros PC, O'Sullivan B, Waldron J, Huang SH, Chen EX, Gilbert R, Liu FF. Identification of a microRNA signature associated with risk of distant metastasis in nasopharyngeal carcinoma. Oncotarget. 2015;**6**:4537-4550

[146] Hess AK, Muer A, Mairinger FD, Weichert W, Stenzinger A, Hummel M, Budach V, Tinhofer I. MiR-200b and miR-155 as predictive biomarkers for the efficacy of chemoradiation in locally advanced head and neck squamous cell carcinoma. European Journal of Cancer. 2017;**77**:3-12

[147] Arantes LM, Laus AC, Melendez ME, de Carvalho AC, Sorroche BP, De Marchi PR, Evangelista AF, Scapulatempo-Neto C, de S, V, Carvalho AL. MiR-21 as prognostic biomarker in head and neck squamous cell carcinoma patients undergoing an organ preservation protocol. Oncotarget. 2017;**8**:9911-9921

[148] Chen HC, Tseng YK, Chi CC, Chen YH, Yang CM, Huang SJ, Lee YC, Liou HH, Tsai KW, Ger LP. Genetic variants in microRNA-146a (C>G) and microRNA-1269b (G>C) are associated with the decreased risk of oral premalignant lesions, oral cancer, and pharyngeal cancer. Archives of Oral Biology. 2016;**72**:21-32

[149] Hudcova K, Raudenska M, Gumulec J, Binkova H, Horakova Z, Kostrica R, Babula P, Adam V, Masarik M. Expression profiles of miR-29c, miR-200b and miR-375 in tumour and tumour-adjacent tissues of head and neck cancers. Tumour Biology. 2016;**37**:12627-12633

[150] Wang L, Jiang H, Li W, Jia C, Zhang H, Sun Y, Chen X, Song X. Overexpression of TP53 mutation-associated microRNA-182 promotes tumor cell proliferation and migration in head and neck squamous cell carcinoma. Archives of Oral Biology. 2017;**73**:105-112

[151] Wang R, Li H, Guo X, Wang Z, Liang S, Dang C. IGF-I induces Epithelial-to-Mesenchymal transition via the IGF-IR-Src-MicroRNA-30a-E-Cadherin pathway in nasopharyngeal carcinoma cells. Oncology Research. 2016;**24**:225-231

[152] Wu Y, Yu J, Ma Y, Wang F, Liu H. miR-148a and miR-375 may serve as predictive biomarkers for early diagnosis of laryngeal carcinoma. Oncology Letters. 2016;**12**:871-878

[153] Ebert MS, Neilson JR, Sharp PA. MicroRNA sponges: Competitive inhibitors of small RNAs in mammalian cells. Nature Methods. 2007;**4**:721-726

[154] Bader AG, Brown D, Winkler M. The promise of microRNA replacement therapy. Cancer Research. 2010;**70**:7027-7030

[155] Rather MI, Nagashri MN, Swamy SS, Gopinath KS, Kumar A. Oncogenic MicroRNA-155 Down-regulates tumor suppressor CDC73 and promotes oral squamous cell carcinoma cell proliferation Implications for Cancer Therapeutics. Journal of Biological Chemistry. 2013;**288**:608-618

[156] Krutzfeldt J, Rajewsky N, Braich R, Rajeev KG, Tuschl T, Manoharan M, Stoffel M. Silencing of microRNAs in vivo with antagomirs. Nature. 2005;**438**:685-689

[157] Janssen HL, Reesink HW, Lawitz EJ, Zeuzem S, Rodriguez-Torres M, Patel K, van der Meer AJ, Patick AK, Chen A, Zhou Y. Treatment of HCV infection by targeting microRNA. New England Journal of Medicine. 2013;**368**:1685-1694

[158] Yan B, Fu Q, Lai L, Tao X, Fei Y, Shen J, Chen Z, Wang Q. Downregulation of microRNA 99a in oral squamous cell carcinomas contributes to the growth and survival of oral cancer cells. Molecular Medicine Reports. 2012;**6**:675-681

[159] Xiao W, Bao ZX, Zhang CY, Zhang XY, Shi LJ, Zhou ZT, Jiang WW. Upregulation of miR-31* is negatively associated with recurrent/newly formed oral leukoplakia. PloS One. 2012;**7**:e38648

[160] Nohata N, Sone Y, Hanazawa T, Fuse M, Kikkawa N, Yoshino H, Chiyomaru T, Kawakami K, Enokida H, Nakagawa M. miR-1 as a tumor suppressive microRNA targeting TAGLN2 in head and neck squamous cell carcinoma. Oncotarget. 2011;**2**:29-42

[161] Lu Z, Liu M, Stribinskis V, Klinge CM, Ramos KS, Colburn NH, Li Y. MicroRNA-21 promotes cell transformation by targeting the programmed cell death 4 gene. Oncogene. 2008;**27**:4373-4379

[162] Yu CC, Chen YW, Chiou GY, Tsai LL, Huang PI, Chang CY, Tseng LM, Chiou SH, Yen SH, Chou MY. MicroRNA let-7a represses chemoresistance and tumourigenicity in head and neck cancer via stem-like properties ablation. Oral Oncology. 2011;**47**:202-210

[163] Hebert C, Norris K, Scheper MA, Nikitakis N, Sauk JJ. High mobility group A2 is a target for miRNA-98 in head and neck squamous cell carcinoma. Molecular Cancer. 2007;**6**:5

[164] Chen Y, Zhu X, Zhang X, Liu B, Huang L. Nanoparticles modified with tumor-targeting scFv deliver siRNA and miRNA for cancer therapy. Molecular Therapy. 2010;**18**:1650-1656

[165] Tazawa H, Tsuchiya N, Izumiya M, Nakagama H. Tumor-suppressive miR-34a induces senescence-like growth arrest through modulation of the E2F pathway in human colon cancer cells. Proceedings of the National Academy of Sciences. 2007;**104**:15472-15477

[166] Esquela-Kerscher A, Trang P, Wiggins JF, Patrawala L, Cheng A, Ford L, Weidhaas JB, Brown D, Bader AG, Slack FJ. The let-7 microRNA reduces tumor growth in mouse models of lung cancer. Cell Cycle. 2008;**7**:759-764

[167] Choi WY, Giraldez AJ, Schier AF. Target protectors reveal dampening and balancing of Nodal agonist and antagonist by miR-430. Science. 2007;**318**:271-274

[168] Weidhaas JB, Babar I, Nallur SM, Trang P, Roush S, Boehm M, Gillespie E, Slack FJ. MicroRNAs as potential agents to alter resistance to cytotoxic anticancer therapy. Cancer Research. 2007;**67**:11111-11116

[169] Nayak S, Herzog RW. Progress and prospects: Immune responses to viral vectors. Gene Therapy 2010;**17**:295-304

[170] Su J, Baigude H, McCarroll J, Rana TM. Silencing microRNA by interfering nanoparticles in mice. Nucleic Acids Research. 2011;**39**:e38

[171] Kumar B, Yadav A, Lang J, Teknos TN, Kumar P. Dysregulation of microRNA-34a expression in head and neck squamous cell carcinoma promotes tumor growth and tumor angiogenesis. PLoS One. 2012;**7**:e37601

[172] Lindenbergh-van der Plas M, Martens-de Kemp SR, de Maaker M, van Wieringen WN, Ylstra B, Agami R, Cerisoli F, Leemans CR, Braakhuis BJ, Brakenhoff RH. Identification of lethal microRNAs specific for head and neck cancer. Clinical Cancer Research. 2013;**19**:5647-5657

[173] Piao L, Zhang M, Datta J, Xie X, Su T, Li H, Teknos TN, Pan Q. Lipid-based nanoparticle delivery of Pre-miR-107 inhibits the tumorigenicity of head and neck squamous cell carcinoma. Molecular Therapy. 2012;**20**:1261-1269

[174] Rahman MA, Amin AR, Wang X, Zuckerman JE, Choi CH, Zhou B, Wang D, Nannapaneni S, Koenig L, Chen Z. Systemic delivery of siRNA nanoparticles targeting RRM2 suppresses head and neck tumor growth. Journal of Controlled Release. 2012;**159**:384-392

Permissions

All chapters in this book were first published in DMHNC, by InTech Open; hereby published with permission under the Creative Commons Attribution License or equivalent. Every chapter published in this book has been scrutinized by our experts. Their significance has been extensively debated. The topics covered herein carry significant findings which will fuel the growth of the discipline. They may even be implemented as practical applications or may be referred to as a beginning point for another development.

The contributors of this book come from diverse backgrounds, making this book a truly international effort. This book will bring forth new frontiers with its revolutionizing research information and detailed analysis of the nascent developments around the world.

We would like to thank all the contributing authors for lending their expertise to make the book truly unique. They have played a crucial role in the development of this book. Without their invaluable contributions this book wouldn't have been possible. They have made vital efforts to compile up to date information on the varied aspects of this subject to make this book a valuable addition to the collection of many professionals and students.

This book was conceptualized with the vision of imparting up-to-date information and advanced data in this field. To ensure the same, a matchless editorial board was set up. Every individual on the board went through rigorous rounds of assessment to prove their worth. After which they invested a large part of their time researching and compiling the most relevant data for our readers.

The editorial board has been involved in producing this book since its inception. They have spent rigorous hours researching and exploring the diverse topics which have resulted in the successful publishing of this book. They have passed on their knowledge of decades through this book. To expedite this challenging task, the publisher supported the team at every step. A small team of assistant editors was also appointed to further simplify the editing procedure and attain best results for the readers.

Apart from the editorial board, the designing team has also invested a significant amount of their time in understanding the subject and creating the most relevant covers. They scrutinized every image to scout for the most suitable representation of the subject and create an appropriate cover for the book.

The publishing team has been an ardent support to the editorial, designing and production team. Their endless efforts to recruit the best for this project, has resulted in the accomplishment of this book. They are a veteran in the field of academics and their pool of knowledge is as vast as their experience in printing. Their expertise and guidance has proved useful at every step. Their uncompromising quality standards have made this book an exceptional effort. Their encouragement from time to time has been an inspiration for everyone.

The publisher and the editorial board hope that this book will prove to be a valuable piece of knowledge for researchers, students, practitioners and scholars across the globe.

List of Contributors

Julio Cesar Osorio
School of Biomedical Sciences, Universidad del Valle, Cali, Colombia

Andres Castillo
Biology Department, Faculty of Exact and Natural Sciences of Universidad del Valle, Cali, Colombia

Kadriye Peker
Department of Dental Public Health, Faculty of Dentistry, Istanbul University, Capa Istanbul, Turkey

Mohammad Hossein Khosravi
Student Research Committee (SRC), Baqiyatallah University of Medical Sciences, Tehran, Iran International Otorhinolaryngology Research Association (IORA), Universal Scientific

Ali Kouhi
International Otorhinolaryngology Research Association (IORA), Universal Scientific Education and Research Network (USERN), Tehran, Iran Department of Otolaryngology-Head and Neck Surgery, Otorhinolaryngology Research Center, Tehran University of Medical Sciences, Tehran, Iran

Ali Bagherihagh and Masoumeh Saeedi
International Otorhinolaryngology Research Association (IORA), Universal Scientific Department of Otorhinolaryngology-Head and Neck Surgery, Faculty of Medicine, Baqiatallah University of Medical Sciences, Tehran, Iran

Payman Dabirmoghaddam
Tehran University of Medical Sciences, Tehran, Iran

Mohammad Hosein Amirzade-Iranaq
International Otorhinolaryngology Research Association (IORA), Universal Scientific Student Research Committee, Shahid Sadoughi University of Medical Sciences, Yazd, Iran

Kaveh Karimnejad, Nathan Lindquist and Reigh-Yi Lin
Department of Otolaryngology – Head and Neck Surgery, Saint Louis University School of Medicine, Saint Louis, Missouri, USA

Ana Andabak Rogulj and Božana Lončar Brzak
Department of Oral Medicine, School of Dental Medicine, University of Zagreb, Zagreb, Croatia

Vlaho Brailo, Vanja Vučićević Boras and Danica Vidović Juras Ivan Alajbeg
Department of Oral Medicine, School of Dental Medicine, University of Zagreb, Zagreb, Croatia Oral Medicine Unit, Dental Clinic, University Clinical Hospital Zagreb, Zagreb, Croatia

Makbule Tambas
Department of Radiation Oncology, Okmeydani Training and Research Hospital, Istanbul, Turkey

Musa Altun
Department of Radiation Oncology, Istanbul Faculty of Medicine, Istanbul University, Istanbul, Turkey

Deniz Tural
Department of Medical Oncology, Bakirkoy Dr. Sadi Konuk Education and Research Hospital, Istanbul, Turkey

Victor M. Silva Ortíz and Fernando Cantú Flores
Pain Management and Palliative Care Department, Hospital Zambrano Hellion, Monterrey, Mexico

Guillermo E. Aréchiga Ornelas
Pain Management and Palliative Care Department, Hospital General Occidente, Guadalajara, Mexico

José A. Flores Cantisani
Pain and P alliative Care, ISSSTELEON, Monterrey, Mexico

Juan Ignacio Reyes Torres
Pain Management and P alliative Care Department, ISSSTE, Saltillo, Mexico

Mohammad Hossein Khosravi
Student Research Committee (SRC), Baqiyatallah University of Medical Sciences, Tehran, Iran International Otorhinolaryngology Research Association (IORA), Universal Scientific Education and Research Network (USERN), Tehran, Iran

Ali Kouhi
International Otorhinolaryngology Research Association (IORA), Universal Scientific Education and Research Network (USERN), Tehran, Iran Department of Otolaryngology Head and Neck Surgery, Otorhinolaryngology Research Center, Tehran University of Medical Sciences, Tehran, Iran

Masoumeh Saeedi and Ali Bagherihagh
International Otorhinolaryngology Research

Association (IORA), Universal Scientific Education and Research Network (USERN), Tehran, Iran Department of Otorhinolaryngology-Head and Neck Surgery, Faculty of Medicine, Baqiyatallah University of Medical Sciences, Tehran, Iran

Mohammad Hosein Amirzade-Iranaq
International Otorhinolaryngology Research Association (IORA), Universal Scientific Education and Research Network (USERN), Tehran, Iran Student Research Committee, Shahid Sadoughi University of Medical Sciences, Yazd, Iran

Andrei Cismaru and Iulia Coroian
Oncology Department, "Iuliu Hatieganu" University of Medicine and Pharmacy, Cluj- Napoca, Romania Medisprof Oncology Clinic, Cluj-Napoca, Romania

Adrian Udrea
Medisprof Oncology Clinic, Cluj-Napoca, Romania

Gabriel Cismaru
5th Department of Internal Medicine, Cardiac Rehabilitation, "Iuliu Hatieganu" University of Medicine and Pharmacy, Cluj-Napoca, Romania

Muhammad Babar Khawar, Naz Fatima, Rabia Mehmood and Saira Kainat Suqaina
Cell & Molecular Biology Lab, Department of Zoology, University of the Punjab, Lahore, Pakistan

Nadeem Sheikh
Cell & Molecular Biology Lab, Department of Zoology, University of the Punjab, Lahore, Pakistan Centre of Applied Molecular Biology, University of the Punjab, Lahore, Pakistan

Muddasir Hassan Abbasi
Cell & Molecular Biology Lab, Department of Zoology, University of the Punjab, Lahore, Pakistan
Department of Zoology, Govt. College of Science, Lahore, Pakistan

Index

P

R

S

T

X

www.ingramcontent.com/pod-product-compliance
Lightning Source LLC
LaVergne TN
LVHW060526210926
848485LV00005B/1158
* 9 7 8 1 6 3 9 8 9 0 9 4 1 *